AF483532

MCQs in
Pharmaceutical Sciences
for GPAT and NIPER

Second Edition

MCQs in Pharmaceutical Sciences for GPAT and NIPER

Second Edition

by

Prof. Prabhakar Reddy Veerareddy

B.Pharm (KU)., M.Pharm (AU)., Ph.D (KU)., PDF (USA)., LLB

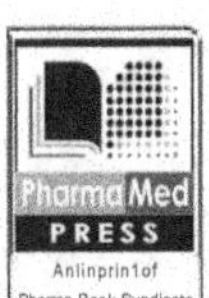

PharmaMed Press

An imprint of Pharma Book Syndicate

A Unit of BSP Books Pvt. Ltd.

4-4-316, Giriraj Lane,

Sultan Bazar, Hyderabad - 500 095.

MCQs in Pharmaceutical Sciences for GPAT and NIPER, Second Edition

by *Prof. Prabhakar Reddy Veerareddy*

© 2019, 2013 *by Publisher*

First Edition 2013
Second Edition 2019

Published by

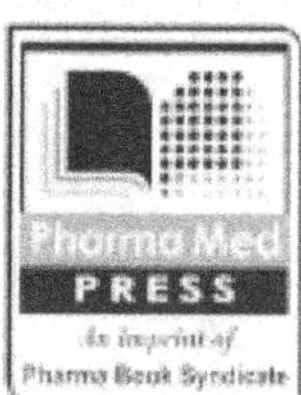

PharmaMed Press

An imprint of Pharma Book Syndicate

A unit of BSP Books Pvt. Ltd.
4-4-309/316, Giriraj Lane, Sultan Bazar, Hyderabad - 500 095.
Phone:040-23445688,23445600; Fax:91+40-23445611
e-mail: info@pharmamedpress.com
www.pharmamedpress.com/pharmamedpress.net

ISBN: 978-93-88305-97-6

About GPAT and NIPER

GRADUATE PHARMACY APTITUDE TEST (GPAT) is a national level entrance examination for entry into M.Pharm programmes. Till 2018, it was conducted by All India Council for Technical Education (AICTE) every year as per the directions of Ministry of Human Resource Development (MHRD), Government of India. The Test will now be conducted by the National Testing Agency (NTA).This test facilitates institutions to select suitable Pharmacy graduates for admission into the Master's (M.Pharm) program. The GPAT is a three hour computer based online test which is conducted in a single session. The GPAT score is accepted by all AICTE-Approved Institutions / University Departments I Constituent Colleges / Affiliated Colleges. A few scholarships and other financial assistance in the field of Pharmacy are also given on the basis of the GPAT score. GPAT qualified candidates are eligible to write NIPER JEE. NIPER JEE (NIPER Joint Entrance Exam) is a national level entrance exam conducted by National Institute of Pharmaceutical Education and Research (NIPER). It is conducted to test the aptitude of candidates seeking admission to various Postgraduate and Doctorate level courses in the field of Pharmacy.

NIPER JEE Exam Pattern

Question Paper Type	MCQ (Multiple Choice Questions)
Total Marks	200 marks
Exam duration	2 hours

CONTENTS

I   PHARMACEUTICAL TECHNOLOGY

1. The ability of a substance dissolves in a given solvent system is depends on
   (a) Nature and intensity of the forces present in the solute
   (b) Nature and intensity of the forces present in the solvent
   (c) Interactions between solute and solvent
   (d) All the above

2. Which of the following substances having poor water solubility
   (a) Weak electrolytes
   (b) Non-polar molecules
   (c) Both
   (d) None

3. The solubility of weak electrolytes & non-polar substances can be increased by adding water miscible solvents. This process is known as
   (a) Co-solvency
   (b) Complexation
   (c) Both
   (d) None

4. How co-solvents increase the solubility of poorly soluble drugs?
   (a) By reducing the interfacial tension between the predominant aqueous solution and hydro-phobic solute
   (b) By reducing the interfacial tension between solute and solvent
   (c) Both
   (d) None

5. Which of the following co - solvents are used to increase the solubility of a drug
   (a) Ethanol
   (b) Sorbitol
   (c) Glycerin
   (d) All the above

6. Which of the following co - solvent is accepted as a co - solvent in parenteral products, but its use in oral liquids is limited
   (a) Glycerol formal
   (b) Glycerol
   (c) Dimethyl acetamide
   (d) None

7. Due to which factor, dimethyl acetamide is not been used as a co-solvent in oral liquids
   (a) Due to objectionable odor
   (b) Due to objectionable taste
   (c) Both
   (d) None

8. Thiomersal ls belongs to which category preservative
   (a) Acidic
   (b) Neutral
   (c) Mercurial
   (d) Quaternary ammonium compounds

9. Which of the following are widely used and excellent preservatives
   (a) Mercurial
   (b) Quaternary ammonium compounds
   (c) Both
   (d) Acidic

10. Benzalkonium chloride is categorized as
    (a) Acidic preservative
    (b) Neutral preservative
    (c) Mercurial preservative
    (d) Quaternary ammonium compounds

11. At which concentration, phenol act as preservative
    (a) 0.2 - 0.5   (b) 0.5 - 0.8
    (c) 0.05 - 0.1   (d) None

12. Which of the following sugar has bitter taste
    (a) Glucose   (b) Sucrose
    (c) Saccharine   (d) None

13. Which of the following is a synthetic sweetener
    (a) Glucose   (b) Sucrose
    (c) Sorbitol   (d) Aspartame

14. To increase the viscosity of liquid, which of the following agents are used
    (a) PVP
    (b) Methyl Cellulose
    (c) Sodium Carboxy Methyl Cellulose
    (d) All the above

15. Which of the following agents are used as flavoring agents
    (a) Menthol   (b) Chloroform
    (c) Both   (d) None

16. Most widely used flavoring agent in food industry
    (a) Menthol
    (b) Chloroform
    (c) Mono sodium glutamate
    (d) None

17. Which of the following flavor is not responsible for sour taste
    (a) Citrus flavors   (b) Liquorice
    (c) Raspberry   (d) Mint spice

18. The filling method of a pharmaceutical liquid depends on the following factors
    (a) Viscosity of the liquid
    (b) Surface tension of the liquid
    (c) Compatibility with the materials used in the construction of the filling machine
    (d) All the above

19. Which of the following methods are generally used in liquid filling
    (a) Gravimetric
    (b) Volumetric
    (c) Constant level method
    (d) All the above

20. In the formulation of suspensions, generally which types of drugs are selected?
    (a) Hydrophilic   (b) Hydrophobic
    (c) Both   (d) None

21. In the formulation, to facilitate the wetting of insoluble solids, which of the following agents used
    (a) Suspending agents
    (b) Flavoring agents
    (c) Wetting agents
    (d) None

22. How surfactants will facilitate or aid wetting of hydrophobic materials in liquid
    (a) By decreasing the solid-liquid interfacial tension
    (b) By increasing the solid-liquid interfacial tension
    (c) Both
    (d) None

23. Stoke's equation is expressed as

    (a) $V = \dfrac{2r^2(d1-dz)g}{9\eta t}$

    (b) $V = \dfrac{2r^2(dl - dz)g}{18\eta t}$

    (c) Both
    (d) None

24. The stability of suspensions can be evaluated by
    (a) Sedimentation volume
    (b) Degree of flocculation
    (c) Re-dispersibility
    (d) All

25. To identify the emulsion type, which of the following tests are conducted?
    (a) Dilution test
    (b) Dye test
    (c) Conductivity test
    (d) All

26. The temperature at which the inversion occurs depends on emulsifier concentration is known as
    (a) Phage temperature
    (b) Inversion temperature
    (c) Phase inversion temperature
    (d) All

27. Which of the following mechanical equipment can be used for emulsification?
    (a) Homogenizers
    (b) Mechanical stirrers
    (c) Ultra sonifiers
    (d) All

28. Which of the following is not used as a emulsifying agent?
    (a) Surfactant
    (b) Hydrophilic colloids
    (c) Electrolytes
    (d) Finely divided solids

29. HLB system was developed by
    (a) Griffin   (b) Stock's
    (c) Dalla Valle   (d) None

30. Gum Arabic is a
    (a) Anionic polysaccharide
    (b) Cationic polysaccharide
    (c) Neutral polysaccharide
    (d) None

31. Which of the following is not a semisolid dosage form
    (a) Paste   (b) Creams
    (c) Ointments   (d) Suspensions

32. Generally pastes contain
    (a) High percentage of insoluble solids
    (b) Low percentage of insoluble solids
    (c) Both
    (d) None

33. Most widely used hydrocarbon in semi-solid dosage forms
    (a) Petrolatum   (b) Mineral oil
    (c) Both   (d) None

34. Which of the following hydrocarbon waxes are employed in the manufacture of creams and ointments?
    (a) Paraffin wax   (b) Ceresin
    (c) Both   (d) None

35. Which of the following Is not a vegetable oil
    (a) Peanut oil   **(b) Almond oil**
    (c) Olive oil   (d) Petrolatum

36. Which of the following fatty acid used in water removable creams as emulsifier
    (a) Stearic acid   (b) Palmitic acid
    (c) Both   (d) None

37. Combination of a surfactant with oil-soluble auxiliary emulsifier is known as
    (a) Simple emulsifier system
    (b) Mixed emulsifier system
    (c) Both
    (d) None

38. Promulgen means
    (a) Anionic emulsifiers composed of fatty alcohols & their ethoxylates
    (b) Non-ionic emulsifiers com-posed of fatty alcohols & their ethoxylates
    (c) Cationic emulsifiers composed of fatty alcohols & their ethoxylates
    (d) All the above

39. Promulgen **D** contains
    (a) Cetyl alcohol & Ceteareth-20
    (b) Stearyl alcohol & Ceteareth-20
    (c) Both
    (d) None

40. Promulgen G contains
    (a) Cetyl alcohol & Ceteareth-20
    (b) Stearyl alcohol & Ceteareth-20
    (c) Both
    (d) None

41. With promulgen D, which type of emulsion generally obtained?
    (a) Liquid emulsion
    (b) Thick consistency emulsion
    (c) Both
    (d) None

42. With promulgen G, which type of emulsion generally obtained?
    (a) Liquid emulsion
    (b) Thick consistency emulsion
    (c) Both
    (d) None

43. Which of the following polyols used as humectants in creams
    (a) Glycerine
    (b) Propylene glycol
    (c) Sorbitol 70%
    (d) All the above

44. The choice of humectants is based on
    (a) Rate of moisture exchange
    (b) Viscosity and texture of preparation
    (c) Both
    (d) None

45. Which of the following Is more hygroscopic at low concentration?
    (a) Sorbitol 70%   (b) Glycerine
    (c) Both   (d) None

46. Due to which factors, petrolatum is most widely used as a hydrocarbon basic in ointments
    (a) Its consistency
    (b) Its neutral characteristics
    (c) Its ability to spread easily on the skin
    (d) All

47. Water number means
    (a) Maximum amount of water that can be added to 100 g of a base at given temperature
    (b) Maximum amount of water that can be added to 10 g of a base at given temperature
    (c) Maximum amount of water that can be added to 5 g of a base at given temperature
    (d) All

48. Lanolin is which type of base
    (a) Hydrocarbon base
    (b) Absorption base
    (c) Both
    (d) None

49. In the preparation of vanishing creams, which types of bases are used generally?
    (a) Absorption bases
    (b) Water removable bases
    (c) Hydrocarbon bases
    (d) None

50. In the preparation of cold creams, which types of bases are used generally?
    (a) Absorption bases
    (b) Water removable bases
    (c) Hydrocarbon bases
    (d) None

51. Water soluble bases are also known as
    (a) Greasy ointment bases
    (b) Greaseless ointment bases
    (c) Both
    (d) None

52. In pastes, the concentration of insoluble powder substances in
    (a) 20%-50%
    (b) 50%-100%
    (c) 50%-75%
    (d) None

53. Jellies are generally
    (a) Water-soluble bases
    (b) Water-insoluble bases
    (c) Both
    (d) None

54. As per USP XX, the term "objectionable" means
    (a) An organism can cause disease or the presence may interrupt the function of the drug or lead to deterioration of the product
    (b) Pathogens if they produce disease or infection, in the newborn or debilitated persons
    (c) Organisms or their toxins that are responsible for human disease or infection
    (d) None

55. The success or failure of a preservative in protecting a formulation against microbial spoilage depends on
    (a) Interaction between preservative with surfactant
    (b) Interaction between preservative with active substances
    (c) Sorption by packaging materials
    (d) All the above

56. A suppository is generally intended for use in
    (a) Rectum
    (b) Vagina
    (c) Urethra
    (d) All the above

57. Vaginal suppositories also called as
    (a) Pessaries
    (b) Simple suppositories
    (c) Bougies
    (d) None

58. "Oleum theobromae" was first recommended by
    (a) A.B. Taylor   (b) Griffin
    (c) Stocks's   (d) None

59. Weight of rectal suppository for adults is
    (a) 1 g   (b) 2 g
    (c) 5 g   (d) None

60. Weight of rectal suppository for children is
    (a) 1 g   (b) 2 g
    (c) 5 g   (d) None

61. Urethral suppositories also called as
    (a) Pessaries   (b) Bougies
    (c) Both   (d) None

62. Urethral suppositories having which shape
    (a) Oviform shape
    (b) Torpedo shape
    (c) Pencil shape
    (d) None

63. Weight of urethral suppository for males & females respectively
    (a) 4 & 2   (b) 2 & 4
    (c) 4 & 6   (d) 6 & 4

64. Shape of vaginal suppositories is
    (a) Oviform shape
    (b) Torpedo shape
    (c) Pencil shape
    (d) None

65. Rectal suppositories mainly used for the treatment of
    (a) Constipation   (b) Hemorrhoids
    (c) Both   (d) None

66. The number of milligrams of **KOH** required neutralizing free acids & saponify the esters contained in 1 g of fat is known as
    (a) Iodine value
    (b) Saponification value
    (c) Water number
    (d) Acid value

67. The number of grams of iodine that reacts with 100 g of fat is known as
    (a) Iodine value
    (b) Saponification value
    (c) Water number
    (d) Acid value

68. The number of milligrams of KOH required neutralizing free acids in 1 g of fat is known as
    (a) Iodine value
    (b) Saponification value
    (c) Hydroxil value
    (d) Acid value

69. The number of milligrams of KOH required neutralize the acetic acid used to acetylate 1 g of fat is known as
    (a) Iodine value
    (b) Saponification value
    (c) Hydroxil value
    (d) Acid value

70. Which of the following method is used to manufacture suppositories
    (a) Hand molding
    (b) Compression molding
    (c) Pour molding
    (d) All the above

71. Which of the following is most commonly used suppository base
    (a) Cocoa butter
    (b) PEG 1000
    (c) PEG $^+$ Hexanetriol
    (d) None

72. Cocoa butter available in following forms
    (a) a-form   (b) -form
    (c) y-form   (d) All

73. The solidification point of cocoa butter lies between
    (a) $12 - 13^{\circ}$ (b) $20 - 30^{\circ}$
    (c) $5 - 10^{\circ}$ (d) None

74. Which of the following method is simple & oldest method of preparation of suppositories?
    (a) Hand molding
    (b) Compression molding
    (c) Pour molding
    (d) All the above

75. Most commonly used method for producing suppositories on both a small & large scale is
    (a) Hand molding
    (b) Compression molding
    (c) Pour molding
    (d) All the above

76. Which formula can be used to calculate the amount of base that is replaced by active ingredients?
    (a) $f = \dfrac{100(G-E)}{(G)(X)} + 1$

    (b) $f = \dfrac{100(E-G)}{(G)(X)} + 100$

    (c) $f = \dfrac{100(E-G)}{(G)(X)} + 1$

    (d) $f = \dfrac{100(E-G)}{(G)(X)} + 10$

77. Rancidity generally results from
    (a) Auto oxidation
    (b) Decomposition of unsaturated fats
    (c) Both
    (d) None

78. Which of the following is not antioxidant
    (a) BHT   (b) BHA
    (c) Tocopherol   (d) Theobroma oil

79. Suppositories are generally evaluated by
    (a) Melting range test
    (b) Breaking test
    (c) Liquefaction
    (d) All the above

80. Which of the following materials are used in pharmaceutical packaging?
    (a) Glass
    (b) Plastic
    (c) Metal
    (d) All the above

81. Which of the following packaging material is protect the drug content against light
    (a) Plastic containers
    (b) Amber colored glass containers
    (c) Both
    (d) None

82. Major disadvantages of glass as a packing material are
    (a) Fragility   (b) Weight
    (c) Both   (d) None

83. Composition of glass is
    (a) Sand
    (b) Soda ash
    (c) Lime stone & Cullet
    (d) All the above

84. Soda ash also known as
    (a) Pure silica
    (b) Sodium carbonate
    (c) Lime stone
    (d) Calcium carbonate

85. Which of the following one is a broken glass & acts as fusion agent
    (a) Cullet   (b) Soda ash
    (c) Lime stone   (d) Sand

86. Which of the following methods are used in the production of glass
    (a) Blowing
    (b) Drawing
    (c) Pressing & casting
    (d) All the above

87. To produce molten glass, which of the following method is used
    (a) Blowing   (b) Drawing
    (c) Pressing   (d) Casting

88. To protect the contents of a bottle from the effects of sunlight by UV rays, which glass is used?
    (a) Amber glass   (b) Red glass
    (c) Both   (d) None

89. To evaluate the chemical resistance of glass, which of the following tests are conducted?
    (a) Powder glass
    (b) Water attack test
    (c) Both
    (d) None

90. Which of the following test is performed on crushed grains, to evaluate the chemical resistance of glass?
    (a) Powder glass
    (b) Water attack test
    (c) Both
    (d) None

91. Which of the following test is performed on whole container?
    (a) Powder glass
    (b) Water attack test
    (c) Both
    (d) None

92. Type I glass is also known as
    (a) Borosilicate glass
    (b) Regular soda-lime glass
    (c) Treated soda-lime glass
    (d) None

93. The advantages of plastic containers over glass containers are
    (a) Easy formation
    (b) Resistance to breakage
    (c) Freedom of design
    (d) All the above

94. Plastic containers are generally made from the following material
    - (a) Polyethylene
    - (b) Polypropylene
    - (c) Polystyrene
    - (d) All the above

95. Which of the following ingredients are present in rubber stopper?
    - (a) Vulcanizing agent
    - (b) Softner
    - (c) Antioxidant
    - (d) All the above

96. Which of the following packaging systems are identified by the FDA?
    - (a) Blister pack
    - (b) Strip pack
    - (c) Bubble pack
    - (d) All the above

97. Which of the following packaging is commonly used for packaging of tablets & capsules?
    - (a) Blister pack   (b) Strip pack
    - (c) Both   (d) None

98. Which of the following materials offer moisture barrier properties?
    - (a) Aclar
    - (b) Cellophane
    - (c) Polyester
    - (d) All the above

99. Which of the following mechanism is responsible for release of encapsulated core materials?
    - (a) By disrupting the coating by pressure

- (b) By offering permeability facilities
- (c) By leaching of permanent fluid
- (d) All the above

100. Pre - formulation studies mainly focus on
    - (a) Physical properties of new compound
    - (b) Chemical properties of new compound
    - (c) Physico-chemical properties of new compound
    - (d) None

101. Which of the following information is helpful in designing the pre-formulation evaluation of a new drug?
    - (a) Structure of a compound
    - (b) Formula & molecular weight of a compound
    - (c) Therapeutic indication of a new compound
    - (d) All the above

102. Which of the following problems commonly encountered in evaluating salt forms are
    - (a) Poor crystallinity
    - (b) Hygroscopicity
    - (c) Instability
    - (d) All the above

103. Which of the following salts generally used in pharmaceutical products?
    - (a) Acetate
    - (b) Gluconate
    - (c) Lactate
    - (d) All the above

104. Description of the outer appearance of a crystal is known as
    (a) Crystal habit
    (b) Internal structure
    (c) Both
    (d) None

105. Which of the following techniques used to prepare amorphous forms?
    (a) Rapid precipitation
    (b) Lyophilization
    (c) Rapid cooling
    (d) All the above

106. Amorphous forms generally having
    (a) Low thermodynamic energy & low solubility
    (b) High thermodynamic energy & high solubility
    (c) Both
    (d) None

107. Which of the following compound possess high aqueous solubility's?
    (a) Hydrates
    (b) Anhydrates
    (c) Both
    (d) None

108. Which of the following properties may change with changing of the internal structure of a solid?
    (a) Melting point
    (b) Density
    (c) Optical properties
    (d) All the above

109. Which of the following methods generally used for studying solid forms?
    (a) DSC
    (b) XRD
    (c) TGA
    (d) All the above

110. Which of the following methods generally used to measure heat loss or gain within a sample?
    (a) DSC
    (b) DTA
    (c) Both
    (d) None

111. Which of the following co-solvent can be used to increase the solubility of poor soluble drugs?
    (a) Ethanol
    (b) Propylene glycol
    (c) Glycerin
    (d) All the above

112. Partition co-efficient generally measures
    (a) Drug's lipophilicity
    (b) Ability of drug to cross cell membrane
    (c) Both
    (d) None

113. Dissolution of a drug particle is described by
    (a) Noyes-Whitney equation
    (b) Stock's equation
    (c) Drag's equation
    (d) None

114. The effect of temperature on drug stability can be described by
    (a) Noyes-Whitney equation
    (b) Stock's equation
    (c) Arheneous equation
    (d) None

115. Unequal distribution of color on a tablet, refers to
    (a) Picking
    (b) Mottling
    (c) Capping
    (d) Sticking

116. Match the following and find out the correct combination
   1. Capping
      (P) Separation of a tablet into 2 or more layers
   2. Lamination
      (Q) Unequal distribution of color on a tablet
   3. Mottling
      (R) Separation of top/bottom crowns of a tablet from the main body
   4. Sticking
      (S) Adherence of tablet material to the die wall
   (a) 2-P, 3-Q, 1-R, 4-S
   (b) 1-P, 2-Q, 3-R, 4-S
   (c) 3-P, 1-Q, 2-R, 4-S
   (d) 4-P, 1-Q, 3-R, 2-S

117. Which of the following one is responsible for sticking?
   (a) Excessive moisture
   (b) Low moisture
   (c) Both
   (d) None

118. Which of the following mixer is a first high shear powder blender/mixer
   (a) Diosna mixer
   (b) Littleford lodige mixer
   (c) Plow mixer
   (d) Gral mixer

119. If the dose of a drug is inadequate, then it generally requires the following one, to make up its bulk
   (a) Binders
   (b) Disintegrants
   (c) Lubricants
   (d) Diluents

120. The first and most widely used diluent in tablet formulation is
   (a) Dextrose   (b) Lactose
   (c) MCC   (d) Starch

121. Anhydrous lactose has the advantage over hydrous lactose
   (a) Improved flow
   (b) Absence of millard reaction
   (c) Improved compressibility
   (d) High microbial load

122. Which of the following is not a commercially available starch product?
   (a) Sta-Rx 1500   (b) Celutab
   (c) Emdex   (d) Sugar tab

123. Which of the following is a synthetic adhesive?
   (a) PVP   (b) MC
   (c) HPMC   (d) HPC

124. Which of the following is a water soluble lubricant?
   (a) Stearic acid
   (b) Mineral oil
   (c) PEG
   (d) Magnesium stearate

125. Find out the correct statements regarding a sweetener, saccharin
   (P) It is 500 times sweeter than sucrose, but it is carcinogenic
   (Q) It is 500 times sweeter than sucrose, but it has bitter taste
   (R) It is sweeter than sucrose, but it is safe

(S) It is sweeter than sucrose, but it is unstable

(a) P, S   (b) P, R

(c) P, Q   (d) R, S

126. Aerosil is used as

(a) Glidant   (b) Lubricant

(c) Antiadherant   (d) None

127. What is the pH of duodenum?

(a) 2-3   (b) 7-8

(c) 4-6   (d) 10

128. Tablets, which are placed between cheek and teeth, are known as

(a) Buccal   (b) Sublingual

(c) Lozenges   (d) Troches

129. Which statement is not correct?

(a) Buccal routes avoids first pass metabolism

(b) Parenteral route avoids first pass metabolism

(c) Sublingual route avoids first pass metabolism

(d) Oral route avoids first pass metabolism

130. Match the following ingredients according to their purpose in the formulation of tablets and find out the correct set

1. Glidant

   (P) Pre- gelatinized starch

2. Diluent

   (Q) Pyramine

3. Adherent

   (R) Colloidal silica

4. Disintegrant

   (S) Calcium sulphate

   (T) Sodium alginate

(a) 1-R, 2-S, 3-P, 4-T

(b) 1-S' 2-R' 3-Q' 4-P

(c) 1-R, 2-S, 3-T, 4-Q

(d) 1-Q' 2-T' 3-R' 4-P

131. Enteric coating is achieved by using

(a) HPMC   (b) CMC

(c) CAP   (d) Povidine

132. The disintegration time for sugar coated tablets is

(a) 30 minutes   (b) 45 minutes

(c) 60 minutes   (d) 75 minutes

133. Flow rate of granules from the hopper can be improved by adding

(a) Disintegrant   (b) Glidant

(c) Binder   (d) Lubricant

134. Given below are equipment used in the manufacture of following products P-T. Match them and find out correct answer

1. Zenasi

   (P) Tablet granules

2. Hepa filter

   (Q) Tablet coating

3. Chilsonator

   (R) Emulsion

4. Accela cota

   (S) Injectables

   (T) Capsule

(a) 1-T, 2-S, 3-P, 4-Q

(b) 1-P' 2-Q' 3-S' 4-R

(c) 1-T' 2-R' 3-Q' 4-P

(d) 1-S, 2-R, 3-P, 4-Q

135. Match the ingredients according to their purpose in the formulation and find out correct set

    1. Film coating

        (P) Sodium benzoate

    2. Syrups

        (Q) Ethyl cellulose

    3. Emulsification

        (R) Eudragit

    4. Enteric coating

        (S) Sucrose

        (T) Sodium oleate

    (a) 1-P, 2-Q, 3-R, 4-S
    (b) 1-R, 2-S, 3-T, 4-Q
    (c) 1-T, 2-P, 3-S, 4-Q
    (d) 1-R, 2-S, 3-Q, 4-T

136. Match the following regions in GIT with the pH levels indicated from P-T and find out correct answer

    1. Mouth

        (P) 5-6

    2. Stomach

        (Q) 6.8-7.5

    3. Deodenum

        (R) 6.8-7

    4. Large intestine

        (S) 3-5

        (T) 1.5-3

    (a) **1-Q,** 2-T, 3-S, 4-R
    (b) 1-P, 2-R, 3-S, 4-T
    (c) 1-S, 2-T, 3-Q, 4-R
    (d) 1-R, 2-S, 3-T, 4-P

137. In sugar coating of tablets, sub- coating is done

    (a) To prevent moisture absorption
    (b) To round the edge & build tablet size
    (c) To smoothen the surface
    (d) To prevent the tablet from breaking due to vibration

138. Some possible causes are mentioned in P-T, for the following defects during the film coating of tablets. Match them

    1. Chipping

        (P) Poor spreading during spraying

    2. Cracking

        (Q) Over heating during spraying

    3. Orange peel

        (R) Higher internal stresses in film

    4. Blistering

        (S) Excessive coating process

        (T) Precipitation of polymer due to high temperature/poor solvent

    (a) 1-S, 2-R, 3-P, 4-Q
    (b) 1-T, 2-S, 3-R, 4-P
    (c) 1-P, 2-Q, 3-R, 4-S
    (d) 1-R, 2-P, 3-Q, 4-T

139. Sub coating is given to the tablets

    (a) To increase the bulkiness
    (b) To avoid deterioration due to microbial attack
    (c) To prevent the solubility in acidic medium
    (d) To avoid stickness

140. The following ingredients are commonly used as coating agents for film coating except

    (a) CAP
    (b) Camauba wax
    (c) HEC
    (d) Sodium CMC

141. The ingredients mentioned in P-S are used in various stages of sugar coating of tablets. Match them and find out correct answer
    1. Seal coating
        (P) Gelatin
    2. Sub coating
        (Q) Camauba wax
    3. Syrup coating
        (R) PEG 4000
    4. Polyshing
        (S) Cane sugar
    (a) 1-S, 2-P, 3-R, 4-Q
    (b) 1-Q, 2-S, 3-R, 4-P
    (c) 1-P, 2-Q, 3-R, 4-S
    (d) 1-R, 2-P, 3-Q, 4-S

142. The courster process can be used to
    (a) Coat tablets
    (b) Determine the disintegration time
    (c) Gas sterilize parenteral solution
    (d) Automatic filling of capsules

143. Which of the following is the first process that must occur before a drug can become available for absorption from a tablet dosage form?
    (a) Dissolution of the drug in GI fluids
    (b) Dissolution of the drug in epithelium
    (c) Ionization of the drug
    (d) Disintegration of the drug

144. Tablets are placed into coating chamber & hot air is introduced through the bottom of the chamber. Coating solution is applied through an atomizing nozzle from the upper end of the chamber. This technique is called
    (a) Sealing before sugar coating
    (b) Coating by air suspension
    (c) Spray-pan coating
    (d) Chamber coating

145. A synthetic sweetening agent which is approximately 200 times sweeter than sucrose & has no taste is
    (a) Saccharin   (b) Aspartame
    (c) Cyclamate   (d) Sorbitol

146. Shellac is used the purpose of coating tablets as
    (a) Polishing agent
    (b) Film coating agent
    (c) Enteric coating agent
    (d) Sub-coating agent for sugar coating

147. Dose dumping is a problem in the formulation of
    (a) Compressed tab
    (b) Suppository
    (c) Soft gelatin capsules
    (d) Controlled release drug products

148. Select the equation that gives the rate of drug dissolution from a tablet
    (a) Fick's law
    (b) Henderson-Hasselbatch equation
    (c) Noyes-Whitney equation
    (d) Michelis Menton equation

149. Which of the following substance is used as muco adhesive
    (a) Acacia
    (b) Sodium CMC
    (c) Burnt sugar
    (d) Saccharin

150. In the preparation of multi layer tablets, one of the following is used for hydrophilic matrix coating
    (a) Shellac
    (b) CMC
    (c) Stearyl alcohol
    (d) Bees wax

151. The diameter of the mesh aperture in the LP. disintegration apparatus is given below. Choose the correct size
    (a) 2 mm   (b) 4 mm
    (c) 1mm   (d) 1.50 mm

152. Diclofenac tablet with CAP has been administered to a patient. Where do you expect the drug to be released?
    (a) Stomach   (b) Oral cavity
    (c) Small intestine (d) Liver

153. Which of the following flavor is used in a formulation containing sour taste?
    (a) Wild cherry   (b) Vanilla
    (c) Citrus   (d) Chocolate

154. Durability of a tablet to combined effects of shock & abrasion is evaluated by using
    (a) Hardness tester
    (b) Disintegration test apparatus
    (c) Friabilator
    (d) Screw guage

155. A retardant material that forms a hydrophilic matrix in the formulation of matrix tablets is
    (a) HPMC
    (b) CAP
    (c) Polyethylene
    (d) Camauba wax

156. A water soluble substance used as coating material in micro encapsulation process is
    (a) Polyethylene   (b) Silicone
    (c) HEC   (d) Paraffin

157. One of the following is used as a p^H dependant controlled release excipient
    (a) Camauba wax
    (b) HPMCP
    (c) MC
    (d) Glyceryl mono stearate

158. In the tablet coating process, inadequate spreading of coating solution before drying causes
    (a) Orange peel effect
    (b) Sticking effect
    (c) Blistering effect
    (d) Picking effect

159. Crown thickness of a tablet is measured by
    (a) Micrometer
    (b) Pychnometer
    (c) Hydrometer
    (d) All the above

160. Friabilator is operated at
    (a) 100 RPM   (b) 75 RPM
    (c) 50 RPM   (d) 25 RPM

161. Enteric coated tablet disintegrate in ……hours in simulated intestinal fluid
    (a) 1   (b) 2
    (c) 3   (d) 4

162. In dissolution test, flask is maintained at
    (a) $37^\circ C \pm 0.5^\circ C$ (b) $41^\circ C \pm 1^\circ C$
    (c) $39^\circ C \pm 0.6^\circ C$ (d) $40^\circ C \pm 1^\circ C$

163. Capping is prevented by using one of the following punches
(a) Flat
(b) Circular
(c) Square
(d) Rectangular

164. Plating of punch faces are done by
(a) Chromium
(b) Zinc
(c) Iron
(d) All

165. Sta-Rx-1500 contains ......% of moisture
(a) 15
(b) 10
(c) 18
(d) 50

166. Acacia trgacanth ls used in the concentration of
(a) 10%-25 %
(b) 60%-70 %
(c) 40%-50 %
(d) 90%

167. Starch on heating hydrolyze into
(a) Glucose
(b) Fructose & Sorbose
(c) Fructose & Mannose
(d) Dextrin & Glucose

168. p^H of the small intestine is
(a) 1-2
(b) 3-4
(c) 6
(d) 7-8

169. Aqua coat is a
(a) 30% w/v of ethyl cellulose dispersion
(b) Solution of HPMC
(c) 2% w/v of methyl cellulose dispersion
(d) None

170. Lozenges were originally named as
(a) Capsule
(b) ODT
(c) Pastillies
(d) Sustained axn tab

171. Implantation tab are NMT........mm in length
(a) 20
(b) 100
(c) 40
(d) 8

172. Seal coating is done by using
(a) Shellac
(b) Acacia
(c) Gelatin
(d) None

173. Sub coating is done to
(a) Round the edges
(b) Increase the bulk of tablet
(c) Both a & b
(d) Make water resistant

174. CAP dissolves at p^H
(a) Above 6
(b) Below 6
(c) 4
(d) 2

175. Which of the following one is used as opacifier
(a) TiO2
(b) Mgo
(c) Siliactes
(d) All of the above

176. Green bone is a source of
(a) Type A Gelatin
(b) Type B Gelatin
(c) Both
(d) None

177. Empty capsule has moisture content in the range of
(a) 60%
(b) 12%-15 %
(c) 50%- 70%
(d) 30%

178. Which treatment is used for solubility of gelatin
(a) Heat
(b) Formalin
(c) Water
(d) Alcohol

179. Which of the following is used to fill powdered dry solid into soft gelatin capsule
    (a) Acea gel   (b) Rotobil
    (c) Rotosort   (d) Rotoweigh

180. Sealing of capsule is achieved by
    (a) 100°c   (b) 20°c
    (c) 37°C-40°C   (d) 70°C

181. Moisture content is determined by
    (a) Gas Chromatography
    (b) K-F Method
    (c) Both
    (d) None

182. Foam stability is measured by
    (a) IR Spectroscopy
    (b) UV Spectroscopy
    (c) Rotational viscometers
    (d) All

183. Particle size is determined by
    (a) Gas Chromatography
    (b) Cascade i_{mp} actor
    (c) Light scatter decay
    (d) Both b & c

184. Chewable tablet contains the following base
    (a) Manito!   (b) Glucose
    (c) Lactose   (d) None

185. Which of the following is not added in lozenges?
    (a) Sweetener   (b) Binder
    (c) Disintegrant   (d) All

186. Enteric coated tablet is disintegrated in
    (a) Stomach   (b) Liver
    (c) Intestine   (d) Mouth

187. Department of Transport Test (DOT) is performed for which of the following?
    (a) Aerosols
    (b) Glass containers
    (c) Capsules
    (d) None

188. Measurement of particle size in pharmaceutical aerosol is by
    (P) Cascade impactor
    (Q) Light scatter decay
    (R) K-F method
    (S) IR
    (a) P, Q   (b) Q, R
    (c) R, S   (d) P, S

189. Identify the correct non-flammable propellant
    (a) Trichloro monofluoro methane
    (b) Dichloro monofluoro methane
    (c) Di methyl ether
    (d) Di fluoro methane

190. The dip tube in an aerosol container is made from one of the following
    (a) Poly propylene
    (b) Glass
    (c) Al
    (d) Stainless steel

191. Which one of the following device is used to increase the efficiency of drug delivery via aerosols?
    (a) Tube spacers
    (b) Metered valves
    (c) Actuator
    (d) Pressure valve

192. The first aerosol insecticide was developed by
    (a) Good-hue & Sullivan
    (b) Good-hue
    (c) Sullivan
    (d) Franklin

193. The first pharmaceutical aerosol was developed in the year of
    (a) 1945   (b) 1949
    (c) 1955   (d) 1960

194. Which drug is formulated as first pharmaceutical aerosol?
    (a) Epinephrine
    (b) Codeine
    (c) Chloropromazine
    (d) Probenecid

195. To dispense inhalation aerosols, which containers are used?
    (a) Stain less steel containers
    (b) Tin plate containers
    (c) Glass containers
    (d) Al containers

196. The valve body /housing in a aerosol bottle valve assembly, is made from one of the following
    (a) Nylon
    (b) Poly propylene
    (c) Poly ethylene
    (d) Stain less steel

197. The equipment listed P-T is used for the identification of properties of aerosol mentioned below. Match them.
    1. Particle size determination
        (P) Pycnometer
    2. Identification of propellants
        (Q) Rotaional viscometer
    3. Stability of foam
        (R) Tag open cap apparatus
    4. Flash point
        (S) IR spectroscopy
        (T) Cascade $i_{m\,p}$ action
    (a) 1-P, 2-Q, 3-R, 4-S
    (b) 1-Q, 2-P, 3-S, 4-T
    (c) 1-T, 2-S, 3-Q, 4-R
    (d) 1-R, 2-S, 3-P, 4-Q

198. Match the coatings given below with their corresponding techniques listed P-T
    1. Compression coating
        (P) Air in the coating pan is replaced with Nitrogen
    2. Dip coating
        (Q) Application of coating to conductive substrates
    3. Electrostatic coating
        (R) Acid insoluble coating
    4. Vacuum film coating
        (S) A tablet within a tablet
        (T) Replaced coating & drying
    (a) 1-T, 2-R, 3-Q, 4-P
    (b) 1-Q, 2-R, 3-S, 4-T
    (c) 1-P, 2-R, 3-T, 4-S
    (d) 1-R, 2-T, 3-P, 4-Q

199. Among the propellants used in aerosols, one of the following is used for topical pharmaceutical aerosols
    (a) Tri chloro monofluoro methane
    (b) Di chloro difluoro methane
    (c) Di chloro tetrafluoro ethane
    (d) Propane

200. Which one of the following propellant is used in the aerosol for oral use
   (a) Propane
   (b) Oxygen
   (c) Methane
   (d) Trichloro monofluoro methane

201. The identification of propellants in pharmaceutical aerosols is carried out by
   (P) Gas chromatography
   (R) Pycnometer
   (Q) Tag open cup apparatus
   (S) IR spectrophotometer
   (a) P,Q
   (b) P,S
   (c) Q, R
   (d) R, S

202. Aerosol packaging container must resist pressure of
   (a) 500 psig
   (b) 140-180 psig
   (c) 40 psig
   (d) 20 psig

203. Gasket is made up of
   (a) Bure-N
   (b) Neoprene rubber
   (c) Both
   (d) All

204. Manufacturing of aerosol involves
   (a) Gas filling
   (b) Pressure filling
   (c) Compressed gas filling
   (d) All the above

205. The nature of propellant is determined by
   (a) R-F method
   (b) Gas Chromatography
   (c) UV
   (d) None

206. Viscosity enhancer in ophthalmic preparation is
   (a) Poly vinyl alcohol
   (b) Povidone
   (c) Dextran
   (d) Macrogol

207. p^H of human tear is
   (a) 7.2
   (b) 8
   (c) 7.6
   (d) 4.6

208. Opthalmic solution is sterilized by
   (a) Autoclave
   (b) Hot air oven
   (c) Both
   (d) Bacterial filters

209. Which of the following one is used to adjust the isotonicity
   (a) Dextrose
   (b) Boric acid
   (c) NaCl
   (d) All the above

210. Freeze drying is used in the manufacturing of
   (a) Heat sensitive drugs
   (b) Heat stable drugs
   (c) Both
   (d) None

211. The temperature above which at irrespective of pressure it is impossible to liquefy a gas is called
   (a) Critical pressure
   (b) Critical temperature
   (c) Both
   (d) None

212. The pressure required to liquefy a gas at its critical temperature is
    (a) Critical pressure
    (b) Critical temperature
    (c) Pressure
    (d) Temperature

213. The critical temperature of water is
    (a) 374°c   (b) 320°c
    (b) 214°c   (d) 390°c

214. Critical pressure for water is
    (a) 100 atm   (b) 150 atm
    (c) 218 atm   (d) 300 atm

215. In the preparation of aerosols __ propellants cause ozone depletion
    (a) Chlorofluorocarbons
    (b) Hydro fluorocarbons
    (c) Both
    (d) None

216. The temperature at which the vapor pressure of the of the liquid equals the external / atmospheric pressure is
    (a) Melting point
    (b) Freezing point
    (c) Boiling point
    (d) None

217. The temperature at which a liquid passes into solid state is
    (a) Melting point
    (b) Freezing point
    (c) Boiling point
    (d) None

218. Different types of liquid crystals are
    (a) Smectic (soap like/grease like)
    (b) Nematic (thread like)
    (c) Both
    (d) None

219. Non aqueous liquid crystals are formed by
    (a) Triethanolamine
    (b) Oleic acid
    (c) Both
    (d) None

220. Which components of bile can form a smectic liquid crystals
    (a) Cholesterol
    (b) Bile acid salt
    (c) Water
    (d) All the above

221. When a mesophase is formed from the gaseous state where the gas is held under a combination of temperatures & pressures that exceed the critical point of a sub is
    (a) Critical pressure
    (b) Super critical fluid
    (c) Critical fluid
    (d) None

222. Thermal analysis can be done by
    (a) Differential scanning calorimetry (DSC)
    (b) Differential thermal analysis (DTA)
    (c) Thermogrvimetric analysis (TGA)
    (d) All the above

223. To determine the amount of water associated with a solid material which method is performed as a potentiometric titration
    (a) Vapor sorption/desorption analysis
    (b) Karl Fisher method
    (c) DSC
    (d) DTA

224. Phase rule is
   (a) $F = C + P + 2$
   (b) $F = C + P - 2$
   (c) $F = C - P + 2$
   (d) $F = C - P - 2$

225. The maximum temperature at which the phase region exists is termed as
   (a) Lower consolute temperature
   (b) Upper consolute temperature
   (c) Both
   (d) None

226. Phenol-water system shows
   (a) Lower consolute temperature
   (b) Upper consolute temperature
   (c) Both
   (d) None

227. Triethanolamine-water system shows
   (a) Lower consolute temperature
   (b) Upper consolute temperature
   (c) Both
   (d) None

228. Nicotine - water system shows
   (a) Lower consolute temperature
   (b) Upper consolute temperature
   (c) Both
   (d) None

229. The point at which liquid and solid phases have the same composition is
   (a) Critical point
   (b) Eutectic point
   (c) Boiling point
   (d) Melting point

230. Which system shows eutectic point
   (a) Nicotine-water
   (b) Phenol-water
   (c) Triethanolamine-water
   (d) Thymol-salol

231. The science and technology of small particles is
   (a) Micromeritics
   (b) Macromeritics
   (c) Both
   (d) None

232. Particle size can be determined by
   (a) Optical microscopy
   (b) Sieving
   (c) Sedimentation
   (d) All the above

233. Optical microscopy is used to determine the particle size in the range of
   (a) $100\ \mu m - 1000\ \mu m$
   (b) $1000\ \mu m - 10000\ \mu m$
   (c) $0.2\ \mu - 100\ \mu m$
   (d) $1A^\circ - 10A^\circ$

234. Andresen apparatus is used for determining particle size by which method
   (a) Optical microscopy
   (b) Sieving
   (c) Sedimentation
   (d) All the above

235. Coulter counter is used to measure
   (a) Particle size
   (b) Particle shape
   (c) Particle volume
   (d) Particle weight

236. Methods for determining surface area
   (a) Adsorption method
   (b) Air permeability method
   (c) Coulter counter method
   (d) a & b

237. Fisher subsieve sizer is used to determine surface area by
    (a) Adsorption method
    (b) Air permeability method
    (c) Both
    (d) None

238. In which type of powders bulk volume is equal to true volume
    (a) Porous
    (b) Non porous
    (c) Both
    (d) None

239. Powder beds of uniform sized spheres can be packed by
    (a) Closet packing
    (b) Cubic packing
    (c) Both
    (d) None

240. The mass of powder divided by the bulk volume is called
    (a) True density
    (b) True volume
    (c) Bulk density
    (d) None

241. Hauser ratio means
    (a) Packed bulk density Vs loose bulk density
    (b) Loose bulk density Vs packed bulk density
    (c) Both
    (d) None

242. Lycopodium shows _____ degree of dustibility
    (a) 57%   (b) 27%
    (c) 100%   (d) 23%

243. Angle of repose is equal to
    (a) $\tan \theta = a$ (b) $\tan \theta = \mu$
    (c) $\cos \theta = \mu$ (d) $\sin \theta = \mu$

244. The glident which increase the flow characteristics of powder are
    (a) Magnesium stearate
    (b) Talc
    (c) Starch
    (d) All the above

245. The surface layer of a liquid posses additional energy. This energy increases when the surface of the same mass of liquid increases and it is known as
    (a) Surface tension
    (b) Surface free energy
    (c) Interfacial tension
    (d) None

246. The surface and interfacial tensions are measured by
    (a) Capillary rise method
    (b) Du Noy ring method
    (c) Both
    (d) None

247. Spreading coefficient of chloroform at $20°c$
    (a) 50.4   (b) 13
    (c) 24.6   (d) -13.4

248. The molecules and ions that are adsorbed at interfaces are
    (a) Surface active agents
    (b) Surfactants
    (c) Diluents
    (d) a&b

249. HLB means
    (a) Hydrophobic lipophilic balance
    (b) Hydrophilic lipophilic balance
    (c) Both
    (d) None

250. In the HLB scale HLB value from 0-3 indicates
    (a) W/O emulsifying agents
    (b) Detergents
    (c) Anti foaming agents
    (d) Wetting agents

251. In the HLB scale HLB value from 3-8 indicates
    (a) W/O emulsifying agents
    (b) O/W emulsifying agents
    (c) Solubilizing agents
    (d) Detergents

252. In the HLB scale HLB value from 8-16 indicates
    (a) W/O emulsifying agents
    (b) O/W emulsifying agents
    (c) Solubilizing agents
    (d) Detergents

253. In the HLB scale HLB value from 16-20 indicates
    (a) W/O emulsifying agents
    (b) O/W emulsifying agents
    (c) Solubilizing agents
    (d) Detergents

254. In the HLB scale HLB value from 13-16 indicates
    (a) W/O emulsifying agents
    (b) O/W emulsifying agents
    (c) Solubilizing agents
    (d) Detergents

255. In the HLB scale HLB value from 6-9 indicates
    (a) W/O emulsifying agents
    (b) Wetting agents
    (c) Solubilizing agents
    (d) Detergents

256. HLB value of sodium lauryl sulphate is
    (a) 4.3   (b) 30
    (c) 40   (d) 1

257. HLB value of methyl cellulose is
    (a) 4.3   (b) 10.5
    (c) 2   (d) 3.8

258. Removal of adsorbate from the adsorbent in solid-gas interface is called as
    (a) Adsorption   (b) Desorption
    (c) Adsorbent   (d) None

259. Langmuir isotherm equation is
    (a) $y = x/m = kp^{1/n}$
    (b) $p/y = 1/ym + 1/ym.p$
    (c) $p/y = 1/b.ym + p/ym$
    (d) None

260. In the electric double layer the anions which are present in the tightly bound layer is called
    (a) Counter ions   (b) Gegenions
    (c) Both   (d) None

261. The difference potential between the actual surface and the electro neutral region of the solution is
    (a) Adsorption isotherm
    (b) Zeta potential
    (c) Electric double layer
    (d) Nemst potential

262. The potential observed at the shear plane in the electric double layer is called as
     (a) Adsorption isotherm
     (b) Zeta potential
     (c) Electric double layer
     (d) Nemst potential

263. The force per unit area which is used to applied to bring about the flow is
     (a) Rate of shear   (b) Shear stress
     (c) Viscosity   (d) Resistence

264. Newton's equation for flow of liquid is represented by
     (a) Rheogram
     (b) Reduced viscosity
     (c) Newtonian flow
     (d) Non-newtonian flow

265. Which type of non-newtonian flow resembles Newtonian flow
     (a) Pseudo plastic flow
     (b) Dilatant flow
     (c) Plastic flow
     (d) None

266. Which type of flow is called as thickening system
     (a) Plastic flow
     (b) Pseudo plastic flow
     (c) Dilatant flow
     (d) All the above

267. An isothermal & comparatively slow recovery, on standing of a material, of a consistency lost through shearing is called as
     (a) Thixotropy
     (b) Shear thinning systems
     (c) a & b
     (d) None

268. Shear thinning systems are _________ transformations
     (a) Gel-sol-gel   (b) Sol-gel-sol
     (c) Gel-gel-sol   (d) Sol-sol-gel

269. Negative thixotropy is observed in
     (a) Flocculated system containing low solid content
     (b) Deflocculated system with high solid content
     (c) Both
     (d) None

270. Degree of thixotropy is estimated by
     (a) Structural break down with time at a constant rate of shear
     (b) determine the structural break down due to increasing shear rate
     (c) both
     (d) none

271. The flow properties of Newtonian fluids is determined by
     (a) Ostwald viscometer
     (b) Falling sphere viscometer
     (c) Both
     (d) None

272. The flow properties of non-newtonian fluids is determined by
     (a) Cup & bob viscometer
     (b) Cone & plate viscometer
     (c) Capillary viscometer
     (d) a & b

273. Ostwald viscometer is applicable for
     (a) Viscous liquids
     (b) Less viscous liquids
     (c) Dilute liquids
     (d) None

274. In which type of viscometer the bob is rotated
    (a) Coquette type
    (b) Capillary
    (c) Falling sphere
    (d) Cone & plate

275. In which type of viscometer the cup is rotated
    (a) Coquette type   (b) Searle type
    (c) Falling sphere   (d) Capillary

276. Plug flow is seen in
    (a) Ostwald viscometer
    (b) Cone & plate viscometer
    (c) Falling sphere viscometer
    (d) Cup & bob viscometer

277. Science that concerns with the flow of liquids and deformation of solids is
    (a) Micromeritics
    (b) Rheology
    (c) Complexation
    (d) Interfacial phenomenon

278. Different types of colloidal dispersions based on interaction of dispersed particles with molecules of the dispersion medium
    (a) Lyophilc
    (b) Lyophobic
    (c) Association
    (d) All the above

279. Lyophilic means
    (a) Solvent hating
    (b) Solvent loving
    (c) Neutral
    (d) None

280. What are the special methods required to prepare lyophobic colloids
    (a) Dispersion methods
    (b) Condensation methods
    (c) Both
    (d) None

281. Particle size, shape & structure can be determined by
    (a) Light microscope
    (b) Electron microscope
    (c) Ultra microscope
    (d) Spectrophotometer

282. Turbidity is used to estimate the concentration of dispersed particles & molecular weights of the solute. Turbidity is measured by
    (a) Spectrophotometer
    (b) Nephelometer
    (c) Both
    (d) None

283. Brownian movement can be determined by
    (a) Light microscope
    (b) Ultra microscope
    (c) Electron microscope
    (d) All the above

284. Zeta potential of a particle is determined by
    (a) Ultra microscope
    (b) Electrophoresis
    (c) HPLC
    (d) TLC

285. The ratio of concentration of the diffusible anion outside & inside the membrane at equilibrium can be calculated by using
    (a) Spectrophotometer
    (b) Electrophoresis
    (c) Donnan membrane equilibrium
    (d) Stokes law

286. Stability of lyophobic colloids can be explained by
(a) DLVO theory
(b) Donnan membrane equilibrium
(c) Turbidity
(d) None

287. According to DLVO theory 2° minimum indicates
(a) Sign of precipitation
(b) Sign of better stability
(c) Sign of aggregation
(d) Vander waals attractive forces

288. Coarse dispersions are
(a) Suspensions
(b) Emulsions
(c) Both
(d) None

289. Based on the nature and behavior of solids, suspensions re classified as
(a) Flocculated
(b) Deflocculated
(c) Both
(d) None

290. In which type of suspensions bio-availability is more
(a) Flocculated
(b) Deflocculated
(c) Both
(d) None

291. In the potential energy curves, the deflocculated system represents
(a) 2° minimum
(b) 1° minimum
(c) Vander waals attraction
(d) Repulsion

292. Factors influencing the settling of particles in suspensions are
(a) Theory of Brownian movement
(b) Theory of sedimentation
(c) Both
(d) None

293. The extent of sedimentation and ease of redispersibility of flocculated suspensions is done by
(a) Sedimentation volume
(b) Brownian movement
(c) Degree of flocculation
(d) a & b

294. Sedimentation volume in suspensions, F = 1 indicates
(a) Complete sedimentation
(b) No sedimentation
(c) Intermediate sedimentation
(d) All the above

295. The dispersion of solids in a vehicle can be achieved by the use of
(a) Diluents
(b) Surfactants
(c) Detergents
(d) Cations

296. HLB range of wetting agents is
(a) 1-3
(b) 5-7
(c) 7-9
(d) 10-12

297. In complexation central atom is connected to surrounding atoms. These surrounding atoms are called as
(a) Ligands
(b) Non metal atoms
(c) Metal atoms
(d) a & b

298. Metal ion complexes are
(a) Chelates
(b) Olefin type
(c) Inorganic type
(d) All the above

299. Organic molecular complexes are
   (a) Quinhydrone type
   (b) Picric acid type
   (c) Polymer type
   (**d**) All the above

300. Inclusion/occlusion compounds are
   (a) Channel lattice
   (b) Clathrates
   (c) Macro molecular type
   (**d**) All the above

301. A substance containing one I more donar groups may combine with a metal to form a special type of complex is known as
   (a) Channel lattice (b) Chelates
   (c) Clathrates   (d) None

302. In chelates when the ligand provides one group for attachment to the central ion , is called as
   (a) Monodentate
   (b) Bidentate
   (c) Tridentate
   (**d**) All the above

303. When the complex contains constituents held together by weak forces of the donar-acceptor type I by hydrogen bonds called as
   (a) Inorganic complex
   (b) Organic complex
   (c) Inclusion
   (**d**) None

304. When one of the constituents of the complex is trapped in the open lattice/ cage like crystal structure of other to yield a stable arrangement is known as
   (a) Inorganic complex
   (b) Organic complex
   (c) Inclusion
   (d) None

305. The entrapment of a single guest molecule in the cavity of one host molecule in the inclusion compounds called as
   (a) Mono molecular inclusion compounds
   (b) Macro molecular inclusion compounds
   (c) Both
   (**d**) None

306. Mono molecular inclusion host structures are represented by
   (a) Bacillus
   (b) Deoxycholic acid
   (c) Cyclodextrins
   (d) Bile acids

307. A determination of stoichiometric ratio of ligand to metal/ donor to acceptor is done by
   (a) Method of continuous variation
   (b) pH titration method
   (c) Solubility method
   (d) All the above

308. Equilibrium dialysis method is used in determining
   (a) Extent of protein binding of drugs
   (b) Complexation of metal ions with macro molecules
   (c) Both
   (**d**) None

309. The study of the rate of a chemical process is called as
(a) Pharmacokinetics
(b) Chemical kinetics
(c) Clinical kinetics
(d) Nonlinear kinetics

310. The agents which are present in and doesn't have any therapeutic activity and they undergo chemical / enzymatic reaction and converted into active drugs are
(a) Parent drugs   (b) Prodrugs
(c) Both   (d) None

311. In which order the rate does not depend on the concentration terms of the reactants
(a) First order
(b) Zero order
(c) Pseudo zero order
(d) Pseudo first order

312. The time required for the concen-tration of reactant to reduce as t90 is
(a) Half life
(b) Manufacturing date
(c) Shelf life
(d) Expiry date

313. The drug degradation in suspensions follows
(a) Zero order
(b) Pseudo zero order
(c) First order
(d) Pseudo first order

314. Reaction in which the rate depends on the concentration terms of two reactants each raised to the power one
(a) First order
(b) Pseudo first order
(c) Second order
(d) Zero order

315. Order of a reaction can be determined by
(a) Graphic method
(b) Substitution method
(c) Half life method
(d) All the above

316. When a catalyst decreases the velocity of a reaction it is called as
(a) - v e catalyst   (b) + ve catalyst
(c) Catalyst   (d) None

317. When the catalyst and reactants from the same phase in the mixture ____ catalysis occur
(a) Heterogeneous
(b) Homogeneous
(c) Both
(d) None

318. The substance poisoned the catalysts is
(a) Carbon monoxide
(b) Cupric ions
(c) Both
(d) None

319. In cortisone acetate suspension during storage cortisone acetate form II is converted into form IV, leads to caking. This condition is called as
(a) Crystal growth
(b) Polymorphism
(c) Hydrolysis
(d) Oxidation

320. Indigo carmine dye tends to fade in the presence of
   (a) Lactose
   (b) Dextrose
   (c) Both
   (d) None

321. Climatic conditions of temperate zone is
   (a) $21°C$, 45%RH
   (b) $25°C$, 60%RH
   (c) $30°C$, 70%RH
   (d) $30°C$, 35%RH

322. Addition of excess quantity of drug that must be added to the preparation to maintain 100% of the labeled amount is
   (a) Overages
   (b) Averages
   (c) Stability
   (d) Shelflife

323. Cold conditions are
   (a) $30°C - 40°C$
   (b) $8°C - 25°C$
   (c) $2°C - 8°C$
   (d) $40°C-50°C$

324. Cool conditions
   (a) $30°c - 40°c$
   (b) $8°C - 25°C$
   (c) $2°C - 8°C$
   (d) $40°C-50°C$

325. In evaporation process the solvent must have following nature
   (a) It must be volatile
   (b) It must be non-volatile
   (c) Both
   (d) None

326. In evaporation process the final product or residue will be
   (a) Solid
   (b) Concentrated liquid
   (c) Aqueous liquid
   (d) None

327. Evaporation rate is expressed as
   (a) $M = KSP/(b-b*)$
   (b) $M = KS(b-b*)$ IP
   (c) $M = K(b-b*)/SP$
   (d) $M = KSP/(b-b*)$

328. In the surface area of evaporating pan is large, the rate of evaporation is
   (a) More
   (b) Less
   (c) Both
   (d) None

329. In the evaporation process is carryout for a long time, then the rate of evaporation will be
   (a) More
   (b) Less
   (c) Both
   (d) None

330. Liquor ice extract Is evaporated by using
   (a) Evaporating pan
   (b) Triple effect evaporator
   (c) Vertical tube evaporator
   (d) None

331. Evaporating pan is not suitable for heat sensitive materials because of
   (a) Long duration of exposure
   (b) Short duration of exposure
   (c) Both
   (d) None

332. Which evaporator is best suitable for non-viscous solutions like cascara extract
   (a) Vertical tube evaporator
   (b) Horizontal tube evaporator
   (c) Climbing film evaporator
   (d) None

333. Which evaporator is best suitable for foam forming liquids
   (a) Vertical tube evaporator
   (b) Horizontal tube evaporator
   (c) Climbing film evaporator
   (d) None

334. Acidic and corrosive materials can be evaporated by using
    (a) Climbing film evaporator
    (c) Both
    (b) Falling film evaporator
    (d) None

335. Highly viscous liquids are concen-trated by
    (a) Climbing film evaporator
    (b) Falling film evaporator
    (c) Both
    (d) None

336. In multiple effect evaporator, feed is introduced into evaporator by
    (a) Parallel feed method
    (b) Forward feed method
    (c) Backward feed method
    (d) None

337. Which of the following method is mostly used in the concentration of salt solutions
    (a) Parallel feed method
    (b) Forward feed method
    (c) Backward feed method
    (d) None

338. Entrainment separator in climbing evaporator acts as
    (a) Only foam breaks
    (b) Only entrainment separator
    (c) Both
    (d) None

339. In climbing film evaporator, the liquid residue time in the heater and evaporator respectively
    (a) 1 second and 20 seconds
    (b) 5 seconds and 25 seconds
    (c) 10 seconds and 30 seconds
    (d) 15 seconds and 35 seconds

340. In forced circulation evaporator, how the liquid is circulated through the tubes
    (a) With the help of pump
    (b) Without the pump
    (c) Both
    (d) None

341. In evaporation process, the solute must be
    (a) Volatile   (b) Non-volatile
    (c) Both   (d) None

342. If the vapor pressure of the liquid is more, the evaporation rate is
    (a) High   (b) Low
    (c) Medium   (d) Too low

343. Which of the following liquids evaporate quickly
    (a) Liquids with low boiling points
    (b) Liquids with high boiling points
    (c) Both
    (d) None

344. Climbing film evaporator also called as
    (a) Falling film evaporator
    (b) Rising film evaporator
    (c) Forced circulation evaporator
    (d) Triple effect evaporator

345. Generally the crystals are obtained from which of the following condition?
    (a) Saturated solution
    (b) Super saturated solution
    (c) Un-saturated solution
    (d) All of the above

346. Super saturation can be achieved through one of the following mechanism
     (a) By evaporating the solvent from solution
     (b) By cooling of the hot solution
     (c) By addition of a substance, which is more soluble in solvent than the solid to be crystallized
     (d) All of the above

347. In crystallization mechanism the initially formed crystal is known as
     (a) Embryo
     (b) Nuclei
     (c) Cluster
     (d) All the above

348. Super saturation theory was proposed by
     (a) Meir's
     (b) Stock's
     (c) Henry's
     (d) All of the above

349. The solubility of KNO_3 increases by one of the following method
     (a) By increasing the temperature
     (b) By decreasing the temperature
     (c) By maintaining low temperature
     (d) All the above

350. In the formulation of dosage forms, which of the following one is mostly preferred
     (a) Hydrates   (b) Anhydrates
     (c) Both   (d) None

351. Solvates are also known as
     (a) Pseudomorphs
     (b) Polymorphs

     (c) Amorphous
     (d) All the above

352. If 2 or more substances possess the same crystalline form is known as
     (a) Polymorphs   (b) Isomorphs
     (c) Amorphous   (d) Both a & b

353. If a compound exist in more than one crystalline form, is known as
     (a) Polymorphs   (b) Isomorphs
     (c) Amorphous   (d) None

354. Which of the following is mostly preferred in dosage form formulations
     (a) Stable polymorph
     (b) Unstable polymorph
     (c) Meta stable polymorph
     (d) None

355. In vacuum crystallizer, super saturation is obtained by which of the following mechanism
     (a) By adiabatic cooling
     (b) By evaporating the hot solvent
     (c) Both
     (d) None

356. To obey Meir's theory, the solute and solvent must be
     (a) Pure   (b) Impure
     (c) Both   (d) None

357. Chrome alum and potash alums are
     (a) Polymorphs
     (b) Isomorphs
     (c) Amorphous
     (d) All the above

358. The word "Equant" means
     (a) Particles of similar length
     (b) Particles of similar width

   (c)   Particles of similar thickness

   (d)   All the above

359. The word" Tabular" means
   (a)   Flat particles of similar length
   (b)   Flat particles of similar width
   (c)   Flat particles of similar length, width and thickness
   (d)   Flat particles of similar length, width, but greater thickness

360. The word "Columnar" denotes
   (a)   Rod like particles
   (b)   Needle like particles
   (c)   Both
   (d)   None

361. Nalidixic acid is which type of crystal
   (a)   Blended type   (b)   Acicular
   (c)   Needle type   (d)   None

362. NaCl is having which crystal shape
   (a)   Equant   (b)   Tabular
   (c)   Plate   (d)   Columnar

363. In a diamond, atoms are bonded together by
   (a)   Hydrogen bond
   (b)   Covalent bond
   (c)   Electrostatic charges
   (d)   All the above

364. Space lattice means
   (a)   3-0 arrangement of particles in a crystal
   (b)   2-0 arrangement of particles in a crystal
   (c)   Orderly arrangement of particles in 3-0 space
   (d)   All of the above

365. When drying takes place?
   (a)   When environment is unsaturated with water
   (b)   When environment is saturated with water vapor
   (c)   When environment is super saturated with water vapor
   (d)   None

366. Bound water is having ……. vapor pressure than the pure water
   (a)   Less   (b)   More
   (c)   Equal   (d)   None

367. Unbound moisture ʾs having ……. Vapor pressure to the pure water
   (a)   Less   (b)   More
   (c)   Equal   (d)   None

368. Hygroscopic materials generally contain which type of moisture
   (a)   Bound Moisture
   (b)   Unbound Moisture
   (c)   Both
   (d)   None

369. Non-hygroscopic materials generally contain which type of moisture
   (a)   Bound Moisture
   (b)   Unbound Moisture
   (c)   Both
   (d)   None

370. If wet solid mass looses water, on exposure of hot air is known as
   (a)   Sorption   (b)   Desorption
   (c)   Both   (d)   None

371. If wet solid mass adsorbs water until EMC is reached is known as
   (a)   Sorption   (b)   Desorption
   (c)   Both   (d)   None

372. Amount of water in a wet solid mass is free to evaporate from the solid surface is known as
     (a) FMC
     (b) EMC
     (c) Both
     (d) None

373. If the temperature of air increases the EMC of solid
     (a) Increases
     (b) Decreases
     (c) First increases, then decreases
     (d) All the above

374. FMC is expressed as
     (a) FMC = Total water content- EMC
     (b) FMC = Total water content+ EMC
     (c) FMC= Total water content- EMC/100
     (d) FMC= Total water content+ EMC/100

375. In drying rate curve, the 2nd phase is known as
     (a) Initial adjustment period
     (b) Constant rate period
     (c) Falling rate period
     (d) None

376. In constant rate period, which of the following factors are constant
     (a) Both temperature and rate of drying are constant
     (b) Only temperature is constant
     (c) Only drying rate is constant
     (d) None

377. In which falling rate period, drying rate falls more rapidly
     (a) 1st falling rate period
     (b) 2nd falling rate period
     (c) Both
     (d) None

378. Vaccines and sterile products can be dried by using
     (a) Freeze dryer
     (b) Spray dryer
     (c) Drum dryer
     (d) Both a & b

379. Antibiotics can be dried by using
     (a) Freeze dryer
     (b) Spray dryer
     (c) Drum dryer
     (d) None

380. Blood plasma can be dried by using
     (a) Freeze dryer
     (b) Spray dryer
     (c) Drum dryer
     (d) None

381. Thermo labile materials can be dried by usimg
     (a) Freeze dryer
     (b) Spray dryer
     (c) Drum dryer
     (d) None

382. In spray dryer, to atomize the liquid into liquid droplets, which device is used
     (a) Atomizer
     (b) Cyclone separator
     (c) Vacuum
     (d) All the above

383. Penicillin is dried by using
     (a) FBD
     (b) Freeze dryer
     (c) Spray dryer
     (d) None

384. In spray dryer, the time taken for completion of drying is
     (a) 3-30 Seconds
     (b) 5-50 Seconds
     (c) 0-50 Seconds
     (d) None

385. The feed liquid which is subjected for distillation is known as
     (a) Distillate
     (b) Distilland
     (c) Condensate
     (d) All the above

386. The condensed liquid in distillation process is known as
     (a) Distillate   (b) Distilland
     (c) Both   (d) None

387. Ideal solutions are also known as
     (a) Real solutions
     (b) Perfect solutions
     (c) Both
     (d) None

388. Solutions which obeys Raoults's law are known as
     (a) Real solutions
     (b) Ideal solutions
     (c) Perfect solutions
     (d) Both b & c

389. Solutions which do not obeys Raoult's law are known as
     (a) Real solutions
     (b) Ideal solutions
     (c) Both
     (d) None

390. Raoult's law expresses the relation-ship between
     (a) Concentration & partial vapor pressure
     (b) Concentration & vapor pressure
     (c) Both
     (d) None

391. Benzene & Toluene are which type of solutions
     (a) Real solutions
     (b) Ideal solutions
     (c) Both
     (d) None

392. Chloroform & Acetone are which type of solutions
     (a) Real solutions
     (b) Ideal solutions
     (c) Both
     (d) None

393. Lie-big condenser is which type of condenser
     (a) Double-surface condenser
     (b) Single-surface condenser
     (c) Multi-tubular condenser
     (d) None

394. Which type of the following condenser increases the efficiency of the condensation
     (a) Single-surface condenser
     (b) Double-surface condenser
     (c) Multi-tubular condenser
     (d) All

395. In the preparation of distilled water & water for injection, which condenser is used
     (a) Single-surface condenser
     (b) Double-surface condenser
     (c) Multi-tubular condenser
     (d) None

396. Florentine receivers are used for
     (a) Separation of oils only
     (b) Separation of oil & water
     (c) Both
     (d) None

397. Florentine receiver Type-I is used for
     (a) Separation of oil heavier than water
     (b) Separation of oil lighter than water
     (c) Both
     (d) None

398. Florentine receiver Type-II is used for
     (a) Separation of oil heavier than water
     (b) Separation of oil lighter than water
     (c) Both
     (d) None

399. Simple distillation process based on
     (a) Differences in volatilities only
     (b) Difference in vapor pressure only
     (c) Both a & b
     (d) None

400. When liquid starts boiling?
     (a) When its vapor pressure is equal to atmospheric pressure
     (b) When its vapor pressure is less than to the atmospheric pressure
     (c) When its vapor pressure is more than to the atmospheric pressure
     (d) All the above

401. Flash distillation is also called as
     (a) Equilibrium distillation
     (b) Differential distillation
     (c) Both
     (d) None

402. Which method is used to separate miscible volatile liquids
     (a) Simple distillation
     (b) Fractional distillation
     (c) Steam distillation
     (d) None

403. If the length of the fractionating column is long, separation of mixture will be
     (a) High   (b) Low
     (c) Medium   (d) None

404. In packed columns, the height of packing is equivalent to how many theoretical plates
     (a) 1   (b) 2
     (c) 3   (d) 4

405. When the boiling points of the constituents in a mixture are close together, which fractionating column is used
     (a) Short   (b) Long
     (c) Both   (d) None

406. When the boiling points of the constituents in a mixture are different, which fractionating column is used
     (a) Short   (b) Long
     (c) Both   (d) None

407. Widmer column is an example of
     (a) Packed column
     (b) Plate column
     (c) Both a & b
     (d) None

408. Solutions which are having constant boiling points can be separated completely by
     (a) Simple distillation
     (b) Fractional distillation
     (c) Azeotopic distillation
     (d) None

409. Absolute alcohol can be prepared by
    (a) Simple distillation
    (b) Fractional distillation
    (c) Azeotopic distillation
    (d) None

410. Process of separation of solids from liquids is known as
    (a) Filtration
    (b) Crystallization
    (c) Clarification
    (d) None

411. Process of separation of low content of solids from a liquid is known as
    (a) Filtration
    (b) Crystallization
    (c) Clarification
    (d) None

412. Solids which are accumulated on the filter is known as
    (a) Filter cake   (b) Filtrate
    (c) Filter medium (d) None

413. Generally air is filtered by using
    (a) Bag filter
    (b) Drum filter
    (c) HEPA filter
    (d) All the above

414. According to Kozeny-Carman equation, the rate of filtration is...........to specific surface area
    (a) Directly proportional
    (b) Inversely proportional
    (c) Both
    (d) None

415. How the rate of filtration can be increased
    (a) By using large size filter
    (b) By applying pressure across filter medium & cake
    (c) By reducing the viscosity of the filtrate
    (d) All the above

416. Which of the following is a filter media
    (a) Talc   (b) Charcoal
    (c) Bentonite   (d) Cotton cloth

417. Which of the following is not a filter aid
    (a) Talc   (b) Charcoal
    (c) Bentonite   (d) Cotton cloth

418. Filter leaf is which type of filter
    (a) Vacuum filter
    (b) Pressure filter
    (c) Both
    (d) None

419. Rotary drum filter is a
    (a) Continuous filter
    (b) Batch filter
    (c) Both
    (d) None

420. Among the following filters, which filter is continuous filter
    (a) Plate, Frame filter
    (b) Rotary drum filter
    (c) Filter leaf
    (d) All the above

421. Meta filter is also known as
    (a) Cartridge filter (b) Edge filter
    (c) Both   (d) None

422. Plate & frame filter press works on the principle of
    (a) Surface filtration
    (b) Depth filtration
    (c) Both
    (d) None

423. Centrifugation is mainly used to separate
    (a) Two immiscible liquids
    (b) A solid from a liquid
    (c) Both
    (d) None

424. Super centrifuge is which type of centrifuge
    (a) Sedimentation centrifuge
    (b) Filtration centrifuge
    (c) Both
    (d) None

425. Ultra centrifuge makes how many revolutions per minute
    (a) 1000 rpm
    (b) 10,000 rpm
    (c) 50,000 rpm
    (d) 1,00,000 rpm

426. Which of the following is a continuous centrifuge
    (a) Perforated basket centrifuge
    (b) Short-cycle batch centrifuge
    (c) Super centrifuge
    (d) None

427. Which of the following centrifuge is a semi continuous centrifuge
    (a) Perforated basket centrifuge
    (b) Short-cycle batch centrifuge
    (c) Super centrifuge
    (d) None

428. To separate two immiscible liquids, which centrifuge is used
    (a) Super centrifuge
    (b) Perforated basket centrifuge
    (c) Both
    (d) None

429. Conical disc centrifuge also called as
    (a) De laval clarifier
    (b) Super centrifuge
    (c) Perforated basket centrifuge
    (d) None

430. Convective mixing is also known as
    (a) Micro mixing
    (b) Macro mixing
    (c) Shear mixing
    (d) None

431. Diffusing mixing also known as
    (a) Micro mixing
    (b) Macro mixing
    (c) Shear mixing
    (d) None

432. Planetary mixer is used to mix
    (a) Cohesive solids
    (b) Free flow solids
    (c) Both
    (d) None

433. V - cone blender is used to mix
    (a) Cohesive solids
    (b) Free flow solids
    (c) Both
    (d) None

434. In a V - cone blender, how mixing of solids can be takes place
    (a) By trituration
    (b) By tumbling action
    (c) Both
    (d) None

435. To break down agglomerates rapidly, which mixer is used
    (a) Planetary mixer
    (b) Sigma blade mixer
    (c) Both
    (d) None

436. Which of the following mixer is a continuous mixer
   (a) Planetary mixer
   (b) Sigma blade mixer
   (c) Zig - zag mixer
   (d) All the above

437. Impellers/ propellers are used to mix
   (a) Liquids   (b) Solids
   (c) Both   (d) None

438. In which type of mixing, vortex formation takes place
   (a) Solid-Solid mixing
   (b) Liquid-Liquid mixing
   (c) Both
   (d) None

439. To prevent vortex formation, which of the following method is used
   (a) By avoid the symmetry
   (b) By using baffled containers
   (c) By mounting 2 or more impellers on same shaft
   (d) All the above

440. What is the effect of vortex formation in liquid mixing
   (a) It increases the mixing intensity
   (b) It reduces the mixing intensity
   (c) Both
   (d) None

441. Silverson mixer is used to mix
   (a) Miscible liquids
   (b) Immiscible liquids
   (c) Both
   (d) None

442. Which of the following mixer is used as both mixer and milling equipment
   (a) Colloid mill
   (b) Silverson mixer
   (c) Rapisonic mixer
   (d) None

443. Which of the following mixer is used to mix semisolids
   (a) Triple roller mill
   (b) Colloidal mill
   (c) Sigma mixer
   (d) All the above

444. In which case, mixing must be done at lower speeds
   (a) In mixing of plastic materials
   (b) In mixing of thixotropic materials
   (c) In mixing of dilatant materials
   (d) All the above

445. Main disadvantage of colloid mill is
   (a) Heat is generated during mixing
   (b) Heat is not generated during mlxing
   (c) Sometimes heat generated
   (d) None

446. Which of the following mixer is used as either batch or continuous mixer in liquid mixing
   (a) Rapisonic homogenizer
   (b) Silverson mixer
   (c) Both
   (d) None

447. Triple roller mill works on the principle of
   (a) Agitation   (b) Shearing
   (c) Both   (d) None

448. In the preparation of emulsion, which mixer is used
 (a) Rapisonic homogenizer
 (b) Sigma mixer
 (c) Planetary mixer
 (d) All the above

449. In the preparation of ointments, which mixer is used
 (a) Triple roller mill
 (b) Rapisonic homogenizer
 (c) Silverson mixer
 (d) None

450. Poly disperse" means
 (a) Consist of different size of particles
 (b) Consist of same size particles
 (c) Both
 (d) None

451. In the production of dosage forms, which type of powder particles generally used
 (a) Mono disperse
 (b) Poly disperse
 (c) Both
 (d) None

452. Size reduction also known as
 (a) Comminution
 (b) Deminution
 (c) Pulverization
 (d) All

453. Which of the following is not a advantage of size reduction
 (a) Improved dissolution rate
 (b) Improved physical stability
 (c) Improved absorption rate
 (d) Drug degradation

454. Fluid energy mill will work on the principle of
 (a) Attrition   (b) Impaction
 (c) Both   (d) None

455. Hammer mill will work on the principle of
 (a) Attrition   (b) impaction
 (c) Both   (d) None

456. Ball mill will work on the principle of
 (a) Impaction   (b) Attrition
 (c) Both   (d) None

457. Ball mill also called as
 (a) Tumbling mill
 (b) Pebble mill
 (c) Both
 (d) None

458. Which of the following mill is used to reduce the size of heat labile substances
 (a) Ball mill
 (b) Fluid energy mill
 (c) Colloid mill
 (d) None

459. Fluid energy mill also called as
 (a) Micronizer
 (b) Jet mill
 (c) Ultrafine grinder
 (d) None

460. Which of the following mill is used in the production of sterile products
 (a) Colloid mill
 (b) Ball mill
 (c) Hammer mill
 (d) All the above

461. Which mill is used for both wet & dry grinder processes
    (a) Ball mill
    (b) Colloid mill
    (c) Fluid energy mill
    (d) All the above

462. To produce the size of toxic substances, which of the following mill is used
    (a) Fluid energy mill
    (b) Colloid mill
    (c) Ball mill
    (d) None

463. To mill the sticky materials, which of the following mill is used
    (a) Fluid energy mill
    (b) Colloid mill
    (c) Rod mill
    (d) None

464. An arrangement for feeding material in a size reduction equipment is known as
    (a) Receiver
    (b) Hopper
    (c) Milling chamber
    (d) None

465. Amount of water vapor present in air is known as
    (a) Humidity
    (b) Relative humidity
    (c) Both
    (d) None

466. Efflorescent substances generally have a tendency
    (a) To lost water
    (b) To absorb water
    (c) Both
    (d) None

467. Substances which absorb moisture are known as
    (a) Efflorescent substances
    (b) Deliquescent substances
    (c) Hygroscopic substances
    (d) None

468. When calcium chloride exposed to atmospheric conditions, if it absorbs moisture & get liquefy, then it is known as
    (a) Hygroscopic
    (b) Deliquescent
    (c) Efflorescent
    (d) None

469. When hard gelatin capsules exposed to low humid conditions, then it
    (a) It loose water & become dry
    (b) It absorb water & become sticky
    (c) Both
    (d) None

470. Humidification is the process of
    (a) Increasing the moisture in the air
    (b) Decreasing the moisture in the air
    (c) Both
    (d) None

471. Dehumidification means
    (a) Increasing the moisture in the air
    (b) Decreasing the moisture in the air
    (c) Both
    (d) None

472. Which of the following is not a liquid adsorbent
    (a) Silica gel
    (b) Ethylene glycol
    (c) Lithium chloride
    (d) Brine

473. Which of the following Is a solid adsorbent
(a) Silica gel
(b) Brine
(c) Lithium chloride
(d) Ethylene glycol

474. Which of the following is not a primary refrigerant
(a) Trichlorofluoro methane
(b) Dichloro tetra fluoro ethane
(c) Ethylene
(d) Brin

475. The vapor pressure of refrigerant liquid in the evaporator section must be
(a) $-20°C$
(b) $-15°C$
(c) $-10°c$
(d) $-5°C$

476. The refrigeration cycle is also called as
(a) Compression cycle
(b) Vapor compression cycle
(c) Both
(d) None

477. Main applications of air conditioning are
(a) In granulation section
(b) In the manufacture of soft gelatin capsules
(c) In Coating
(d) All the above

478. The temperature at which dew is formed is known as
(a) Dew point temperature
(b) Wet bulb temperature
(c) D_{ry} bulb temperature
(d) All the above

479. Enthalpy is expressed as
(a) Kilo Joules per Kg of d_{ry} air
(b) Joules per Kg of d_{ry} air
(c) Kilo Joules Per gram of dry air
(d) None

480. What is the percentage of carbon in cast iron
(a) 1%
(b) 1.5%
(c) 0.5%
(d) 2%

481. Aluminium is which type of metal
(a) Ferrous metal
(b) Non- ferrous metal
(c) Non- metal
(d) None

482. Glass is composed of
(a) Sand
(b) Soda ash
(c) Limestone
(d) All the above

483. Which of the following one is acts as fusion agent
(a) Sand
(b) Soda ash
(c) Cullet
(d) All the above

484. Which of the following glass is used in the manufacture of laboratory glassware
(a) Pyrex glass
(b) Flint glass
(c) Hard glass
(d) None

485. Flint glass also known as
(a) Potash glass
(b) Potash lead glass
(c) Soda glass
(d) All the above

486. Which of the following is a a-form of stainless steel?
   (a) Austenitic
   (b) Ferritic
   (c) Martensitic
   (d) All the above

487. Stainless steel is most widely used due to
   (a) Heat resistance
   (b) Corrosion resistance
   (c) Cleaning & Sterilization
   (d) All the above

488. Which of the following material act as base material in a glass
   (a) Soda ash   (b) Sand
   (c) Cullet   (d) Lime stone

489. For the use of food & pharma-ceuticals, which grade aluminium is used?
   (a) Low grade   (b) High grade
   (c) Super grade   (d) None

490. Which of the following glass is used in pharmaceutical industry
   (a) Highly resistant borosilicate glass
   (b) Treated soda lime glass
   (c) Soda lime glass
   (d) All the above

491. Flint glass is generally used in optical instruments, because
   (a) Of its resistance to heat
   (b) Of its resistance to acid & alkali
   (c) Of its refractive index
   (d) All the above

492. Hard glass is also known as
   (a) Potash glass
   (b) Potash lead glass

   (c) Soda glass
   (d) All the above

493. Soft glass is also known as
   (a) Potash glass
   (b) Potash lead glass
   (c) Soda glass
   (d) None

494. Which of the following rubber is used in making of gloves & stoppers?
   (a) Soft rubber
   (b) Hard rubber
   (c) Synthetic rubber
   (d) None

495. Hard rubber is the combination of
   (a) Soft rubber with sulfur
   (b) Soft rubber with carbon
   (c) Soft rubber with carbon black
   (d) None

496. Synthetic rubber has an advantage over natural rubber is due to
   (a) Resistance to oxidation
   (b) Resistance to oil
   (c) Resistance to solvent
   (d) All the above

497. What is the other name for Neoprene
   (a) Poly chloroprene
   (b) Poly isoprene
   (c) Poly siloranes
   (d) None

498. Which of the following one is not a "Thermoplastic material"
   (a) Polyethylene
   (b) Polypropylene
   (c) PVC
   (d) Urea

499. To prepare gaskets, which of the following thermoplastic plastic is used
    (a) Polyethylene
    (b) Polypropylene
    (c) PVC
    (d) Teflon

500. Dry corrosion means
    (a) Direct attack of dry gases on metals
    (b) Direct attack of aqueous media on metals
    (c) Both
    (d) None

501. Wet corrosion means
    (a) Direct attack of dry gases on metals
    (b) Direct attack of aqueous media on metals
    (c) Both
    (d) None

502. The compound which is formed during corrosion
    (a) Corroded
    (b) Corrosion product
    (c) Corrosion media
    (d) None

503. If the temperature increases, the rate of corrosion is
    (a) Increases   (b) Decreases
    (c) Both   (d) None

504. If corrosion is generally confined to a metal surface, then it is known as
    (a) Fluid corrosion, General
    (b) Fluid corrosion, Structural
    (c) Fluid corrosion, Localized
    (d) Fluid corrosion, Biological

505. If fluid corrosion occurs on different locations
    (a) General corrosion
    (b) Localized corrosion
    (c) Structural corrosion
    (d) Biological corrosion

506. If a metal is destructed by abrasion & attrition caused by the flow of liquid gas, is known as
    (a) Corrosion   (b) Erosion
    (c) Both   (d) None

507. The ability of a metal surface to withstand repeated cycles of corrosion is known as
    (a) Corrosion
    (b) Erosion
    (c) Corrosion fatigue
    (d) None

508. Impingement corrosion is also known as
    (a) Erosion-Corrosion
    (b) Velocity accelerated corrosion
    (c) Both
    (d) None

509. Graphite corrosion generally occurs in
    (a) Iron
    (b) Graphite
    (c) Cast iron
    (d) Gray cast iron

510. Graphite corrosion is an example for
    (a) General fluid corrosion
    (b) Structural fluid corrosion
    (c) Biological fluid corrosion
    (d) None

511. Which of the following method is used to prevent corrosion
     (a) By applying coating
     (b) By altering environment
     (c) By selecting proper material
     (d) All the above

512. Which of the following coating methods are used to control corrosion?
     (a) Electroplating
     (b) Cladding
     (c) Organic coatings
     (d) All the above

513. Which of the following inhibitors are added to the environment to decrease corrosion of materials?
     (a) Chromates
     (b) Phosphates
     (c) Silicates
     (d) All the above

514. What is the concentration of inhibitors used to control corrosion?
     (a) 1%
     (b) 0.5%
     (c) 0.1 %
     (d) All the above

515. Which of the following factors will influence the selection of a plant location?
     (a) Primary factor
     (b) Secondary factor
     (c) Both
     (d) None

516. To control water pollution, which of the following methods are used?
     (a) Physical treatment
     (b) Chemical treatment

     (c) Both
     (d) None

517. Which of the following method is used for controlling dust in the pharmaceutical industry?
     (a) Filtration
     (b) Inertial separation
     (c) Electrostatic precipitation
     (d) All the above

518. Which of the following devices are used to prevent fire hazards?
     (a) Fire alarms
     (b) Fire fighting equipments
     (c) Sprinkler system
     (d) All the above

519. Factories act was enacted in the year of
     (a) 1948   (b) 1950
     (c) 1952   (d) 1954

520. Arrangement of machinery in a department is known as
     (a) Plant layout
     (b) Plant location
     (c) Both
     (d) None

521. Process layout also known as
     (a) Product layout
     (b) Functional layout
     (c) Straight line layout
     (d) None

522. In a layout, if machines performing same work is placed in one department. Then this type of layout is known as
     (a) Product layout
     (b) Functional layout
     (c) Straight line layout
     (d) All the above

523. Which of the following method is used to remove gaseous pollutants from air streams?
    (a) Absorption
    (b) Adsorption
    (c) Incineration
    (d) All the above

524. Which of the following method is used to remove sub - micron particles
    (a) Bag filters
    (b) Electrostatic precipitators
    (c) Venturi scrubbers
    (d) All the above

525. Heat is generally flow from which of the following mechanisms
    (a) Conduction
    (b) Convection
    (c) Radiation
    (d) All the above

526. If the heat flow is achieved by mixing of warmer portions with cooler portions, that process is known as
    (a) Conduction   (b) Convection
    (c) Radiation   (d) None

527. If the heat flows through space by means of electromagnetic waves, is called as
    (a) Conduction   (b) Convection
    (c) Radiation   (d) None

528. If the mixing of liquid is obtained by the use of stirrer, is known as
    (a) Forced convection
    (b) Natural convection
    (c) Both
    (d) None

529. Which of the following device is used for transferring heat from one fluid to another fluid is known as
    (a) Heat interchanger
    (b) Heat exchanger
    (c) Both
    (d) None

530. Multi pass heater is an example of
    (a) Heat interchanger
    (b) Heat exchanger
    (c) Both
    (d) None

531. Which of the following devices used for transferring heat from one liquid to another liquid or from one gas to another gas is known as
    (a) Heat interchanger
    (b) Heat exchanger
    (c) Both
    (d) None

532. In a two pass heater, how many times the liquid is passed through the tubes
    (a) One time   (b) Two times
    (c) Many times   (d) None

533. In a multi pass heater, how many times the liquid is passed through the tubes
    (a) One time   (b) Two times
    (c) Many times   (d) None

534. Double pipe heat interchanger is an example of
    (a) Heat exchanger
    (b) Heat interchanger
    (c) Both
    (d) None

535. A body, whose absorptivity is constant at all wavelengths of radiation, ls known as
    (a) Black body   (b) Grey body
    (c) Both   (d) None

536. A body, which radiates maximum possible amount of energy at a given temperature is known as
    (a) Black body   (b) Grey body
    (c) Both   (d) None

537. Amount of radiation is emitted by black body is expressed by
    (a) Fourier's Law
    (b) Stefan-Boltzmann law
    (c) Thermal radiation law
    (d) None

538. Emmissivity means
    (a) $\dfrac{\text{Energy emitted by actual body}}{\text{Energy emitted by black body}}$
    (b) $\dfrac{\text{Energy emitted by black body}}{\text{Energy emitted by actual body}}$
    (c) $\dfrac{\text{Energy emitted by actual body}}{\text{Energy emitted by grey body}}$
    (d) None

539. Emmissivity is denoted by
    (a) E   (b) a
    (c) p   (d) T

540. Which device is used to measure pressure of the liquid
    (a) Manometer
    (b) Hygrometer
    (c) Hydrometer
    (d) All the above

541. Fluid statics deals with
    (a) Fluids at rest
    (b) Fluids in motion
    (c) Both a & b
    (d) None

542. Fluid dynamics deals with
    (a) Fluids at rest
    (b) Fluids in motion
    (c) Both a & b
    (d) None

543. Which of the following manometer is most commonly used
    (a) Simple manometer
    (b) Differential manometer
    (c) Inclined manometer
    (d) All the above

544. Which of the following manometer is used to measure small pressure differences in a liquid is known as
    (a) Simple manometer
    (b) Differential manometer
    (c) Inclined manometer
    (d) All the above

545. The type of flow of liquid through a pipeline can be determined by
    (a) Ostwald's experiment
    (b) Reynold's experiment
    (c) Both
    (d) All the above

546. In Reynold's experiment, the flow conditions are affected by which of the following factors
    (a) Diameter of pipe
    (b) Density of liquid
    (c) Average velocity of liquid
    (d) All the above

547. Reynold's number can be expressed by which of the following formula
    (a) Re = Dup/11
    (b) Re = 2Dup/11
    (c) Re = 3Dup/11
    (d) Re = Dup/211

548. If Reynold's number is less than 2000, then the flow type is
    (a) Laminar
    (b) Turbulent
    (c) Laminar to turbulent
    (d) All the above

549. If Reynold's number is greater than 4000, then the flow type is
    (a) Laminar
    (b) Turbulent
    (c) Laminar to turbulent
    (d) All the above

550. Which method is used to measure the rate of flow of fluids
    (a) Direct weighing methods
    (b) Hydrodynamic methods
    (c) Direct displacement methods
    (d) All the above

551. Pitot tube also known as
    (a) Variable head meter
    (b) Insertion meter
    (c) Area meter
    (d) None

552. Rota meter is also known as
    (a) Variable head meter
    (b) Insertion meter
    (c) Area meter
    (d) None

553. Rota meter generally measures
    (a) The area of flow
    (b) The velocity head of the flow
    (c) Both
    (d) None

554. Pitot tube generally measures
    (a) The area of flow
    (b) The velocity head of the flow
    (c) Both
    (d) None

555. When two or more ingredients prescribed which are antagonistic in nature and an undesirable product is formed which may affect the safety, purpose or appearance of the preparation is called as
    (a) Idiosyncrasy
    (b) Incompatibility
    (c) Accumulation
    (d) Antagonism

556. Causes for therapeutic incompatibility are
    (a) Over dose
    (b) Wrong dose
    (c) Contra indicated drugs
    (d) All the above

557. Which type of incompatibility is observed in the following prescription Rx Codeine phosphate-0.6 gm powder
    (a) Physical incompatibility
    (b) Chemical incompatibility
    (c) Therapeutic incompatibility
    (d) None

558. Which type of incompatibility is observed in the following prescription Rx Diazepam-0.5 gm
    (a) Physical incompatibility
    (b) Chemical incompatibility
    (c) Therapeutic incompatibility
    (d) None

559. Which type of incompatibility ls observed in the following prescription Rx Ispaghula granules-3.5 gm
     (a) Physical incompatibility
     (b) Chemical incompatibility
     (c) Therapeutic incompatibility
     (d) None

560. The combination of penicillin and probenecid shows
     (a) Additive effect
     (b) Antagonism
     (c) Synergism
     (d) All the above

561. Which type of incompatibility ls observed in the following prescription
     Rx
     Acetophenatidin
     Acetyl salicylic acid
     Caffeine
     (a) Physical incompatibility
     (b) Chemical incompatibility
     (c) Therapeutic incompatibility
     (d) None

562. Reasons for physical incompatibility
     (a) Immiscibility
     (b) Insolubility
     (c) Liquefaction
     (d) All the above

563. Physical incompatibility can be corrected by
     (a) Order of mixing
     (b) Alteration of solvents
     (c) Change in the form of ingredient
     (d) None

564. which type of incompatibility ls observed in the following prescription
     Rx
     Phenacitin
     Caffeine
     Orange syrup
     Water
     (a) Physical incompatibility
     (b) Chemical incompatibility
     (c) Therapeutic incompatibility
     (d) All the above

565. Which type of incompatibility is observed in the following prescription
     Rx
     Menthol
     Camphor
     Ammonium chloride
     Light magnesium carbonate
     (a) Physical incompatibility
     (b) Chemical incompatibility
     (c) Therapeutic incompatibility
     (d) All the above

566. Causes for chemical incompatibility
     (a) Oxidation-reduction
     (b) Acid-base reaction
     (c) Hydrolysis
     (d) All the above

567. The incompatibility observed between strychnine and soluble iodides are
     (a) Physical incompatibility
     (b) Chemical incompatibility
     (c) Therapeutic incompatibility
     (d) All the above

568. Which type of incompatibility is observed in the following prescription

    Rx

    Quinine HCl

    Sodium salicylates

    Water

    (a) Physical incompatibility

    (b) Chemical incompatibility

    (c) Therapeutic incompatibility

    (d) All the above

569. Which type of incompatibility is observed in the following prescription

    Rx

    Sodium salicylate

    Caffeine citrate

    Water

    (a) Tolerated chemical incompatibility

    (b) Adjusted chemical incompatibility

    (c) Physical incompatibility

    (d) Therapeutic incompatibility

570. Which type of incompatibility is observed in the following prescription

    Rx

    Sodium salicylate-1 gm

    $NaHCO_3$-1 gm

    Sodium meta bisulphate-up to 15 mL

    (a) Physical incompatibility

    (b) Chemical incompatibility

    (c) Therapeutic incompatibility

    (d) None

571. Which type of incompatibility is observed in the following prescription

    Rx

    Sodium salicylate-5 gm

    Syrup of lemon-20 mL

    Water-up to 75 mL

    (a) Tolerated chemical incompatibility

    (b) Adjusted chemical incompatibility

    (c) Physical incompatibility

    (d) Therapeutic incompatibility

572. Liquid extract of liquorice should not be used as flavoring agent in

    (a) Acidic solution

    (b) Neutral solution

    (c) Alkaline solution

    (d) All the above

573. When soluble barbiturates prescribed with ammonium bromide, to get a clear solution ammonium bromide is replaced with chemically equivalent amount of

    (a) NaBr   (b) K.Br

    (c) Both   (d) None

574. The term prescription is derived from

    (a) Latin   (b) Greek

    (c) English   (d) French

575. Prescription means

    (a) To write

    (b) To write before

    (c) To write later

    (d) All the above

576. Superscription is represented by

    (a) K   (b) P

    (c) Rx   (d) S

577. Rx means

    (a) You take

    (b) You give

    (c) You bring

    (d) All the above

578. Rx symbol represents _ _ _ _ god.
    (a) Venus   (b) Jupiter
    (c) Mars   (d) Saturn

579. Inscription includes
    (a) Base
    (b) Adjuvant
    (c) Vehicle
    (d) All the above

580. Subscription means
    (a) Directions for pharmacist
    (b) Directions for patient
    (c) Directions for physician
    (d) Directions for nurse

581. _______ indicates Instructions for patients
    (a) Transcription   (b) Signatura
    (c) Both   (d) None

582. Handling of prescription includes
    (a) Receiving, reading & checking
    (b) Collecting & weighing materials
    (c) Compounding, labeling & packaging
    (d) All the above

583. Identify the source of error in the prescription
    (a) Abbreviation
    (b) Dose
    (c) Incompatibility
    (d) All the above

584. For dusting powders which type of containers are used for packing
    (a) Strip packing
    (b) Sifted top containers
    (c) Dropper bottles
    (d) Collapsible tubes

585. What is the caution on the label when emulsion is dispensed
    (a) For external use only
    (b) Shake well before use
    (c) Dilute well before use
    (d) None

586. What is the label condition for throat paint
    (a) To be sipped & swallowed slowly without addition of water
    (b) Shake well before use
    (c) Not to be swallowed in large quantity
    (d) All the above

587. What is the label condition for eye lotion
    (a) Discard 24 hours after first opening
    (b) Discard 30 days after first opening
    (c) Discard 1 year after first opening
    (d) Discard 5 years after first opening

588. What is the label condition for eye drops
    (a) Discard 24 hours after first opening
    (b) Discard 30 days after first opening
    (c) Discard 1 year after first opening
    (d) Discard 5 years after first opening

589. 1 pound is equal to
    (a) 10 ounces   (b) 12 ounces
    (c) 14 ounces   (d) 16 ounces

590. 1 gallon is equal to
    (a) 1 quart   (b) 1 pint
    (c) 160 Fl.oz   (d) 480 minims

591. 1 quart =
    (a) 1000mL   (b) 500 mL
    (c) 200 mL   (d) 100 mL

592. 1 pint =
    (a) 1000 mL   (b) 500 mL
    (c) 200 mL   (d) 100mL

593. 1 table spoonful =
    (a) 4 mL   (b) 8 mL
    (c) 15 mL   (d) 20 mL

594. 1 teaspoonful =
    (a) 4 mL   (b) 8 mL
    (c) 15 mL   (d) 20 mL

595. 1 desert spoonful=
    (a) 4 mL   (b) 8 mL
    (c) 15 mL   (d) 20 mL

596. 1 minim is equal to
    (a) 1 drop   (b) 0.06 mL
    (c) both   (d) 2 drops

597. Prepare 100 mL of a 1in 4000 solution of potassium permanganate
    (a) 0.025 gm   (b) 0.05 gm
    (c) 0.075 gm   (d) 0.1 gm

598. Calculate the volume of 95% alcohol required to prepare 600mL of 70% alcohol
    (a) 757.90 mL   (b) 442.10 mL
    (c) 780 mL   (d) 450 mL

599. Calculate the volume of water to prepare 1000 ml dilute acetic acid 4% from 33% dilute acetic acid
    (a) 878.8 mL   (b) 121.2 mL
    (c) 890 mL   (d) 885.2 mL

600. $100°$ proof contains ... absolute alcohol
    (a) 59.1 %v/v   (b) 58.1¾v/v
    (c) 57.1 %v/v   (d) 56.1 %v/v

601. What is the real strength of $30°$ OP
    (a) 74.15%   (b) 67.15%
    (c) 88.15%   (d) 54.15%

602. Solutions for IM injection should be
    (a) Isotonic   (b) Hypertonic
    (c) Hypotonic   (d) Paratonic

603. The solutions which are not having the same osmotic pressure as that of body fluids are known as
    (a) Isotonic   (b) Hypertonic
    (c) Hypotonic   (d) Paratonic

604. Find out the proportion of procaine hydrochloride which will yield a solution iso osmotic with blood plasma. (freezing point of 1% w/v solution of procane HCl is $0.122°C$)
    (a) 5.26% w/v   (b) 4.26%w/v
    (c) 4.75%w/v   (d) 3.75%w/v

605. Find the concentration ofNacl required to make 1% solution of boric acid is isoosmotic with blood plasma. (freezing point of 1%w/v solution ofboric acid is $0.288°C$, freezing point of 1%w/v solution ofNacl is $0.576°C$)
    (a) 0.1 %w/v   (b) 0.326%w/v
    (c) 0.402%w/v   (d) 0.502%w/v

606. Convert $120°F$ into $°C$
(a) $37°c$
(b) $47°c$
(c) $48.9°C$
(d) $50.2°c$

607. Convert $100°C$ into $°F$
(a) $120°F$
(b) $180°F$
(c) $200°F$
(d) $212°F$

608. The quantity of drug which displaces one part of the base is called as
(a) Displacement value
(b) Isotonicity
(c) Proof spirit
(d) Allegation

609. Displacement value of zinc oxide is
(a) 3
(b) 4
(c) 5
(d) 1

610. Displacement value of iodoform is
(a) 3
(b) 4
(c) 5
(d) 1

611. The term posology was derived from
(a) Greek
(b) Latin
(c) French
(d) English

612. The word posos means
(a) How many
(b) How much
(c) How about
(d) Amount

613. Reasons for accumulation
(a) Slow excretion
(b) Defective degradation
(c) More absorption
(d) All the above

614. Which formula is used to calculate the dose of a child according to their age
(a) Dillings
(b) Cowling's
(c) Fried's
(d) All the above

615. Clark's formula is
(a) Child's weight in k g / 70 X adult dose
(b) Child's weight in pounds/ 150 X adult dose
(c) Both
(d) None

616. Catzel's rule is
(a) S.A of child (m^2) I 1.73 X adult dose
(b) Child weight in k g / 70 X adult dose
(c) Age in years/ age in years+ 12 X adult dose
(d) Age in years I 20 X adult dose

617. Vanishing creams come under which type of emulsion
(a) 0 / W
(b) W / 0
(c) **W/0/W**
(d) None of the above

618. Example for 0 / W type of emulsions
(a) Vanishing cream
(b) Foundation cream
(c) Cleansing cream
(d) Both a and b

619. Cleansing cream comes under which type of emulsion
(a) W / 0
(b) 0 / W
(c) W / 0 / W
(d) 0 / W / 0

620. For dry skins which type of creams are used
(a) Foundation cream
(b) Vanishing cream
(c) Moistening cream
(d) Night cream

621. Which of the following comes under hydrocarbons?
    (a) Vegetable oils   (b) Mineral Oils
    (c) Palm oil   (d) Arachis oil

622. Which of the following do not contains hydrocarbons
    (a) Petrolatum   (b) Paraffin wax
    (c) Palm oil   (d) Ceresin

623. Which of the following are the examples of mineral waxes?
    (a) Ozokerite
    (b) Ceresin
    (c) Both a and b
    (d) None of the above

624. Ceresin is produced by mixing refined Ozokerite wax with
    (a) Paraffin
    (b) Different portions of paraffin
    (c) Paraffin and oil
    (d) Paraffin, waxes and oil

625. Which of the following is not an example for fatty acid?
    (a) Laurie acid
    (b) Palmitic acid
    (c) Stearic acid
    (d) Acetic acid

626. Which of the following is a most popular fatty acid?
    (a) Oleic acid   (b) Stearic acid
    (c) Palmitic acid   (d) Laurie acid

627. What is the other name for wool fat?
    (a) Ceresin   (b) Ozokerite
    (c) Lanolin   (d) Mineral oil

628. Which of the following waxes comes under the animal origin?
    (a) Bees wax   (b) Spermaceti
    (c) Both a and b   (d) Japan wax

629. Which of the following is not commonly used wax in skin cosmetic production?
    (a) Bees wax   (b) Ceresin
    (c) Spermaceti   (d) Monton wax

630. Which comes under which type of agents?
    (a) Soap   (b) Humectants
    (c) Fatty acids   (d) Waxes

631. What is the chemical name for carbitol?
    (a) Tri ethylene glycol Mono ethyl ether
    (b) Di methylene glycol Mono ethyl ether
    (c) Di ethylene glycol Mono ethyl ether
    (d) Di propylene glycol Mono ethyl ether

632. Which of the following is not used as a binding agent?
    (a) Methyl cellulose
    (b) Ceresin
    (c) Japan wax
    (d) Fatty acids

633. Which of the following compounds possess both germicidal and fungicidal properties?
    (a) Triethanolamine
    (b) Quatamium ammonium compounds
    (c) Morpholine
    (d) Polyhydric alcohol

634. Perfumes are added at which temperature in cosmetic technology
   (a) 60° C
   (b) 75° C
   (c) 40° C
   (d) 80° C

635. Which of the following ingredients used to produce white cream?
   (a) TiO2
   (b) SiO2
   (c) $Fe2O_3$
   (d) ZnO

636. Which of the following creams are used to remove dust on the skin?
   (a) Vanishing cream
   (b) Cleansing cream
   (c) Moisturising cream
   (d) Cold cream

637. Which of the following is not example for preservatives?
   (a) Borax
   (b) Methyl paraben
   (c) Propyl paraben
   (d) Triethanolamine

638. For skin diseases like eczema, the skin creams should also contain
   (a) Triethanolamine
   (b) Uric acid
   (c) Urea
   (d) Ammonia

639. Which of the following ingredients are used for defatting of skin?
   (a) Waxes, Fats
   (b) Emollients
   (c) Thickening agents
   (d) Cleansing agents

640. Which of the following chemicals are used in preparation of sunscreen lotion?
   (a) Para amino benzoate

   (b) Ethyl para amino benzoate
   (c) Amino benzoate
   (d) Benzoate

641. What is the other name for sun protection factor?
   (a) Light protection factor
   (b) Proteccion solar
   (c) Both A and B
   (d) Light factor

642. Which of the following is not an example for semi permanent dyes?
   (a) Nitro amino phenes
   (b) Amino phenes
   (c) Nitrophenylene diamines
   (d) Amino anthraquinone

643. Which of the following is an example of temporary hair dye?
   (a) Crystal violet
   (b) Bromophenol blue
   (c) Crystal blue
   (d) All of the above

644. Semi permanent colorants gives its characters due to its
   (a) Neutral affinity
   (b) Amphoteric affinity
   (c) Cationic affinity
   (d) Anionic affinity

645. Which of the following is the example of solvent, used in the preparation of semi permanent colorants?
   (a) Benzyl alcohol
   (b) Ethyl alcohol
   (c) Propyl alcohol
   (d) Butyl alcohol

646. In order to increase penetration of colorants which of the following ingredients are used?
   (a) Uric acid   (b) Urea
   (c) Methyl alcohol (d) Ammonia

647. In permanent hair dyes, products along with a dye intermediate, which of the following is used?
   (a) Oxidising agent
   (b) Reducing agent
   (c) Complexing agent
   (d) Diazotising agents

648. Which of the following is not the example of water soluble reducing agent?
   (a) Sulphites   (b) Sulphates
   (c) Bisulphites   (d) Dithiourites

649. Chemically the hair can be removed by
   (a) Epilitory
   (b) Biplitory
   (c) Deplitory
   (d) All the above

650. Which of the following is an example for sulphide used in depilatories?
   (a) Strontium sulphide
   (b) Barium sulphide
   (c) Propyl sulphide
   (d) Benzyl sulphide

651. Which of the following is an example for film former in nail lacquer?
   (a) Ethyl stearates
   (b) Zinc oxide
   (c) Nitro cellulose
   (d) titanium dioxide

652. Which of the following agents are added to provide hard film for nail lacquers?
   (a) Resins   (b) Solvents
   (c) Plasticizers   (d) Diluents

653. Which of the following is an example for natural resins?
   (a) Dammer
   (b) Ethyl alcohol
   (c) Zinc oxide
   (d) Nitrocellulose

654. Which of the following resins are not most commonly used one?
   (a) Shellac
   (b) Benzoin
   (c) Ployaryl sulphion amides
   (d) Sandarac

655. In order to regulate the drying time which agents are used?
   (a) Solvents   (b) Resins
   (c) Sulphides   (d) Plasticizer

656. Which of the following agents are used to increase the strength?
   (a) Plasticizer   (b) Diluents
   (c) Latent solvents (d) Resins

657. Which of the following agents are used to reduce the hardness of enamel film?
   (a) Resins   (b) Solvents
   (c) Plasticizers   (d) Diluents

658. Which of the following is an opacifier?
   (a) Ethyl alcohol
   (b) Nitrocellulose
   (c) Dammer
   (d) Titanium dioxide

659. Which of the following is an example for UV absorbent?
(a) Bismuth oxychloride
(b) Sodium oxychloride
(c) Zinc oxychloride
(d) Bismuth chloride

660. Which of the following is an example for suspending agents?
(a) ZnO
(b) TiO2
(c) Bentonite
(d) Ethyl alcohol

661. Which of the following is not an example for paraffin?
(a) Hard paraffin
(b) Bees wax
(c) Ethyl alcohol
(d) Ozokerite wax

662. Which of the following is a microcrystalline wax?
(a) Ozokerite wax   (b) Ceresin
(c) Both a and b   (d) Bees wax

663. Which of the following is an example for hard wax?
(a) Bees wax   (b) Candellite
(c) Ozokerite wax   (d) Ceresin

664. Which of the following is an example for softening agents?
(a) Hard paraffin
(b) Bees wax
(c) Wool fat
(d) Ozokerite wax

665. Which of the following oils cannot be used in preparation of lipsticks?
(a) Castor oil   (b) Palm oil
(c) Mineral oil   (d) Olive oil

666. Which of the following agents are the examples for pearlescent agent?
(a) Bismuth oxychloride
(b) Bismuth chloride
(c) Oxychloride
(d) Chloride

667. Which of the following is an example for anti oxidant?
(a) Bismuth oxychloride
(b) Ceresine
(c) Butylated hydroxy touline
(d) Benzoate

668. Which of the following is an example for mould releasers?
(a) Dimethyl silicone
(b) Dimethyl sulphate
(c) Diethyl silicone
(d) Trimethyl silicone

669. Which of the following is used as UV filter in lipstick preparations?
(a) Dimethyl silicone
(b) Benzo phenone
(c) Olive oil
(d) Bismuth oxychloride

670. Rancidity is done by determining its
(a) Breaking load number
(b) Softening point
(c) Peroxide number
(d) Melting point

671. Which of the following is not an example for dentifrices?
(a) Precipitated $CaCO_3$
(b) Calcium sulphate
(c) Calcium phosphate
(d) Dicalcium phosphate

672. Which of the following is polishing agent used in preparation of fluoride tooth paste?
    (a) Precipitated CaCo3
    (b) Di calcium pyrophosphate
    (c) Tetra calcium pyrophosphate
    (d) Tri calcium pyrophosphate

673. What is the other name for abrasive silica?
    (a) Xerogels   (b) Cresols
    (c) Crogels   (d) Pumice

674. Which of the following surfactants is used in the preparation of dentifrices?
    (a) Sodium lauryl sarcosinate
    (b) Barium lauryl sarcosinate
    (c) Sodium ethyl sarcosinate
    (d) Sodium lauryl sulphosuccinate sodium ethyl

675. Which of the following is the most popular binder in tooth pastes?
    (a) Sodium carboxy methyl cellulose
    (b) Barium carboxy methyl cellulose
    (c) Sodium carboxy ethyl cellulose
    (d) None of the above

676. Which of the following humectants provide sweetness taste?
    (a) Glycerol
    (b) Propylene glycol
    (c) Sorbitol
    (d) Benzoates

677. Which of the following agents are used in acid balanced shampoos?
    (a) Ammonium sulphate
    (b) Ammonium lauryl ether sulphate
    (c) Ammonium lauryl sulphate
    (d) Ammonium lauryl propyl sulphate

678. Which of the following cationic agents all used in low p^H shampoos?
    (a) Quaternary ammonium compounds
    (b) Fatty acids
    (c) Fatty alcohols
    (d) Glycol stearate

679. What is the other name for eye irritatory test?
    (a) Pyrogen test
    (b) Draize test
    (c) Ames test
    (d) All of the above

680. Medicinal and toilet preparation act, 1955 is effectively implemented throughout India from
    (a) 2nd may, 1956
    (b) 5th June 1957
    (C) 2nd April, 1952
    (d) 5th June, 1957

681. Narcotics producing in human
    (a) Dependence
    (b) Dependence, tolerance
    (c) Tolerance
    (d) Dependence, tolerance and withdraw! syndrome

682. Bonded manufactory/laboratory
    (a) Drug has not been paid
    (b) Duty has been paid
    (c) Both a and b
    (d) None of these

683. Medicinal and toilet preparation (Excise duty) Act was passed in
    (a) 1955   (b) 1975
    (c) 1965   (d) 1976

684. Non-bonded laboratories
    (a) Licensed for the manufacture and storage of medicinal preparations
    (b) Licensed for the manufacture of medicinal and toilet preparations
    (c) Licensed for the manufacture and storage of medicinal and toilet preparations
    (d) None of the above

685. Spirit store means
    (a) Storage of alcohol
    (b) Storage of opium and Indian hemp
    (c) Both a and b
    (d) None of the above

686. Objectives of medicinal and toilet preparations Act
    (a) To establish uniformity of excise duties throughout the country
    (b) Levy and collection of excise duties on medicinal and toilet preparations containing alcohol and other narcotic drugs
    (c) Both a and b
    (d) None of the above

687. Manufacture outside the bond is also called as
    (a) Manufacture in bond
    (b) Manufacture without the bond
    (c) Bonded laboratories
    (d) Non-bonded laboratories

688. Which of the following is not a power of excise officer?
    (a) Inspection
    (b) Search
    (c) Suspension of licence
    (d) Countersign the indent

689. The excise officer in case of offence forwards the articles seized to the officer incharge of police station? What is the excise officer performing in this act?
    (a) Duties   (b) Power
    (c) Responsibility (d) None

690. Inspection is must in
    (a) Bonded laboratories
    (b) Non-Bonded laboratories
    (c) Both A and B
    (d) None of the above

691. In which of the following case alcoholic preparations can be exported from India?
    (a) Export under bond
    (b) Export after payment of duty
    (c) Both A and B
    (d) None of the above

692. Medicinal and Toilet preparations are stored in bulk jars or bottles. Each containing
    (a) Not less than 2,200 mL
    (b) Not less than 2,273 mL
    (c) Not less than 2,500 mL
    (d) None of the above

693. Rectified spirit is
    (a) Undenaturated alcohol of a strength not less than 50.0° over proof
    (b) Undenaturated alcohol of a strength not more than 50.0° over proof
    (c) Both a and b
    (d) None of the above

694. The percentage of wastage in the production of medicinal or toilet preparation is fixed by
    (a) State government
    (b) Central government
    (c) Both State and centralgovemment
    (d) None of the above

695. Issue of alcoholic preparations from the bonded laboratory can be taken out by manufacturers by making an application to
    (a) Officer-in charge
    (b) Excise officer
    (c) Excise-commissioner
    (d) None of the above

696. Objectives of drug (price control) order
    (a) To ensure equitable distribution of essential bulk drugs
    (b) To fix the maximum retail price for drug formulation in order to meet profit
    (c) Both a and b
    (d) None of the above

697. Scheduled bulk drug
    (a) A bulk drug specified in the first schedule
    (b) A bulk drug specified in the second schedule
    (c) Both a and b
    (d) None of the above

698. Provisions of the drug (price control) order
    (a) Fix prices of bulk drugs in first scheduled
    (b) Fix prices of wholesaler and retailer

    (c) Both a and b
    (d) None of the above

699. In order to fix the maximum sale price of bulk drug central government established national pharmaceutical pricing authority (NPPa) in
    (a) August 1998
    (b) August 1997
    (c) September 1997
    (d) August 1999

700. Drug (price control) order contains
    (a) Schedule I
    (b) Schedule II
    (c) Schedule III
    (d) All the above

701. For the purpose of enquiries the details in form I are furnished by the manufacturer
    (a) Once in six months
    (b) Once in a year
    (c) Once in two years
    (d) Twice in month

702. In fixing price of bulk drug government considers the following thing
    (a) A post tax return of 14% on net worth (18% if the production is from basic stage)
    (b) A return of 22% on capital employed (26% if production is from basic stage)
    (c) Internal rate return of 12% based on long term marginal costing for a new product
    (d) Any one of the above

703. M.A.P.E
    (a) Minimum allowable packing expenses
    (b) Minimum allowable purchasing expenses
    (c) Maximum allowable post-manufacturing expenses
    (d) Maximum allowable pre-manufacturing expenses

704. For a scheduled formulation, the manufacturer selling price for
    (a) R.P-20%   (b) R.P-16%
    (c) R.P-12%   (d) R.P-10%

705. In august 1997, which authority did the central government establish in order to enquire and fix the price for the bulk drugs?
    (a) National Pharmaceutical packing authority
    (b) National Pharmaceutical pricing authority
    (c) National Pharmaceutical purchasing authority
    (d) National Pharmaceutical processing authority

706. Drug price (display and control) order was passed in
    (a) 1970   (b) 1987
    (c) 1966   (d) 1995

707. Which of the following member is not an ex-officio member?
    (a) Drug controller of India
    (b) Director of CDA
    (c) President of MCI
    (d) Govt analyst

708. DTAB means
    (a) Drug transport advisory board
    (b) Drug transport administration board
    (c) Drug technical advisory board
    (d) None of the above

709. Functions of drug consultative committee include?
    (a) To advise central government
    (b) To advise state government
    (c) To advise DTAB
    (d) All the above

710. Central drug laboratory situated at
    (a) Kasauli
    (b) Izathnagar
    (c) Calcutta
    (d) All the Above

711. Indian veterinary research situated at?
    (a) Kasauli
    (b) Izathnagar
    (c) Calcutta
    (d) All the Above

712. Central research institute situated at?
    (a) Kasauli
    (b) Izathnagar
    (c) Calcutta
    (d) All the Above

713. For analysis of biological for veterinary use, a person/ govt analyst should have following qualifications?
    (a) A graduate in veterinary science and with 5 years experience of testing
    (b) A post graduate in veterinary science and with 3 years experience of testing
    (c) Both a and b
    (d) Either a or b

714. Every inspector shall be deemed to be public servant under which section of IPC
    (a) Section 20   (b) Section 21
    (c) Section 22   (d) Sections 22

715. To inspect pretnIses manufacturing biological drug inspector should have the following qualifications?
    (a) A graduate in veterinary science and 18 months experience in manufacturing or testing of veterinary biologicals
    (b) A post graduate in veterinary science and with 3 years experience in the inspection of firm manufacturing veterinary biologicals
    (c) Both a and b
    (d) Either a or B

716. The process of movement of drug from its site of administration to systemic circulation is called as
    (a) Absorption
    (b) Distribution
    (c) Metabolism
    (d) Excretion

717. The movement of drug between one compartment and the other (blood & extra vascular tissues) is referred to as drug
    (a) Absorption
    (b) Distribution
    (c) Metabolism
    (d) Excretion

718. Distribution and elimination together called as
    (a) Absorption
    (b) Elimination
    (c) Drug disposition
    (d) None

719. Kinetics of ADME is called as
    (a) Pharmacokinetics
    (b) Pharmacodynamics
    (c) Clinical pharmacokinetics
    (d) Drug disposition

720. The loss of drug that occurs after oral administration is called
    (a) Presystemic metabolism
    (b) First pass effect
    (c) Both a & b
    (d) None

721. Passive diffusion is also called as
    (a) Nonionic diffusion
    (b) Ionic diffusion
    (c) Cationic diffusion
    (d) All the above

722. Concentration gradient ls the driving force for
    (a) Passive diffusion
    (b) Active transport
    (c) Pore transport
    (d) Endocytosis

723. Passive diffusion is expressed by
    (a) Noyes whitney equation
    (b) Fick's 2nd law of diffusion
    (c) Modified Noyes whitney equation
    (d) Fick's 1st law of diffusion

724. Passive diffusion follows
    (a) Zero order kinetics
    (b) First order kinetics
    (c) Second order kinetics
    (d) None

725. The area in which the carrier system is most dense is called
    (a) Active transport
    (b) Passive diffusion
    (c) Endocytosis
    (d) Absorption window

726. At a given pH the rate of permeation is in the following order
    (a) Anions> cations> unionized molecules
    b) Unionized molecules > anions > cations
    (c) Cations > anions > unionized molecules
    (d) Cations = anions = unionized molecules

727. Phagocytosis means
    (a) Cell drinking
    (b) Cell eating
    (c) Electro chemical diffusion
    (d) None

728. Pinocytosis means
    (a) Cell drinking
    (b) Cell eating
    (c) Electro chemical diffusion
    (d) None

729. Orally administered sabin polio vaccine is absorbed by
    (a) Cell drinking
    (b) Cell eating
    (c) Electro chemical diffusion
    (d) None

730. Mass transfer from the solid surface to the liquid phase is called
    (a) Dispersion
    (b) Diffusion
    (c) Dissolution
    (d) Disintegration

731. Drug dissolution can be explained by
    (a) Diffusion layer model
    (b) Surface renewal theory
    (c) Interfacial barrier model
    (d) All the above

732. Diffusion layer model or film theory can be explained by
    (a) Fick's 1st law of diffusion
    (b) Modified noyes -whitney's equation
    (c) Both a & b
    (d) None

733. The area of solid surface exposed to the dissolution medium is called as
    (a) Absolute surface area
    (b) Effective surface area
    (c) Both a & b
    (d) None

734. Example for hydrophilic diluent
    (a) PEG
    (b) PVP
    (c) Dextrose
    (d) All the above

735. The relative amount of ionized and unionized drug in solution at a particular pH and the percent of drug ionized at this pH can be determined by
    (a) Henderson-hasselbach equation
    (b) Noyes-whitney's equation
    (c) Modified noyes-whitney's equation
    (d) None

736. Stomach p^H is
     (a) 5-8   (b) >8
     (c) 1-3   (d) None

737. Very weak acids with pKa > 8 their absorption is
     (a) Rapid & independent of GI p^H
     (b) Rapid & dependent of GI p^H
     (c) Slow & independent of GI p^H
     (d) Slow & dependent of GI p^H

738. Which acids with pKa < 2.5 are ionized in the entire p^H range of GIT and poorly absorbed
     (a) Very weak acids
     (b) Strong acids
     (c) Weak bases
     (d) Strong bases

739. Which type of drugs are unionized at all p^H values &their absorption is rapid and p^H independent
     (a) Weak base with pKa range 5-11
     (b) Strong base with pKa <5
     (c) Very weak base with pKa >11
     (d) Very weak base with pKa < 5

740. Stronger bases with pKa > 11 are
     (a) Mecamylamine
     (b) Guanethidine
     (c) Both a & b
     (d) None

741. Limitation of fp^H partition h_{yp}othesis is
     (a) Presence of virtual membrane p^H
     (b) Absorption of ionized drug
     (c) Presence of aqueous unstirred diffusion layer
     (d) All of the above

742. Surfactants acts as
     (a) Wetting agents
     (b) Solubilizers
     (c) Emulsifiers
     (d) All the above

743. Example for precipitation inhibitor is
     (a) PVP
     (b) HPMC
     (c) PEG
     (d) All the above

744. Gastric emptying is a
     (a) Zero order process
     (b) 1st order process
     (c) 2nd order process
     (d) Mixed order process

745. The speed at which the stomach contents empty into the intestine is called
     (a) Gastric emptying time
     (b) Gastric emptying half life
     (c) Gastric emptying rate
     (d) Distribution

746. The time required for the gastric contents to empty into the small intestine is called
     (a) Gastric emptying time
     (b) Gastric emptying half life
     (c) Gastric emptying rate
     (d) Distribution

747. The time taken for half the stomach contents to empty
     (a) Gastric emptying time
     (b) Gastric emptying half life
     (c) Gastric emptying rate
     (d) Distribution

748. Which is the major site for absorption
 (a) Stomach
 (b) Esophagus
 (c) Small intestine
 (d) Large intestine

749. Which enzyme of stomach mucosa inactivates ethanol
 (a) Digestive enzyme
 (b) Hydrolase
 (c) Hepatic enzyme
 (d) Alcohol dehydrogenase

750. Which drug can undergo first pass hepatic metabolism
 (a) Isoprenaline
 (b) Propranolol
 (c) Nitroglycerine
 (d) All the above

751. Distribution is defined as
 (a) The reversible transfer of a drug between one compartment and another
 (b) Reversible transfer of a drug between the blood & the extra vascular fluids and tissues
 (c) A passive process whose driving force is the concentration gradient between blood & extra vascular tissues
 (d) All the above

752. Distribution of drug present in the systemic circulation to extra vascular tissues involves
 (a) Permeation of free or unbound drug present in the blood through the capillary wall & entry into the extra cellular fluid
 (b) Permeation of drug present in the extra cellular fluid through the membrane of tissue cells & into the intracellular fluid
 (c) Both a & b
 (d) None

753. The special cells pericytes & astrocytes present in
 (a) BBB
 (b) Simple cell membrane barrier
 (c) Blood - cerebrospinal fluid barrier
 (d) Blood - placental barrier

754. Fetal abnormalities caused by administration of drugs during pregnancy is called as
 (a) Cirrhosis
 (b) Teratogenicity
 (c) UTI
 (d) None

755. During teratoginecity what are the harmful effects observed at the time of first 2 weeks of pregnancy
 (a) Mental retardation
 (b) Development & functional abnormalities
 (c) Cleft palate
 (d) Miscarriage

756. During teratogenecity what are the harmful effects observed at the time of 2 - 8 weeks of pregnancy
 (a) Cleft palate
 (b) Mental retardation

(c) Optic atrophy

(d) All the above

757. Blood- testis barrier is located at

(a) Sertoli- sertoli cell junction

(b) Synopsis

(c) Cerebrospinal fluid

(d) Nerve ending

758. Distribution is

(a) Permeability rate limited

(b) Perfusion rate limited

(c) Both

(d) None

759. The volume of blood that flows per unit time per unit volume of the tissue is called

(a) Gastric emptying time

(b) Glomerular filtration rate

(c) Perfusion rate

(d) Transit time

760. Perfusion rate is expressed in

(a) mL/min/mL   (b) mL/min/min

(c) mL/mL/min   (d) min/mL/min

761. The equation for tissue distribution half life is

(a) 0.693+K   (b) 0.693+Ke

(c) 0.693+Kf   (d) 0.693+Kt

762. Total body water is much greater in

(a) Infants   (b) Children

(c) Adults   (d) Elders

763. In which disease state the drugs like penicillin G & ampicillin will cross the **BBB**

(a) Meningitis   (b) Encephalitis

(c) Both   (d) None

764. The hypothetical volume of body fluid into which a drug is dissolved / distributed is called as

(a) Real volume of distribution

(b) Apparent volume of distribution

(c) Plasma volume

(d) Total body water

765. The body water is made up of

(a) Vascular fluid

(b) Extra cellular fluid

(c) Intra cellular fluid

(d) All the above

766. Plasma volume can be determined by high molecular weight substances like

(a) Evans blue

(b) Indocyanine green

(c) I - 131 albumin

(d) All

767. The extra cellular fluid volume is approximately

(a) 5 L   (b) 10 L

(c) 15 L   (d) 20 L

768. The difference between total body water and extra cellular fluid volume is defined as

(a) Plasma volume

(b) Intra cellular fluid volume

(c) Both a & b

(d) None

769. The intracellular fluid volume including those of blood cells is approximately

(a) 7 L   (b) 17 L

(c) 27 L   (d) 37 L

770. The factors which produce alteration in binding of drug to blood components results in
    (a) Increase in V_d
    (b) Decrease in V_d
    (c) Constant V_d
    (d) None

771. The factors which produce alteration in binding tp extra vascular components results in
    (a) Increase in V_d
    (b) Decrease in V_d
    (c) Constant V_d
    (d) None

772. The Vd of various drugs ranges from
    (a) 1 L - 10 L   (b) 2 L - 20 L
    (c) 3 L - 40,000 L   (d) 3 L - 60,000 L

773. V_d is altered when the conditions that affect
    (a) Absorption pattern of the drug
    (b) Distribution pattern of the drug
    (c) Metabolism pattern of the drug
    (d) Excretion pattern of the drug

774. The phenomenon of complex formation with proteins is called as
    (a) Drug binding
    (b) Drug interaction
    (c) Protein binding
    (d) Lipid binding

775. When the drug is bound to a cell protein which may be the drug receptor & this binding elicits a pharmacological response. This type of binding is called as
    (a) Intra cellular binding
    (b) Extra cellular binding

(c) Both
(d) None

776. When the drug bind to an extra cellular protein but the binding does not usually elicit a pharmacological response. This type of binding is called
    (a) Intra cellular binding
    (b) Extra cellular binding
    (c) Both a & b
    (d) None

777. In intracellular binding the receptors with which drug interact to show response are called as
    (a) 1° receptors   (b) 2° receptors
    (c) Both a & b   (d) None

778. In extra cellular binding the receptors does not elicit a pharmacological response. These receptors are called as
    (a) 1° receptors
    (b) Silent receptors
    (c) Both a & b
    (d) None

779. By protein binding of drugs their
    (a) Half life increased
    (b) AUC increased
    (c) Clearance increased
    (d) V_d increased

780. Protein - drug binding generally involves
    (a) Hydrogen bonds
    (b) Hydrophobic bonds
    (c) Vantler waals forces
    (d) All the above

781. The order of binding of drugs to various plasma proteins is
    (a) Globulins> lipoproteins > a1- acid glycoprotein > albumin
    (b) Globulins< lipoproteins < a1- acid glycoprotein < albumin
    (c) Albumin< a1-acid glycoprotein < lipoproteins < globulins
    (d) Albumin> a1-acid glycoprotein > lipoproteins > globulins

782. Molecular weight of human serum albumin is
    (a) 64,000
    (b) 64,500
    (c) 65,000
    (d) 65,500

783. Human serum albumin contain ____ site for drug binding
    (a) Warfarin & azapropazone binding site
    (b) Digitoxin binding site
    (c) Tamoxifen binding site
    (d) All the above

784. a 1- acid glycoprotein is also called as
    (a) LDL
    (b) HDL
    (c) Orosomucoid
    (d) **None**

785. Molecular weight of a1- acid glycoprotein is
    (a) 44,000
    (b) 45,000
    (c) 46,000
    (d) 47,000

786. a1-acid glycoprotein binds to
    (a) Acidic drugs
    (b) Basic drugs
    (c) Neutral drugs
    (d) All the above

787. Very low density lipoproteins (VLDL) is rich in
    (a) Triglycerides
    (b) Apoproteins
    (c) Both a & b
    (d) None

788. High density lipoproteins (HDL) is rich in
    (a) Triglycerides
    (b) Apoproteins
    (c) Both a & b
    (d) None

789. a1-globulin also called as
    (a) Transcortin
    (b) Corticosteroid
    (c) Both a & b
    (d) Ceruloplasmin

790. a2-globulin is also called as
    (a) Transcortin
    (b) Ceruloplasmin
    (c) Transferrin
    (d) Antigen

791. B1- globulin is also called as
    (a) Transcortin
    (b) Ceruloplasmin
    (c) Transferrin
    (d) Antigen

792. B2- globulins binds to
    (a) Carotinoids
    (b) Antigens
    (c) Antibodies
    (d) All the above

793. y-globulins binds to
    (a) Aarotenoids
    (b) Antigens
    (c) Antibodies
    (d) All the above

794. Molecular weight of hemoglobin is
    (a) 64,000
    (b) 64,500
    (c) 65,000
    (d) 65,500

795. The drugs which bind to carbonic anhydrase are
    (a) Acetazolamide
    (b) Chlorthalidone
    (c) Both a & b
    (d) None

796. Which drugs bind to RBC membrane
    (a) Imipramine
    (b) Chlorpromazine
    (c) Both a & b
    (d) None

797. Plasma - protein binding results in
    (a) Increase in V_d
    (b) Decrease in V_d
    (c) Increase in clearance
    (d) Decrease in clearance

798. Tissue - drug binding results in
    (a) Increase in V_d
    (b) Decrease in V_d
    (c) Increase in clearance
    (d) Decrease in clearance

799. The order of tissue binding of drugs is
    (a) Liver >kidney> lung> muscles
    (b) Liver < kidney < lung < muscles
    (c) Liver = kidney = lung = muscles
    (d) None

800. Epoxides of a number of halogenated hydro carbons & paracetamol bind irreversibly to liver tissues resulting in
    (a) Teratogenecity
    (b) Carcinogenicity
    (c) Hepatotoxicity
    (d) Retinopathy

801. By which method we can determine protein - drug binding
    (a) Indirect techniques
    (b) Direct techniques
    (c) Both a & b
    (d) None

802. In protein - drug binding when lipophilicity of drug increases
    (a) Extent of drug binding increases
    (b) Extent of drug binding decreases
    (c) Extent of drug binding is equal
    (d) None

803. Identify the anionic / acidic drug which bind more to human serum albumin
    (a) Penicillins
    (b) Sulphonamides
    (c) Both a & b
    (d) None

804. Identify the cationic/ basic drug which bind more to lipoproteins
    (a) Imipramine   (b) Alprenolol
    (c) Ibuprofen   (d) a & b

805. Which has greater affinity for al-acid glycoprotein (AAG) than for human serum albumin (HSA)
    (a) Penicillins   (b) Ibuprofen
    (c) Verapamil   (d) Lidocaine

806. When a drug has 99% bound, a displacement of just 1% of the bound drug results in
    (a) 50% raise in free drug concentration
    (b) 1% raise in free drug concentration
    (c) 100% raise in free drug concentration
    (d) No effect

807. The free bilirubin is not conjugated by the liver of neonates and thus crosses BBB and precipitates. This condition is called as
(a) Teratogenicity   (b) Kernicterus
(c) Both a & b   (d) None

808. Equation for fraction of drug unbound in plasma is
(a) $\overline{vd} = X/C$
(b) $fu = Cu/C$
(c) $fut = Cut/Ct$
(d) $vd = Vp+Vtfu/fut$

809. Equation for fraction of drug unbound to tissues is
(a) $\overline{vd} = X/C$
(b) $fu = Cu/C$
(c) $fut = Cut/Ct$
(d) $Vd = Vp+Vtfu/fut$

810. Kernicterus disorder in infants is caused by displacement of bilirubin from albumin binding sites by
(a) NSAIDs
(b) Sulphonamides
(c) Both a & b
(d) Penicillins

811. The value of association rate constant (Ka) & number of binding sites (N) can be obtained by
(a) Scatchard plot
(b) Line weaver - Burke plot
(c) Hitchcock plot
(d) All the above

812. When the pharmacological activity of a drug is altered by the concomitant use of another drug / by the presence of some other substance is called
(a) Pharmacokinetics
(b) Pharmacodynamics
(c) Drug interactions
(d) C_{max}

813. The drug whose activity is affected by an interaction is called as
(a) Object drug   (b) Precipitant
(c) Both   (d) None

814. The agent which precipitates an interaction is called as
(a) Object drug   (b) Precipitant
(c) Both   (d) None

815. The absorption interaction may result in a change in the
(a) Rate of absorption
(b) Amount of drug absorbed
(c) Both
(d) All the above

816. The frequency of administration of a drug in a particular dose is called
(a) Therapeutic index
(b) Pharmacokinetics
(c) Pharmacodynamics
(d) Dosage regimen

817. The ratio of maximum safe concentration to truillllum effective concentration of the drug is called
(a) Therapeutic index
(b) Pharmacokinetics
(c) Pharmacodynamics
(d) Dosage regimen

818. The application of pharmacokinetic principles in the safe & effective management of individual patient is called as
(a) Population pharmacokinetics
(b) Toxic kinetics
(c) Clinical pharmacokinetics
(d) bio pharmaceutics

819. The study of pharmacokinetic differences of drugs in various population groups is called as
(a) Population pharmacokinetics
(b) Toxicokinetics
(c) Clinical pharmacokinetics
(d) Bio pharmaceutics

820. The application of pharmacokinetic principles to the design, conduct and inter pretation of drug safety evaluation studies called as
(a) Population pharmacokinetics
(b) Toxicokinetics
(c) Clinical pharmacokinetics
(d) Bio pharmaceutics

821. The concentration of drug at peak is known as
(a) Peak plasma concentration
(b) Peak height concentration
(c) Maximum drug concentration
(d) All the above

822. The time for drug to reach peak concentration in plasma is called
(a) C_{max} (b) T_{max}
(c) $t\frac{1}{2}$ (d) AUC

823. C_{max} is expressed in
(a) mg/mL   (b) mg/hr
(c) µg/mL   (d) µg/sec

824. t_{max} is expressed in
(a) µg/mL   (b) hrs
(c) µg/mL.hrs   (d) L

825. Which represents the total integrated area under the plasma level-time profile and expresses the total amount of drug that comes into the systemic circulation after its administration.
(a) Cmax   (b) Imax
(c) $t\frac{1}{2}$ (d) AUC

826. AUC is expressed in
(a) µg/mL   (b) hrs
(c) µg/mL.hrs   (d) No units

827. The minimum concentration of drug in plasma required to produce the therapeutic effect is defined as
(a) MEC
(b) MSC
(c) AUC
(d) Onset of action

828. The concentration of drug in plasma above which adverse / unwanted effects are precipitated is called as
(a) MEC
(b) MSC
(c) AUC
(d) Onset of action

829. The beginning of pharmacological response is called as
(a) Onset of action
(b) Intensity of action
(c) Therapeutic index
(d) Duration of action

830. The time required for the drug to start producing pharmacological response is called as
    (a) Onsetofaction
    (b) Onset time
    (c) Duration of action
    (d) Intensity of action

831. The time period for which the plasma concentration of drug remains above the MEC level is called
    (a) Onset of action
    (b) Onset time
    (c) Duration of action
    (d) Intensity of action

832. The maxinnum pharmacological response produced by the peak plasma concentration of drug is called
    (a) Therapeutic range
    (b) Intensity of action
    (c) Duration of action
    (d) Therapeutic index

833. The drug concentration between MEC & MSC represents
    (a) Intensity of action
    (b) Duration of action
    (c) Therapeutic range
    (d) Therapeutic index

834. The manner in which the concentration of drug influences the rate of reaction is defined as
    (a) Order of reaction
    (b) Zero order kinetics
    (c) First order kinetics
    (d) Mixed order kinetics

835. The rate of reaction cannot be increased further by increasing the concentration of reactants is defined as
    (a) Order of reaction
    (b) Zero order kinetics
    (c) First order kinetics
    (d) Mixed order kinetics

836. Equation for zero order half- life is
    (a) $t\frac{1}{2} = 0.693/K$
    (b) $t\frac{1}{2} = 0.5C/ K$
    (c) $t\frac{1}{2} = K/2C$
    (d) None

837. Esxample for zero - order process is
    (a) Protein - drug binding
    (b) IV infusion
    (c) Osmotic pumps
    (d) All the above

838. When rate is directly proportional to the concentration of drug undergoing reaction is defined as
    (a) Zero order process
    (b) First order process
    (c) Linear kinetics
    (d) both b & c

839. Equation for first order halflife
    (a) $t\frac{1}{2} = 0.693+K$
    (b) $t\frac{1}{2} = 0.5C+ k$
    (c) $C = C - k t$
    (d) None

840. When the kinetics of a pharmacokinetic process changes from first order to zero order with increasing dose is called as
    (a) Mixed order kinetics
    (b) Nonlinear kinetics
    (c) Dose dependent kinetics
    (d) All

841. Nonlinearities in pharmacokinetics can be observed in
     (a) Naproxen   (b) Vitamin C
     (c) Riboflavin   (d) All

842. The kinetics of capacity limited processes can be described by
     (a) Zero order kinetics
     (b) First order kinetics
     (c) Michaelis - menten kinetics
     (d) None

843. When one or more peripheral compartments connected to the central compartment in a manner similar to connection of satellites to a planet known as
     (a) Mammillary model
     (b) Catenary model
     (c) Blood flow rate limited model
     (d) Distributed parameter model

844. When the compartments are joined to one another in a series like compartments of a train that model is known as
     (a) Mammillary model
     (b) Catenary model
     (c) Blood flow rate limited model
     (d) Distributed parameter model

845. Physiological models are also called as
     (a) Mammillary model
     (b) PB-PK models
     (c) Catenary model
     (d) None

846. In which method the drugs *I* metabolites follow linear kinetics & can be applied to any compartment model
     (a) Nonlinear kinetics
     (b) Non compartmental analysis
     (c) Blood flow rate limited model
     (d) Distributed parameter model

847. The average amount of time spent by the drug in the body before being eliminated is called as
     (a) Mean residence time
     (b) Onset of time
     (c) AUC
     (d) AUMC

848. The theoretical volume of body fluid containing drug from which the drug is completely removed in a given period of time is defined as
     (a) Absorption
     (b) Metabolism
     (c) Clearance
     (d) Biliary excretion

849. Clearance by all organs other than kidney is called as
     (a) Renal clearance
     (b) Organ clearance
     (c) Hepatic clearance
     (d) Non renal clearance

850. An index of how efficiently the eliminating organ clears the blood flowing through it of drug is known as
     (a) Rate of extraction
     (b) Extraction ratio
     (c) Systemic availability
     (d) Hepatic clearance

851. Absorption of rate constant can be calculated by method of residuals. This technique is also known as
     (a) Feathering   (b) Peeling
     (c) Stripping   (d) All

852. The time difference between drug administration and start of absorption is called as
   (a) Time lag
   (b) Absorption phase
   (c) Residual curve
   (d) Onset of time

853. First order absorption rate constant (Ka) in extra vascular administration can be determined by
   (a) Curve - fitting method
   (b) Wagner - nelson method
   (c) Both
   (d) None

854. Which method involves determination of Ka from percent unabsorbed -time plot and does not require the assumption of zero / first order absorption
   (a) Curve - fitting method
   (b) Wagner - nelson method
   (c) Both a & b
   (d) None

855. The disadvantage of Wagner nelson method is
   (a) It applies only to drugs with one compartment characteristics
   (b) It applies only to drugs with two compartment characteristics
   (c) It applies only to drugs with both compartment characteristics
   (d) None

856. After the IV bolus of a drug the decline in plasma concentration is biexponential indicating the presence of two disposition processes i.e., distribution and elimination. This model is called as
   (a) One compartment kinetics
   (b) Two compartment kinetics
   (c) Both
   (d) None

857. Nonlinearity in drug absorption can obtained from
   (a) When absorption is solubility/ dissolution rate limited
   (b) When absorption involves carrier mediated transport systems
   (c) When presystemic gut wall / hepatic metabolism attains saturation
   (d) All

858. Nonlinearity in distribution of drugs administered at high doses may be due to
   (a) Saturation of binding sites on plasma proteins
   (b) Saturation of tissue binding sites
   (c) Both
   (d) None

859. Which shows nonlinearity im drug metabolism
   (a) Phenytoin
   (b) Alcohol
   (c) Carbamazepine
   (d) All

860. What is rnichaelis menten equation
   (a) $t^{1/2} = 0.693/K$
   (b) $t^{1/2} = 0.5C/K$
   (c) $-deft = (V_{max} \cdot C)/(Km+C)$
   (d) $C = C- Kt$

861. In michaelis menten equation when $K_m = C$, then the equation becomes
    (a) $-dc/dt = V_{max} \div 2$
    (b) $-dc/dt = V_{max}.C \div K_m$
    (c) $-dc/dt = V_{max}$
    (d) None

862. In michaelis menten equation which plot shows uniformly scattered points
    (a) Hanes - woolf plot
    (b) Woolf- augustinsson-hofstce plot
    (c) a & b
    (d) Line weaver - burke plot

863. Practically the values of K_m & V_{max} can be obtained by
    (a) Graphical method
    (b) Line weaver - burke plot
    (c) Direct linear plot
    (d) All

864. The rate and extent of absorption of unchanged drug from its dosage form is called as
    (a) Bioequivalence
    (b) Bioavailability
    (c) Dissolution
    (d) Disintegration

865. The fraction of administered dose that enters the systemic circulation is called
    (a) Bio available fraction
    (b) Systemic availability
    (c) Relative bioavailability
    (d) Bioequivalence

866. When the systemic availability of a drug administered orally is determined in comparison to its intravenous administration is called as
    (a) Relative bioavailability
    (b) Absolute bioavailability
    (c) Systemic availability
    (d) Bio available fraction

867. When the systemic availability of a drug after oral administration is compared with that of an oral standard of the same drug is called as
    (a) Relative bioavailability
    (b) Absolute bioavailability
    (c) Systemic availability
    (d) Bio available fraction

868. Which type of dissolution apparatus is used for evaluation of transdermal products as well as non-disintegrating controlled release oral preparations
    (a) Cylinder apparatus
    (b) Rotating paddle apparatus
    (c) Reciprocating cylinder apparatus
    (d) Reciprocating disc apparatus

869. Which type of dissolution apparatus is used for evaluation of formulations containing poorly soluble drugs, micro particles & implants
    (a) Flow through cell
    (b) Rotating paddle
    (c) Reciprocating disc
    (d) Cylinder apparatus

870. What is the dissolution methodology for BCS class I drugs
    (a) Single point if NLT 85% Q in 15 min
    (b) Multiple point if Q < 85% in 15 min
    (c) Both a & b
    (d) None

871. The predictive mathematical model that describes the relationship between an *in vitro* property of a dosage form and an *in vivo* response is called as
   (a) IV bolus
   (b) IV infusion
   (c) IVIVC
   (d) IM

872. Why bioequivalence studies are conducted
   (a) If there is a risk of bio-inequivalence
   (b) If there is a risk of pharmacotherapeutic failure
   (c) Both a & b
   (d) None

873. Which is the term compares drug products with respect to a specific characteristic / function / to a defined set of standards.
   (a) Bioavailability
   (b) Bio-pharmaceutics
   (c) Pharmacokinetics
   (d) Equivalence

874. When two / more drug products contain the same labeled chemical substance as an active ingredient in the same amount is defined as
   (a) Chemical equivalence
   (b) Pharmaceutical equivalence
   (c) Bioequivalence
   (d) Therapeutic equivalence

875. When two / more drug products are identical in strength, quality, purity, content uniformity and disintegration & dissolution characteristics are called as
   (a) Chemical equivalence
   (b) Pharmaceutical equivalence
   (c) Bioequivalence
   (d) Therapeutic equivalence

876. When two / more identical dosage forms, reaches the systemic circulation at the same relative rate & to the same relative extent is defined as
   (a) Chemical equivalence
   (b) Pharmaceutical equivalence
   (c) Bioequivalence
   (d) Therapeutic equivalence

877. When two / more drug products that contain the same therapeutically active ingredient elicit identical pharmacological effects & can control the disease to the same extent is called as
   (a) Chemical equivalence
   (b) Pharmaceutical equivalence
   (c) Bioequivalence
   (d) Therapeutic equivalence

878. Administration of two / more treatments one after the other in a specified / random order to the same group of patients is called as
   (a) Cross over design
   (b) Change over design
   (c) Both a & b
   (d) Latin square design

879. According to BCS classification class I drugs shows
   (a) High solubility/ high permeability
   (b) Low solubility / high permeability
   (c) High solubility/ low permeability
   (d) Low solubility / low permeability

880. According to BCS classification class N drugs shows
 (a) High solubility/ high permeability
 (b) Low solubility / high permeability
 (c) High solubility / low permeability
 (d) Low solubility / low permeability

881. Identify the BCS class II drug
 (a) Nifedipine   (b) Diltiazem
 (c) Insulin   (d) Furosemide

882. Identify the BCS class III drug
 (a) Insulin
 (b) Metformin
 (c) Cimetidine
 (d) All the above

883. Which are the drug properties that determine BCS classification
 (a) Solubility
 (b) Dissolution rate
 (c) Permeability
 (d) All the above

884. By micronization process which drugs bioavailability can be increased
 (a) Griseofulvin
 (b) Steroidal drugs
 (c) Sulpha drugs
 (d) All the above

885. For the preparation of nano particles which technology is used
 (a) Pearl milling
 (b) Homogenization in water
 (c) Homogenization in non-aqueous media
 (d) All the above

886. Drug precipitation / crystallization can be prevented by use of inert polymers such as
 (a) HPMC
 (b) PVP
 (c) PEG
 (d) All the above

887. A binary system comprising of a solid solute molecularly dispersed in a solid solvent is called as
 (a) Precipitation
 (b) Solid solution
 (c) Salt form
 (d) Evaporation

888. The bioavailability of a _ _ _ drug is increased by molecular inclusion com
 (a) Barbiturates plex
 (b) Benzodiazepines
 (c) NSAIDs
 (d) All of the above

889. Compounds which facilitate the transport of drugs across the bio membrane are called as
 (a) Penetration
 (b) Permeation enhancers
 (c) Promoters
 (d) All the above

890. Penetration enhancers that have average to strong activity but cause sustained histological changes are
 (a) SLS   (b) EDTA
 (c) Citric acid   (d) All

891. By which method bioavailability of a drug can increased by enhancement of drug stability in the GIT
    (a) Enteric coating
    (b) Complexation
    (c) Use of metabolism inhibitors
    (d) All

892. Identify the powerful inhibitor of enzyme CYP3A4 and enhance the bioavailability of several drugs
    (a) Grape fruit juice
    (b) Mango juice
    (c) Lemon juice
    (d) None

893. When a test product displays an appreciably larger bioavailability than the reference product is called as
    (a) Reference product
    (b) Pharmaceutical alternatives
    (c) Non linear kinetics
    (d) Supra bioavailability

894. If a patient does not suffer from renal impairment, liver diseases / other patho physiologic states which might affect the disposition function. In such case _ _ _ _ can be taken as criteria for calculation of dosage regimen
    (a) Age   (b) Sex
    (c) Surface area   (d) Body weight

895. What ls the therapeutic index of diazepam
    (a) < 5   (b) > 10
    (c) 5 - 10   (d) None

896. The application of pharmacokinetic principles in the dosage regimen design for the safe and effective management of illness in individual patient is called as
    (a) Non compartmental model
    (b) Bio equivalence
    (c) Clinical pharmacokinetics
    (d) Therapeutic bioavailability

897. The manner in which the drug is taken called as
    (a) Frequency of dose
    (b) Dosage regimen
    (c) Dosage form
    (d) Route of administration

898. Which is the one in which the drug is administered in suitable doses with sufficient frequency that ensures maintenance plasma concentration within the therapeutic window for the entire duration of therapy
    (a) Single dosage regimen
    (b) Multiple dosage regimen
    (c) Clinical pharmacokinetics
    (d) Pharmacodynamics

899. Greater the dose size, greater the fluctuations between $C_{ss,max}$ & $C_{ss,min}$ & shows
    (a) Both therapeutic and toxic responses
    (b) Optimum dose therapeutically
    (c) Ineffective therapeutically
    (d) None

900. The ratio of C_{max} & C_{min} is called as
    (a) Dose frequency
    (b) Fluctuation
    (c) Dose size
    (d) Dosing interval

901. How many half lives the drug takes to reach the desired steady state and show therapeutic activity
(a) 3   (b) 5
(c) 9   (d) 10

902. Equation for loading dose is
(a) Xo/C o
(b) An/F
(c) (C $_{ss,avg}$ X Vd)/F
(d) XoL–;- Xo

903. When tie = $t\frac{1}{2}$, the dose ratio should be equal to
(a) < 2   (b) > 2
(c) 2   (d) None

904. The ease / difficulty in maintaining drug concentration within the therapeutic window depends upon
(a) Therapeutic index of drug
(b) $t\frac{1}{2}$ of drug
(c) Convenience of dosing
(d) All the above

905. Which drug has very long $t\frac{1}{2}$
(a) Penicillin   (b) Heparin
(c) Amlodipine   (d) All

906. Which drug is lipid soluble & distribute more in adipose tissues, the Vd is larger per kg body weight in obese patients
(a) Thiopental   (b) Phenytoin
(c) Diazepam   (d) All

907. Mosteller's equation is
(a) (height x weight) $\frac{1}{2} \div 60$
(b) A_m!F
(c) Css,avg. Vd/F
(d) Xo,L–;- Xo

908. Infants & children require larger mg/kg doses than adults because
(a) Their body SA per kg body weight is larger
(b) Larger volume of distribution
(c) Both
(d) None

909. Dosing of drugs in renal disease is adjusted by
(a) Dose adjustment based on total body clearance
(b) Dose adjustment based on elimination rate constant
(c) a & b
(d) None

910. Management of drug therapy in individual patient often requires evaluation of response of the patient to the recommended dosage regimen is called as
(a) Multiple dosage regimen
(b) Monitoring of drug therapy
(c) Both a & b
(d) None

KEY

1. (a)	**2.** (c)	**3.** (a)	**4.** (a)	**5.** (d)
6. (c)	**7.** (c)	**8.** (c)	**9.** (c)	**10.** (d)
11. (a)	**12.** (c)	**13.** (d)	**14.** (d)	**15.** (c)
16. (c)	**17.** (d)	**18.** (d)	**19.** (d)	**20.** (b)
21. (c)	**22.** (a)	**23.** (b)	**24.** (d)	**25.** (d)
26. (c)	**27.** (d)	**28.** (c)	**29.** (a)	**30.** (c)
31. (d)	**32.** (a)	**33.** (c)	**34.** (c)	**35.** (d)
36. (a)	**37.** (b)	**38.** (b)	**39.** (a)	**40.** (b)
41. (b)	**42.** (a)	**43.** (d)	**44.** (c)	**45.** (a)
46. (d)	**47.** (a)	**48.** (c)	**49.** (b)	**50.** (a)
51. (b)	**52.** (a)	**53.** (a)	**54.** (a)	**55.** (d)
31. (d)	**32.** (a)	**33.** (c)	**34.** (c)	**35.** (d)
36. (a)	**37.** (b)	**38.** (b)	**39.** (a)	**40.** (b)
41. (b)	**42.** (a)	**43.** (d)	**44.** (c)	**45.** (a)
46. (d)	**47.** (a)	**48.** (c)	**49.** (b)	**50.** (a)
51. (b)	**52.** (a)	**53.** (a)	**54.** (a)	**55.** (d)
31. (d)	**32.** (a)	**33.** (c)	**34.** (c)	**35.** (d)
36. (a)	**37.** (b)	**38.** (b)	**39.** (a)	**40.** (b)
41. (b)	**42.** (a)	**43.** (d)	**44.** (c)	**45.** (a)
46. (d)	**47.** (a)	**48.** (c)	**49.** (b)	**50.** (a)
51. (b)	**52.** (a)	**53.** (a)	**54.** (a)	**55.** (d)
56. (d)	**57.** (a)	**58.** (a)	**59.** (b)	**60.** (a)
61. (b)	**62.** (c)	**63.** (a)	**64.** (a)	**65.** (c)
66. (b)	**67.** (a)	**68.** (d)	**69.** (c)	**70.** (d)
71. (a)	72. (d)	**73.** (a)	**74.** (a)	**75.** (c)
76. (c)	**77.** (c)	**78.** (d)	**79.** (d)	**80.** (d)
81. (b)	**82.** (c)	**83.** (d)	**84.** (b)	**85.** (a)
86. (d)	**87.** (a)	**88.** (c)	**89.** (c)	**90.** (a)
91. (b)	**92.** (a)	**93.** (d)	**94.** (d)	**95.** (d)
96. (d)	**97.** (b)	**98.** (d)	**99.** (d)	**100.** (c)

101.	(d)	**102.**	(d)	**103.**	(d)	**104.**	(a)	**105.**	(d)
106.	(b)	**107.**	(b)	**108.**	(d)	**109.**	(d)	**110.**	(c)
111.	(d)	**112.**	(c)	**113.**	(a)	**114.**	(d)	**115.**	(b)
116.	(c)	**117.**	(a)	**118.**	(b)	**119.**	(d)	**120.**	(b)
121.	(b)	**122.**	(d)	**123.**	(a)	**124.**	(c)	**125.**	(c)
126.	(a)	**127.**	(c)	**128.**	(a)	**129.**	(d)	**130.**	(a)
131.	(c)	**132.**	(c)	**133.**	(b)	**134.**	(a)	**135.**	(b)
136.	(a)	**137.**	(b)	**138.**	(a)	**139.**	(d)	**140.**	(b)
141.	(a)	**142.**	(a)	**143.**	(d)	**144.**	(b)	**145.**	(b)
146.	(c)	**147.**	(d)	**148.**	(c)	**149.**	(b)	**150.**	(a)
151.	(a)	**152.**	(c)	**153.**	(c)	**154.**	(c)	**155.**	(a)
156.	(c)	**157.**	(d)	**158.**	(a)	**159.**	(b)	**160.**	(a)
161.	(b)	**162.**	(a)	**163.**	(a)	**164.**	(a)	**165.**	(b)
166.	(a)	**167.**	(d)	**168.**	(d)	**169.**	(b)	**170.**	(c)
171.	(c)	**172.**	(a)	**173.**	(c)	**174.**	(a)	**175.**	(a)
176.	(b)	**177.**	(c)	**178.**	(b)	**179.**	(a)	**180.**	(c)
181.	(b)	**182.**	(c)	**183.**	(d)	**184.**	(a)	**185.**	(c)
186.	(c)	**115.**	(b)	**116.**	(c)	**117.**	(a)	**118.**	(b)
119.	(d)	**120.**	(b)	**121.**	(b)	**122.**	(d)	**123.**	(a)
124.	(c)	**125.**	(c)	**126.**	(a)	**127.**	(c)	**128.**	(a)
129.	(d)	**130.**	(a)	**131.**	(c)	**132.**	(c)	**133.**	(b)
134.	(a)	**135.**	(b)	**136.**	(a)	**137.**	(b)	**138.**	(a)
139.	(d)	**140.**	(b)	**141.**	(a)	**142.**	(a)	**143.**	(d)
144.	(b)	**145.**	(b)	**146.**	(c)	**147.**	(d)	**148.**	(c)
149.	(b)	**150.**	(a)	**151.**	(a)	**152.**	(c)	**153.**	(c)
154.	(c)	**155.**	(a)	**156.**	(c)	**157.**	(d)	**158.**	(a)
159.	(b)	**160.**	(a)	**161.**	(b)	**162.**	(a)	**163.**	(a)
164.	(a)	**165.**	(b)	**166.**	(a)	**167.**	(d)	**168.**	(d)
169.	(b)	**170.**	(c)	**171.**	(c)	**172.**	(a)	**173.**	(c)
174.	(a)	**175.**	(a)	**176.**	(b)	**177.**	(c)	**178.**	(b)
179.	(a)	**180.**	(c)	**181.**	(b)	**182.**	(c)	**183.**	(d)
184.	(a)	**185.**	(c)	**186.**	(c)	**187.**	(a)	**188.**	(a)

189. (a)	**190.** (a)	**191.** (b)	**192.** (a)	**193.** (c)
194. (a)	**195.** (a)	**196.** (a)	**197.** (c)	**198.** (a)
199. (d)	**200.** (d)	**201.** (b)	**202.** (b)	**203.** (c)
204. (c)	**205.** (b)	**206.** (d)	**207.** (c)	**208.** (a)
209. (d)	**210.** (a)	**211.** (b)	**212.** (a)	**213.** (a)
214. (c)	**215.** (c)	**216.** (c)	**217.** (b)	**218.** (c)
219. (c)	**220.** (d)	**221.** (b)	**222.** (d)	**223.** (b)
224. (c)	**225.** (b)	**226.** (b)	**227.** (a)	**228.** (c)
229. (b)	**230.** (d)	**231.** (a)	**232.** (d)	**233.** (c)
234. (c)	**235.** (c)	**236.** (d)	**237.** (b)	**238.** (b)
239. (c)	**240.** (c)	**241.** (a)	**242.** (c)	**243.** (b)
244. (d)	**245.** (b)	**246.** (c)	**247.** (b)	**248.** (d)
249. (b)	**250.** (c)	**251.** (a)	**252.** (b)	**253.** (c)
254. (d)	**255.** (b)	**256.** (c)	**257.** (b)	**258.** (b)
259. (c)	**260.** (c)	**261.** (d)	**262.** (b)	**263.** (b)
264. (a)	**265.** (c)	**266.** (c)	**267.** (c)	**268.** (a)
269. (a)	**270.** (c)	**271.** (c)	**272.** (d)	**273.** (b)
274. (a)	**275.** (b)	**276.** (d)	**277.** (b)	**278.** (d)
279. (b)	**280.** (c)	**281.** (b)	**282.** (c)	**283.** (a)
284. (b)	**285.** (c)	**286.** (a)	**287.** (c)	**288.** (c)
289. (c)	**290.** (b)	**291.** (b)	**292.** (c)	**293.** (d)
294. (b)	**295.** (b)	**296.** (c)	**297.** (d)	**298.** (d)
299. (d)	**300.** (d)	**301.** (b)	**302.** (a)	**303.** (b)
304. (c)	**305.** (a)	**306.** (c)	**307.** (d)	**308.** (c)
309. (b)	**310.** (b)	**311.** (b)	**312.** (c)	**313.** (b)
314. (c)	**315.** (d)	**316.** (a)	**317.** (b)	**318.** (a)
319. (b)	**320.** (c)	**321.** (a)	**322.** (a)	**323.** (c)
324. (b)	**325.** (a)	**326.** (b)	**327.** (b)	**328.** (a)
329. (a)	**330.** (a)	**331.** (a)	**332.** (b)	**333.** (c)
334. (b)	**335.** (b)	**336.** (d)	**337.** (a)	**338.** (c)
339. (a)	**340.** (a)	**341.** (b)	**342.** (a)	**343.** (a)
344. (b)	**345.** (b)	**346.** (d)	**347.** (b)	**348.** (a)

349. (a)	350. (b)	351. (a)	352. (b)	353. (a)
354. (c)	355. (a)	356. (a)	357. (b)	358. (d)
359. (d)	360. (a)	361. (b)	362. (a)	363. (b)
364. (a)	365. (a)	366. (a)	367. (c)	368. (a)
369. (b)	370. (b)	371. (a)	372. (a)	373. (b)
374. (a)	375. (b)	376. (a)	377. (b)	378. (b)
379. (a)	380. (a)	381. (a)	382. (a)	383. (c)
384. (a)	385. (b)	386. (a)	387. (b)	388. (d)
389. (a)	390. (b)	391. (b)	392. (a)	393. (b)
394. (b)	395. (c)	396. (b)	397. (a)	398. (b)
399. (c)	400. (a)	401. (a)	402. (c)	403. (a)
404. (a)	405. (b)	406. (a)	407. (a)	408. (c)
409. (c)	410. (a)	411. (c)	412. (a)	413. (c)
414. (b)	415. (d)	416. (d)	417. (d)	418. (a)
419. (a)	420. (b)	421. (b)	422. (a)	423. (c)
424. (a)	425. (d)	426. (c)	427. (b)	428. (a)
429. (a)	430. (b)	431. (a)	432. (a)	433. (b)
434. (b)	435. (a)	436. (c)	437. (a)	438. (b)
439. (d)	440. (b)	441. (b)	442. (a)	443. (d)
444. (c)	445. (a)	446. (c)	447. (b)	448. (a)
449. (a)	450. (a)	451. (a)	452. (d)	453. (d)
454. (c)	455. (b)	456. (a)	457. (c)	458. (b)
469. (d)	460. (a)	461. (a)	462. (c)	463. (c)
464. (b)	465. (a)	466. (a)	467. (c)	468. (b)
469. (a)	470. (a)	471. (b)	472. (a)	473. (a)
474. (d)	475. (b)	476. (b)	477. (d)	478. (a)
479. (a)	480. (b)	481. (b)	482.(d)	483.(c)
484. (a)	485. (b)	486. (b)	487. (d)	488.(b)
489. (c)	490. (d)	491. (c)	492. (a)	493.(c)
494. (b)	495. (a)	496. (d)	497. (a)	498.(d)
499 (d)	500. (a)	501. (b)	502. (b)	503. (a)
504. (a)	505. (b)	506. (b)	507. (c)	508. (c)

509.	(d)	**510.**	(b)	**511.**	(d)	**512.**	(d)	**513.**	(d)
514.	(c)	**515.**	(c)	**516.**	(c)	**517.**	(d)	**518.**	(d)
519.	(a)	**520.**	(a)	**521.**	(b)	**522.**	(b)	**523.**	(d)
524.	(d)	**525.**	(d)	**526.**	(b)	**527.**	(c)	**528.**	(a)
529.	(b)	**530.**	(b)	**531.**	(b)	**532.**	(b)	**533.**	(c)
534.	(b)	**535.**	(b)	**536.**	(a)	**537.**	(b)	**538.**	(a)
539.	(a)	**540.**	(a)	**541.**	(a)	**542.**	(b)	**543.**	(a)
544.	(b)	**545.**	(b)	**546.**	(d)	**547.**	(a)	**548.**	(a)
549.	(b)	**550.**	(d)	**551.**	(b)	**552.**	(c)	**553.**	(a)
554.	(b)	**555.**	(b)	**556.**	(d)	**557.**	(c)	**558.**	(c)
559.	(c)	**560.**	(c)	**561.**	(b)	**562.**	(d)	**563.**	(d)
564.	(a)	**565.**	(a)	**566.**	(d)	**567.**	(b)	**568.**	(b)
569.	(b)	**570.**	(b)	**571.**	(b)	**572.**	(a)	**573.**	(c)
574.	(a)	**575.**	(b)	**576.**	(c)	**577.**	(a)	**578.**	(b)
579.	(d)	**580.**	(a)	**581.**	(c)	**582.**	(d)	**583.**	(d)
584.	(b)	**585.**	(b)	**586.**	(c)	**587.**	(a)	**588.**	(b)
589.	(b)	**590.**	(c)	**591.**	(a)	**592.**	(b)	**593.**	(c)
594.	(a)	**595.**	(b)	**596.**	(c)	**597.**	(a)	**598.**	(b)
599.	(a)	**600.**	(c)	**601.**	(a)	**602.**	(b)	**603.**	(d)
604.	(b)	**605.**	(c)	**666.**	(c)	**607.**	(d)	**608.**	(a)
609.	(c)	**610.**	(a)	**611.**	(a)	**612.**	(b)	**613.**	(d)
614.	(d)	**615.**	(c)	**616.**	(a)	**617.**	(a)	**618.**	(d)
619.	(a)	**620.**	(c)	**621.**	(b)	**622.**	(c)	**623.**	(c)
624.	(b)	**625.**	(d)	**626.**	(a)	**627.**	(c)	**628.**	(c)
629.	(d)	**630.**	(b)	**631.**	(c)	**632.**	(a)	**633.**	(b)
634.	(c)	**635.**	(a)	**636.**	(b)	**637.**	(d)	**638.**	(c)
639.	(b)	**640.**	(b)	**641.**	(c)	**642.**	(b)	**643.**	(a)
644.	(c)	**645.**	(a)	**646.**	(b)	**647.**	(a)	**648.**	(b)
649.	(c)	**650.**	(a)	**651.**	(c)	**652.**	(a)	**653.**	(a)
654.	(c)	**655.**	(a)	**656.**	(c)	**657.**	(c)	**658.**	(d)
659.	(a)	**660.**	(b)	**661.**	(c)	**662.**	(c)	**663.**	(b)
664.	(c)	**665.**	(d)	**666.**	(d)	**667.**	(c)	**668.**	(a)

669.	(b)	**670.**	(c)	**671.**	(b)	**672.**	(c)	**673.**	(a)
674.	(a)	**675.**	(a)	**676.**	(b)	**677.**	(b)	**678.**	(a)
679.	(b)	**680.**	(b)	**681.**	(d)	**682.**	(a)	**683.**	(a)
684.	(c)	**685.**	(c)	**686.**	(c)	**687.**	(b)	**688.**	(d)
689.	(c)	**690.**	(b)	**691.**	(d)	**692.**	(b)	**693.**	(a)
694.	(a)	**695.**	(b)	**696.**	(d)	**697.**	(a)	**698.**	(c)
699.	(b)	**700.**	(d)	**701.**	(a)	**702.**	(d)	**703.**	(c)
704.	(a)	**705.**	(b)	**706.**	(c)	**707.**	(d)	**708.**	(c)
709.	(d)	**710.**	(c)	**711.**	(b)	**712.**	(a)	**713.**	(d)
714.	(b)	**715.**	(d)	**716.**	(a)	**717.**	**(b)**	**718.**	(c)
719.	**(a)**	**720.**	(c)	**716.**	(a)	**717.**	**(b)**	**718.**	(c)
719.	**(a)**	**720.**	(c)	**721.**	(a)	**722.**	(a)	**723.**	(d)
724.	(b)	**725.**	(d)	**726.**	(b)	**727.**	(b)	**728.**	(a)
729.	(a)	**730.**	(c)	**731.**	(d)	**732.**	(b)	**733.**	(b)
734.	(d)	**735.**	(a)	**736.**	(c)	**737.**	(a)	**738.**	(b)
739.	(d)	**740.**	(c)	**741.**	(d)	**742.**	(d)	**743.**	(d)
744.	(b)	**745.**	(c)	**746.**	(a)	**747.**	(b)	**748.**	(c)
749.	(d)	**750.**	(d)	**751.**	(d)	**752.**	(c)	**753.**	(a)
754.	(b)	**755.**	(d)	**756.**	(d)	**757.**	(a)	**758.**	(c)
759.	(c)	**760.**	(a)	**761.**	(d)	**762.**	(a)	**763.**	(c)
764.	(b)	**765.**	(d)	**766.**	(d)	**767.**	(c)	**768.**	(b)
769.	(c)	**770.**	(a)	**771.**	(b)	**772.**	(c)	**773.**	(b)
774.	(c)	**775.**	(a)	**776.**	(b)	**777.**	(a)	**778.**	(b)
779.	(a)	**780.**	(d)	**781.**	(d)	**782.**	(c)	**783.**	(d)
784.	(c)	**785.**	(a)	**786.**	(b)	**787.**	(a)	**788.**	(b)
789.	(c)	**790.**	(b)	**791.**	(c)	**792.**	(a)	**793.**	(b)
794.	(b)	**795.**	(c)	**796.**	(c)	**797.**	(b)	**798.**	(a)
799.	(a)	**800.**	(c)	**801.**	(c)	**802.**	(a)	**803.**	(c)
804.	(d)	**805.**	(d)	**806.**	(c)	**807.**	(b)	**808.**	(b)
809.	(c)	**810.**	(c)	**811.**	(d)	**812.**	(c)	**813.**	(a)
814.	(b)	**815.**	(d)	**816.**	(d)	**817.**	(a)	**818.**	(c)
819.	(a)	**820.**	(b)	**821.**	(d)	**822.**	(b)	**823.**	(c)

824.	(b)	825.	(d)	826.	(c)	827.	(a)	828.	(b)
829.	(a)	830.	(b)	831.	(c)	832.	(b)	833.	(c)
834.	(a)	835.	(b)	836.	(b)	837.	(d)	838.	(d)
839.	(a)	840.	(d)	841.	(d)	842.	(c)	843.	(a)
844.	(b)	845.	(b)	846.	(b)	847.	(a)	848.	(c)
849.	(d)	850.	(b)	851.	(d)	852.	(a)	853.	(c)
854.	(b)	855.	(a)	856.	(b)	857.	(d)	858.	(c)
859.	(d)	860.	(c)	861.	(a)	862.	(c)	863.	(d)
864.	(b)	865.	(a)	866.	(b)	867.	(a)	868.	(d)
869.	(a)	870.	(c)	871.	(c)	872.	(c)	873.	(d)
874.	(a)	875.	(b)	876.	(c)	877.	(d)	878.	(c)
879.	(a)	880.	(d)	881.	(a)	882.	(d)	883.	(d)
884.	(d)	885.	(d)	886.	(d)	887.	(b)	888.	(d)
889.	(d)	890.	(d)	891.	(d)	892.	(a)	893.	(d)
894.	(c)	895.	(c)	896.	(c)	897.	(b)	898.	(d)
899.	(a)	900.	(b)	901.	(b)	902.	(c)	903.	(c)
904.	(d)	905.	(c)	906.	(d)	907.	(a)	908.	(c)
909.	(c)	910.	(b)						

II   PHARMACEUTICAL CHEMISTRY

1. Match the following Term Alkane

   (P) Undecane   (1) 20 C
   (Q) Cetane   (2) 12 C
   (R) Dodecane   (3) 16 C
   (S) Icosane   (4) 11 C

   (a) P-1, Q-3, R-2, S-4
   (b) P-2, Q-3, R-4, S-1
   (c) p-1, Q-4, R-2, S-3
   (d) P-4, Q-3, R-2, S-1

2.

   $H_3C-\overset{H}{\underset{CH_3}{C}}-\overset{H2}{C}-\overset{H2}{C}- \quad =?$

   (a) n-Pentyl   (b) Amyl
   (c) $3^°$-Butyl   (d) $2^°$-Pentyl

3.

   The correct IUPAC name of this molecule
   (a) 2,4,4-trimethyl pentane
   (b) 3,3,2- trimethyl pentane
   (c) 2,2,4- trimethyl pentane
   (d) 1,1,1,3-tetramethyl butane

4. Which of the following are homologues?
   (a) Methane, Ethane
   (b) Methane, Propane
   (c) Ethane, Butane
   (d) Butane, Decane

5. H3C-CHrBr +Mg----?-----> H3C-CHrMgBr
   (a) Wet ether   (b) dil. HCl
   (c) dil. NaOH   (d) Dry ether

6.

   $H_3C-\overset{2}{C}-CH_3 \xrightarrow[\text{light, }121^°c]{1\,Br2}$ Major product?

   (a) 1-Bromopropane
   (b) 1,2-dibromopropane
   (c) 2- Bromopropane
   (d) 1,3- dibromopropane

7. Which of the following statement/s is/are correct regarding the halogenation of alkanes?
   (P) Chlorine is more reactive & less selective
   (Q) Bromine is more reactive & less selective
   (R) Bromine is less reactive & more selective
   (S) Chlorine is less reactive & more selective

   (a) P, R   (b) Q, S
   (c) Only P   (d) R, S

8.

   $H_3C-\overset{H2}{C}-CH_3 \xrightarrow[\text{light, }25^°C]{1\,Cl2}$ Major product?

   (a) 1-Chloropropane
   (b) 2- Chloropropane
   (c) Neither isomer predominates
   (d) None of the above

9. Which of the following is the correct order of stability of free radicals?
   (a) $1^° > 2^° > 3^°$ (b) $2^° > 3^° > 1^°$
   (c) $3^° > 2^° > 1^°$ (d) $1^° > 3^° > 2^°$

10.

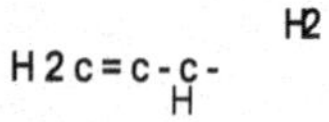

$$H_2C=C-\underset{H}{C}-$$

The common name of the above molecule is

(a) Vinyl   (b) Isopropyl
(c) Allyl   (d) Amyl

11. 2-Bromopentane (Major product?
(a) 1-Pentene   (b) n-Pentene
(c) 2-Pentene   (d) 3-Pentene

12.

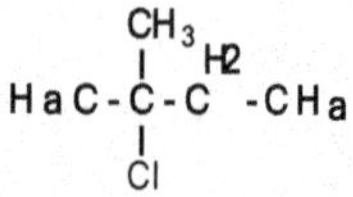

$$H_3C-\underset{Cl}{\overset{CH_3}{C}}-\overset{H_2}{C}-CH_3$$

Which of the following is related to the above reaction?

(a) Satzeff rule
(b) Markovnikov's rule
(c) Huckel's rule
(d) Van't hoff rule

13.

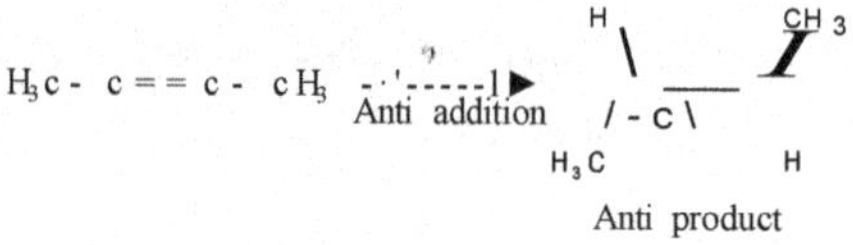

$$H_3C-c==c-cH_3 \xrightarrow{\text{Anti addition}}$$

Anti product

(a) Na or Li in liquid NH_3
(b) H_2, Lindlar's catalyst
(c) $LiAlH_4$
(d) $NaBH_4$

14. Among the following which alkene is less stable?

(a) $RCH=CH_2$ (b) $RCH=CHR$
(c) $R_2C=CHR$ (d) $R_2C=CR_2$

15. Wilkinson's catalyst is? (Used for hydrogenation purpose).

(a) $Zn+Hg/HCl$

(b) H_2/Ni or Pt
(c) $NH_2NH_2.H_2O$
(d) Organic complexes of transition metals like Rhodium or Iridium

16. Effect of peroxide is seen in which of the following hydrogen acids?

(a) HCl   (b) HBr
(c) HI   (d) HF

17.

This reaction is a

(a) Chemoselective reaction
(b) Stereoselective reaction
(c) Stereospecific reaction
(d) Regioselective

18.

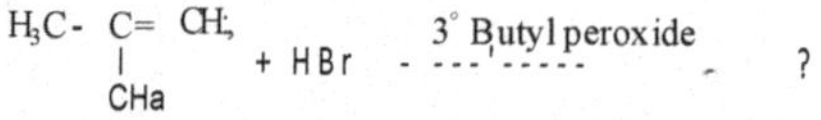

$$H_3C-\underset{CH_3}{\overset{}{C}}=CH_2 + HBr \xrightarrow{3°\text{ Butyl peroxide}} ?$$

(a) 1-Bromo-2-methyl propane
(b) 2-Bromo-2-methyl propane
(c) 1-Bromo n-butane
(d) 2- Bromo butane

19.

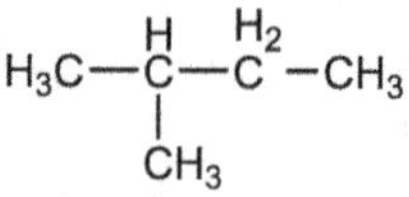

$$H_3C-\underset{CH_3}{\overset{H}{C}}-\overset{H_2}{C}-CH_3$$

The type of carbon atom that is not present in 2-methyl butane

(a) $1°$ (b) $2°$
(c) $3°$ (d) $4°$

20. $A + Br_2 \xrightarrow{Ccl_4}$ Rapid decolorization of bromine solution takes place, then what is A?

(a) 2-Propanol
(b) 2-Bromopentane
(c) 2-Butene
(d) 2-Chlorobutanal

21. A carbocation may
    (P) Combine with -ve ion or other basic molecule
    (Q) Rearrange to a more stable carbocation
    (R) Eliminate a proton to form an alkene
    (S) Abstract a proton to form an alkene
    (a) Only P, R
    (b) Only Q, R, S
    (c) Only P, S
    (d) P, Q, R&S

22. Ethers such as THF or Diglymine are used in which of the following reaction of alkenes?
    (a) Addition of HX
    (b) Hydroboration-Oxidation
    (c) Oxymercuration-demercuration
    (d) Reaction with Br_2/CCl_4

23. H-Br ____peroxide____>?
    (a) Heterolytic cleavage takes place
    (b) Homolytic cleavage takes place
    (c) No cleavage of H-Br bond
    (d) Dimerization takes place

24. n CH_2=CH_2 ____?--------> (-CHz-CHz-)n
    Ethylene Polyethylene
    (a) dil.HCl
    (b) Conc.HCl
    (c) O_2, heat, pressure
    (d) $HNO3+H_2SO_4$

25.

    H3C-C=CH2 ——cold alkaline KMnO4 ▶— ?
       |
       H

    (a) 2-Hydroxy propane
    (b) 1, 3-Dihydroxy propane
    (c) I-Hydroxy propane
    (d) 1,2-Dihydroxy propane

26.

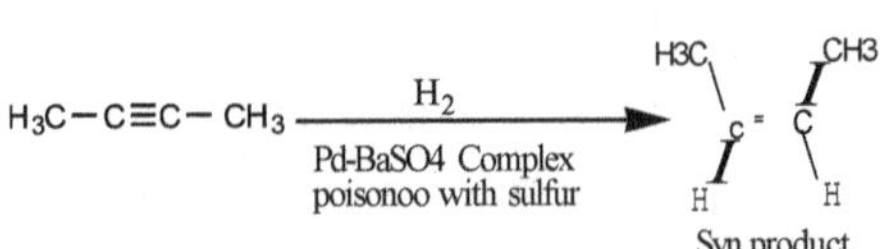

    Why sulfur is used in this reaction?
    (a) Sulphur prevents further reduction of butene into butane.
    (b) Syn product is formed due to sulfur only.
    (c) Sulphur enhances rate of reaction.
    (d) All the above

27. The reaction in the question 26 is a
    (a) Stereoselective reaction
    (b) Chemoselective reaction
    (c) Stereospecific reaction
    (d) Regioselective

28. Which of the following statement is correct regarding keto-enol tautomerism?
    (a) Equilibrium lies very much in favor of keto form
    (b) Equilibrium lies very much in favor of enol form
    (c) Equilibrium favors both the forms equally
    (d) None of the above

29. Compounds whose structures differ markedly in arrangement of atoms, but which exist in rapid equilibrium are called
    (a) Rotamers   (b) Epimers
    (c) Conformers   (d) Tautomers

30. Which of the following statement/s is/are correct about tautomerism?
    (P) Enamine form is more stable
    (Q) Imine form is more stable
    (R) Enol form is more stable
    (S) Keto form is more stable
    (a) Only Q is correct
    (b) Both Q & S are correct
    (c) Both P & R are correct
    (d) Both P & S are correct

31. Which of the following even though it doesn't turn the color of litmus paper, it is acidic
    (a) HCl   (b) HF
    (c) Methane   (d) Acetylene

32. The correct order of relative acidities of the following compounds is
    (a) Ethanol> water> acetylene> ammomia
    (b) Water> ethanol> acetylene> ammomia
    (c) Acetylene>ammonia> ethanol>water
    (d) Ethanol> acetylene> water> ammomia

33. R-X + Mg ____Y____> RMgX (Grignard's reagent). Y= ?
    (a) We tether   (b) Water
    (c) Heating   (d) Dry ether

34. 3,3-dimethyl-l-bromo butane doesn't contains which type of carbon atom
    (a) 2^0 (b) lo
    (c) 3^0 (d) 4^0

35. Which of the following statement is wrong about SN_2 mechanism
    (a) An SN_2 reaction proceeds with complete stereochemical inversion
    (b) It is a second order reaction & a high concentration of Nu:- favours the SN_2 reaction
    (c) Reactivity in SN_2: CH3 W > 1^0> $2^0 > 3^0$
    (d) Rearrangement of carbocations takes place

36. Which of the following statement is wrong about SN_1 mechanism
    (a) It is a 1st order reaction
    (b) Depends upon the concentration of Nu:-
    (c) Doesn't depends upon the concentration of Nu:
    (d) A low concentration favors the SN_1 reaction

37. Which of the following are aprotic solvents?
    (a) 2,2,2-trifluoroethanol, DMF & **DMSO**
    (b) HCOOH, CF3COOH & H_2O
    (c) Hexamethyl phosphorotriamide (HMPT), DMF & DMSO
    (d) Ethanol, water & DMF

38. SN_1 reactions of neutral substrates are faster in
    (a) **DMF**
    (b) **DMSO**
    (c) H_2O
    (d) Hexamethyl phosphorotriamide (HMPT)

39. Which of the following statement is wrong about SN_1 mechanism?
    - (a) Reactants are more polar than transition state
    - (b) Transition state is more polar than reactants
    - (c) Transition state is more stabilized by polar solvents
    - (d) SN_1 reactions are faster in polar solvents

40. Which of the following statement is wrong about SN_2 mechanism
    - (a) Reactants have concentrated charge
    - (b) Transition state has dispersed charge
    - (c) Reactants are more stabilized than transition state by salvation
    - (d) SN_2 reactions are faster in polar solvents

41. $CH_3Br + X- \underline{\quad}_{sN2} -----> CH_3X + Br-$. X= F, Cl, Br or I

    Reactivity of which of the following halide ion is more when the reaction is carried out in a solution of methanol
    - (a) I^-
    - (b) Br^-
    - (c) cl^-
    - (d) F^-

42. Which of the following statement is wrong about E_2 mechanism?
    - (a) Follow 2nd order kinetics
    - (b) Is not accompanied by rearrangements
    - (c) Is accompanied by rearrangements
    - (d) Strong base favors E_2 reaction

43. 2-Bromopentane $--------KOH_{(aic)}------->$ Preferred product?
    - (a) 2-Pentene
    - (b) 1-Pentene
    - (c) Isopentene
    - (d) 1-Bromopentane

44. Which of the following statement is wrong about E_1 mechanism
    - (a) Follow 1st order kinetics
    - (b) Doesn't depends upon the concentration of base
    - (c) Is accompanied by rearrangements
    - (d) Strong base favors E_1 reaction

45. N-methyl aniline is a
    - (a) 1° amine
    - (b) 2° amine
    - (c) 3° amine
    - (d) 4° amine

46.

H_2N--O- OCH_3

    - (a) Anisole
    - (b) Benzidine
    - (c) Toluidine
    - (d) Anisidine

47. GABA is a
    - (a) 1° amine
    - (b) 2° amine
    - (c) 3° amine
    - (d) 4° amine

48.

$$R-\overset{O}{\overset{\|}{C}}-OH \xrightarrow{SOCl_2} R-\overset{O}{\overset{\|}{C}}-Cl$$

    Which of the following statement/s is/are correct?
    - (P) -OH group is a bad leaving group
    - (Q) -OH group is a good leaving group

(R) -Cl group is a bad leaving group
(S) -Cl group is a good leaving group

(a) Q,R
(b) Only R
(c) P,S
(d) Both Q,S

49.

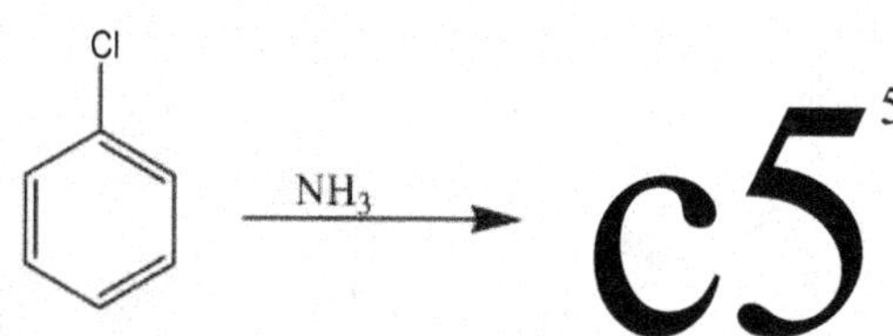

50. Which of the following alkylhalide undergoes elimination reaction when treated with methylamine?
(a) Ethylamine
(b) $3°$ butylamine
(c) Propylamine
(d) Butylamine

51.

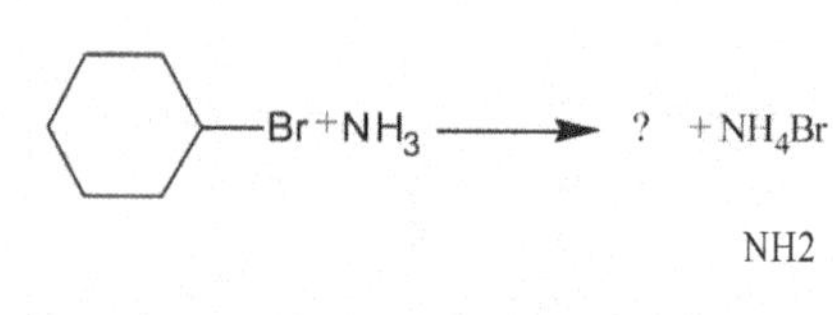

Aryl halide

Under normal conditions this reaction is not feasible. The above reaction takes place when which of the following group is present on chlorobenzene ring?
(a) -CH3
(b) -NO2
(c) -OH
(d) -OCH3

52. HVZ reaction (which is a regioselective reaction) is not shown by
(a) Acetic acid
(b) Butanoic acid
(c) Isobutanoic acid
(d) 2,2-dimethyl propanoic acid

53.

$$H3C-\overset{O}{\overset{\|}{C}}-OH \xrightarrow{\text{Halogen, red P}} Cl-H2C-\overset{O}{\overset{\|}{c}}-OH$$

(a) Simmons-Smith reaction
(b) Pinacol-Pinacolone rearrangement
(c) HVZ reaction
(d) Gattermann-koch reaction

54.

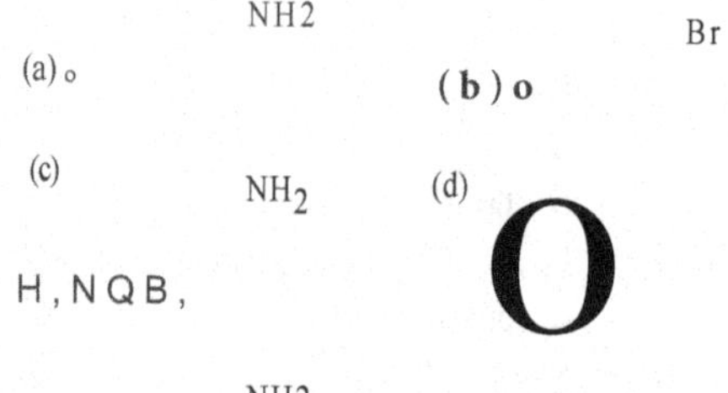

What is X, Y, Z respectively
(a) K2Cr2O1 in H2SO4; NH3; H2/Ni
(b) H2/Ni; NH3; K2Cr2O1 in H2SO4
(c) 02; H2,N2; H2/Ni
(d) NaB ;   NH3; 11 heating

55.

56.

$$H_3C-\overset{H_2}{C}-\overset{O}{\overset{\|}{C}}-NH_2 \xrightarrow{NaOBr} \quad ?$$

(a) $H_3C-\overset{H_2}{C}-\overset{H_2}{C}-NH_2$

(b) $H_3C-\overset{H_2}{C}-NH_2$

(c) $H_3C-\overset{H_2}{C}-\overset{O}{\overset{\|}{C}}-NH_2$

(d) Reaction doesn't takes place

57. Which of the following is more basic?
   (a) Ammonia
   (b) 1° amine
   (c) 2° amine
   (d) 3° amine

58. 3° amines even though contains 3 alkyl groups it is less basic than 2° amines & 1° amines. Why?
   (a) Alkyl groups decreases the electron density on the N atom
   (b) Alkyl groups increases the electron density on the N atom
   (c) Alkyl groups causes the steric hindrance due to which electrons are not easily available
   (d) Alkyl groups decreases the electronegativity of N atom

59.

G^- is electron relea,ing group

Generally electron releasing groups increases the basicity of amines (aniline). But when electron releasing groups are present at which position of phenyl ring of aniline decreases the basicity of it?
   (a) Meta
   (b) Para
   (c) Ortho
   (d) Both (b) and (c)

60.

$$H_3C-\overset{H_2}{C}-\underset{\overset{|}{+N(CH_3)_3}}{\overset{H}{C}}-CH_3 \xrightarrow{\ ^-OH} \quad \text{What is the major product}$$

   (a) 2-Butene
   (b) 1,3-Butadiene
   (c) I-Butene
   (d) 2-Hydroxy butane

61.

$$H_3C-\overset{H_2}{C}-\underset{\overset{|}{X}}{\overset{H}{C}}-CH_3 \xrightarrow[\text{Base}]{\text{alc. KOH}} H_3C-g=g-CH_3 +$$

2-Butene 4%

$$H,c-c-\overset{H,}{\diamond}=CH,$$

I-Butene is the cheif product 96%

$X=$ F or Cl or Br or I

In the dehydrohalogenation of above reaction if I-butene is the chief means what is X
   (a) F
   (b) Cl
   (c) Br
   (d) I

62.

$$O-\overset{O}{\overset{\|}{\diamond}}-Cl$$

Which of the following doesn't react with the above molecule?
   (a) NH3
   (b) CH3-NH2
   (c) CH3-NH-CH3
   (d) N (CH3)3

63.

Name of the above reaction is?
(a) Philips condensation reaction
(b) Schotten-Baumann reaction
(b) Gattermann-Kosch reaction
(d) Knoevenogel reaction

64.

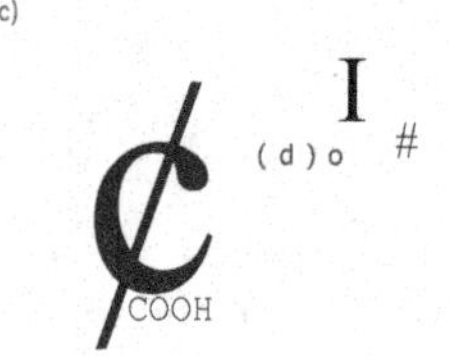

Acidic conditions CW) - ?
$HNO_3 + H_2SO_4$

(a) NH_2, NO_2

(b) NH_2, NO_2

(c) Both a & b

(d) $+NH_3$, NO_2

65.

Oxidatio° ► ?

(a) NO_2, CH_3

(b) NH_2, $COOH$

66.

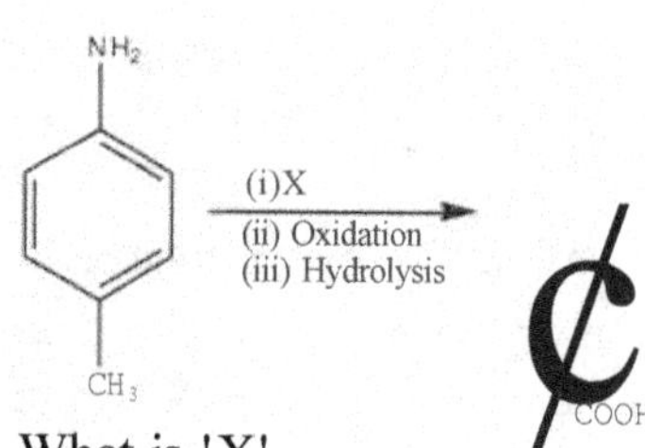

(i)X
(ii) Oxidation
(iii) Hydrolysis

What is 'X'
(a) (CH3CO)2   (b) KMnO4
(c) LiAlH4   (d) dil. HCl

67. 'Sulphanilic acid' is a
(a) Cation   (b) Anion
(c) Zwitter ion   (d) Neutral

68. An amine+ $NaNO_2$ (Sodium nitrite)+
2HCl ----cold, $0°-5°$ c-----> A diazonium
salt In the above reaction the amine is
(a) Methylamine
(b) Dimethylamine
(c) N,N-Dimethylaniline
(d) Aniline

69. An amine+ $NaNO_2$ (Sodium nitrite)+
2HCl ----cold, $0°-5°$ c-----> N_2 gas is
evolved In the above reaction the
amine is
(a) Methylamine
(b) Dimethylamine
(c) N,N-Dimethylaniline
(d) Aniline

70. HNO_2 is
(a) Nitric acid
(b) Nitrous oxide
(c) Nitrous acid
(d) Nitric oxide

71.

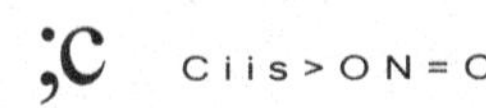

The above reaction is a/an
(a) Nucleophilic substitution
(b) Electrophilic aromatic substitution
(c) Free radical substitution
(d) Nucleophilic addition

72.

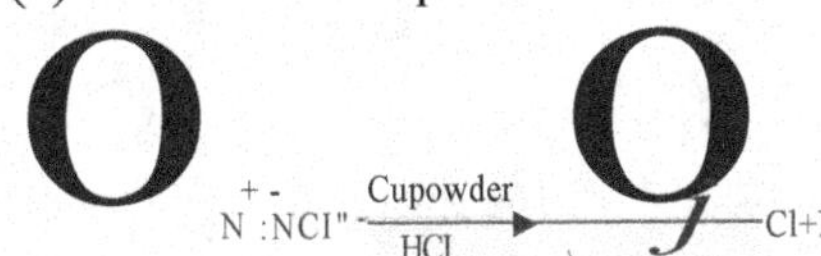

In the above reaction electrophile is
(a) Nitronium ion
(b) Nitrosonium ion
(c) Nitric oxide
(d) Both a & b

73. Nitrosonium ion is
(a) Strong electrophile
(b) Strong nucleophile
(c) Weak nucleophile
(d) Weak electrophile

74.

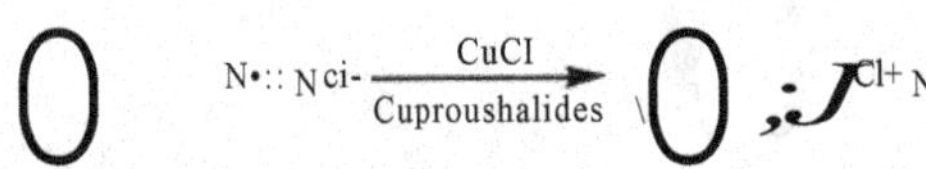

The above reaction is named as
(a) Gattermann reaction
(b) Sandmeyer reaction
(c) Michael reaction
(d) Birch reaction

75.

The above reaction is named as
(a) Gattermann reaction
(b) Sandmeyer reaction
(c) Michael reaction
(d) Birch reaction

76. Phenol+ Diazonium salt----------> an 'azo compound' Phenol can couple with diazonium salts to form an azo compound. Which of the following condition slows down the above reaction?
(a) Basic
(b) Neutral
(c) Acidic
(d) All the above

77.

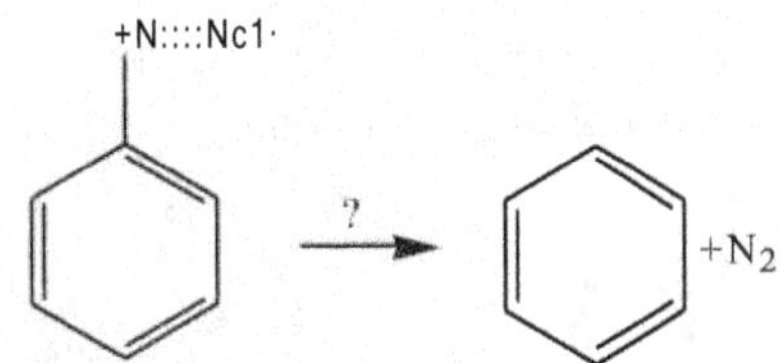

Phenyl diawnium salt

(a) H_2O + ice cold
(b) CuCN
(c) HBF4
(d) H3P03 + H20

78.

The above reaction is a/an
(a) Nucleophilic substitution
(b) Electrophilic aromatic substitution
(c) Free radical substitution
(d) Nucleophilic addition

79.

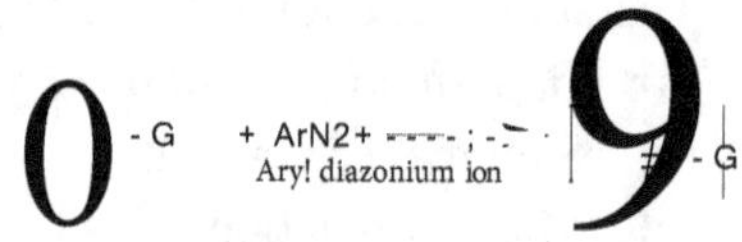

When 'G' is which of the following, the reaction doesn't takes place

(a) -OH
(b) -NHR
(c) -NO$_2$
(d) -NH$_2$

80. Which of the following test is used for the analysis of amines?

(a) Lucas test
(b) Baeyer's test
(c) Tollen's test
(d) Hinsberg test

83. Which of the following molecule is said to be as an arene?

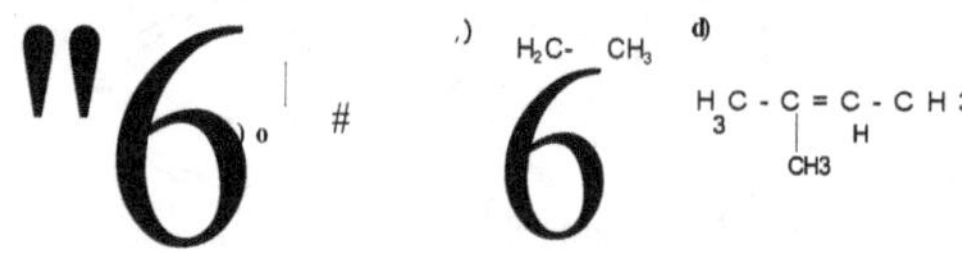

84.

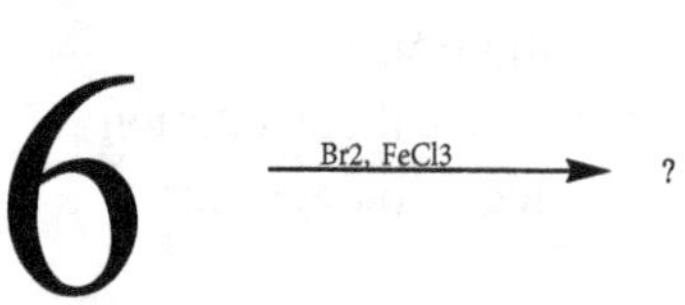

(a) m-Bromo ethylbenzene
(b) 1-Bromo-2-phenyl ethane
(c) 1- Bromo-2-phenyl ethane
(d) p-Bromo ethylbenzene

85.

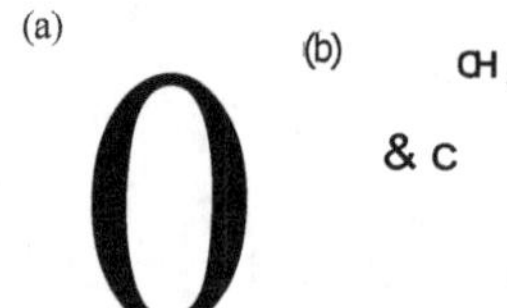

81.

Amine + C$_6$H$_5$SO$_2$Cl $\xrightarrow{OH^-}$ Sulfonamide $\xrightarrow{KOH}$

The above reaction is a reaction of hinsberg test. The sulphonamide which is formed from which of the following amine reaction with KOH & others are not

(a) 1° amine
(b) 2° amine
(c) 3° amine
(d) 4° amine

82. Which of the following is a weaker amine?

(a) Methylamine
(b) Aniline
(c) Ethylamine
(d) Trimethylamine
(a) m-Bromo ethylbenzene
(b) 1-Bromo-2-phenyl ethane
(c) 1- Bromo-2-phenyl ethane
(d) p-Bromo ethylbenzene

86.

OCH,
Name of this molecule is?
(a) Phenyl ethylene
(b) Styrene
(c) Vinyl benzene
(d) All of the above

87. m-Xylene

(c) 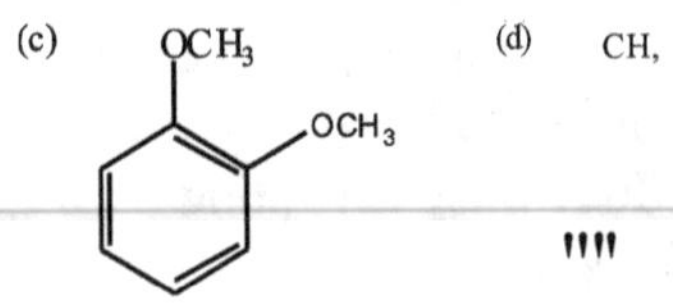

(d)   CH,

(b)

o -

88. Which of the following molecule do not undergo friedel-crafts alkylation (R-X & AlCb) reaction?

(a) 0

(b) 0

(c) 0 |

(d) CN 6

89.

H3C-C- CHB $\xrightarrow[\text{NH}_2\text{NH}_2, \text{Base}]{\text{Zn-Hg \& HCl}}$ or ?

(a) H₃C—CH—CH₃ with OH below C and H above

$$H_3C\!-\!\overset{H}{\underset{OH}{C}}\!-\!CH_3$$

(b) H₃C - C - H

(c) $H_2C\!=\!\overset{}{\underset{H}{C}}\!-\!CH_3$

(d) $H_3C\!-\!\overset{H_2}{C}\!-\!CH_3$

90. Which of the following molecule is benzal?

(a)

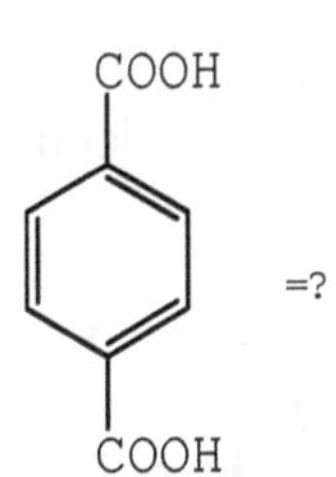

(c)

O-r

(d)

\ j r-

o-

91. Which of the following is the correct decreasing order of stability of free radicals?

(a) $3°>2°>$allylic, benzylic$>1°>CH_3+>$vinylic

(b) $3°>2°>1°>$ allylic, benzylic$>CH_3+>$vinylic

(c) Allylic, benzylic$>3°>2°>1°>CH_3+>$vinylic

(d) Vinylic$> CH/>1°>3°>2°>$ allylic, benzylic

92.

COOH on benzene ring with COOH para

=?

(a) Isophthalic acid
(b) Terephthalic acid
(c) Phthalic anhydride
(d) Phthalic acid

93. Resonance energy of benzene is

(a) 20 Kcal   (b) 36 Kcal
(c) 80 Kcal   (d) 50 Kcal

94. Which of the following statement is correct regarding benzene?
    (a) It has 2 resonance structures
    (b) SP^2 hybridization with $120°$ bond angle
    (c) It is a very symmetrical molecule
    (d) All the above

95. In the 4n+2 Huckel's rule, n indicates?
    (a) Number of n-bonds
    (b) Number of electrons in the molecule
    (c) Number of rings
    (d) Number of atoms

96. Which of the following molecule is an aromatic according to Huckel's rule?
    (a) Cyclopentadiene
    (b) Cyclohexene
    (c) Pyrrole
    (d) None of the above

97. Which of the following molecule is more aromatic?
    (a) Pyrroline
    (b) Pyrrole
    (c) Furan
    (d) Thiophene

98. Which of the following is the correct decreasing order of aromaticity of the following compounds?
    (a) Furan > pyrrole > thiophene
    (b) Pyrrole > furan > thiophene
    (c) Thiophene > furan > pyrrole
    (d) Thiophene > pyrrole > furan

99. Which of the following molecule is not aromatic according Huckel's rule?
    (a) Pyrroline
    (b) Pyrrole
    (c) Furan
    (d) Thiophene

100. Match the following (effect of substitution on benzene ring)
    (P) Moderately activating
    (Q) Weakly activating
    (R) Strongly activating
    (S) Deactivating ortho, para
    (1) -NH2
    (2) $-CH_3$ directors
    (3) -Cl
    (4) $-NHCOCH_3$
    (a) R-4, Q-2, S-3, P-1
    (b) R-3, Q-1, S-2, P-4
    (c) R-1, Q-2, S-3, P-4
    (d) R-3, Q-4, S-1, P-2

101. Which of the following is a deactivating, meta director
    (a) -CN   (b) -OC2Hs
    (c) -Br   (d) -OH

102.

rn,CI $\underline{A\_|Cl_3}$?

& N O :
(a) NH2

9' N O ;
    CH$_3$
(b)   NH2

C h N O ;

(c) 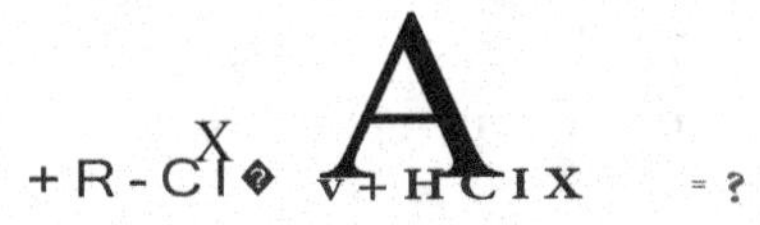

NHCH₃

NO₂

(d)

NH₂

H₃C

NO₂

CH₃

103. In the nitration of benzene, the electrophile is

(a) $\overset{+}{N}O$

(b) $\overset{+}{N}O2$

(c) $\overset{-}{N}O3$

(d) $\overset{+}{N}O3$

104. Which of the following electrophilic aromatic substitution reaction is reversible?

(a) Nitration
(b) Sulphonation
(c) Halogenation
(d) Friedel-Craft alkylation

105. Which of the following even though it doesn't contain a +ve charge it will acts as electrophile in the electrophilic aromatic substitution reaction of benzene?

(a) Sulphur trioxide
(b) Nitronium ion
(c) Halonium ion
(d) Acylonium ion

106.

$+ R-Cl \quad \xrightarrow{} \quad + HClX \quad = ?$

0

(a) Lewis acid
(b) Lewis base
(c) HCl
(d) NaOH

107. Which of the following statement/s is/are correct?

(P) Electron releasing groups stabilizes carbocation
(Q) Electron withdrawing groups destabilizes carbocation
(R) Electron withdrawing groups stabilizes carbocation
(S) Electron releasing groups destabilizes carbocation

(a) P,Q
(b) R,S
(c) P,R
(d) Any of the above

108. Which of the following group when present on benzene ring releases electrons through its inductive effect?

(a) -NHCOCH₃
(b) -OCH₃
(c) -NH2
(d) -C2Hs

109. -N\CH₃)₃ trimethyl ammonium group when present on benzene ring acts as a powerful deactivating group due to the presence of

(a) Three methyl groups
(b) Electronegative N atom
(c) Full-fledged +ve charge on N atom
(d) Lone pair of electrons on N atom

110. Which of the following group is/are activating group of benzene ring?

(a) -CN
(b) -SO₃H
(c) -CHO
(d) -OCH₃

111. Which of the following statement/s is/are correct when halogens are present on benzene ring?
     (P) They deactivate by inductive effect
     (Q) They acts as ortho & para directors due to resonance
     (R) They activate by inductive effect
     (S) They are deactivating, meta directors
     (a) R, S (b) P, Q
     (c) Q, S (d) Q, R

112. Which of the following statement/s is/are correct when halogens are present on benzene ring?
     (P) Reactivity is controlled by the resonance effect
     (Q) Reactivity is controlled by the stronger inductive effect
     (R) Orientation is controlled by the resonance effect
     (S) Orientation is controlled by the stronger inductive effect
     (a) P,R (b) R,S
     (c) Q,R (d) P,Q

113.

In the electrophilic aromatic substitution (halogenation) reactions of naphthalene attack by electrophile occur almost exclusively at .... position

(a)
(b) a
(c) Both a & equally
(d) Naphthalene doesn't undergo electrophilic aromatic substitution reactions

114. During the electrophilic aromatic substitution reactions of naphthalene attack occurs at a-position preferentially than at -position because
     (a) a-attack results in the formation of 2 more stable carbocation
     (b) - attack results in the formation of 2 more stable carbocation
     (c) a-attack results in the formation of 1 more stable carbocation
     (d) - attack results in the formation of 1 more stable carbocation

115. Which of the following is an unsaturated carboxylic acid?
     (a) Laurie acid
     (b) Myristic acid
     (c) Oleic acid
     (d) Stearic acid

116.

     (a) Anthranilic acid
     (b) Phthalic acid
     (c) Isophthalic acid
     (d) Terephthalic acid

117. Propionic acid (Mwt 74), n-Butyl alcohol (Mwt 74). Boiling point of propionic acid is greater than n-butyl alcohol, this is because of
    (a) Intermolecular hydrogen bonding with water
    (b) Intramolecular hydrogen bonding with other propionic acid units
    (c) The presence of -COOR group at one end
    (d) The presence of 3 carbon atoms

118. A pair of carboxylic acid molecules are held together by .... number of hydrogen bonds
    (a) 1   (b) 2
    (c) 3   (d) 4

119. Salts of carboxylic acids are
    (a) Crystalline
    (b) Non-volatile
    (c) Solid
    (d) All the above

120. Which of the following salt of carboxylic acid is insoluble in water & in organic solvents?
    (a) Ethanoic acid
    (b) Propanoic acid
    (c) Butanoic acid
    (d) Pentanoic acid

121.

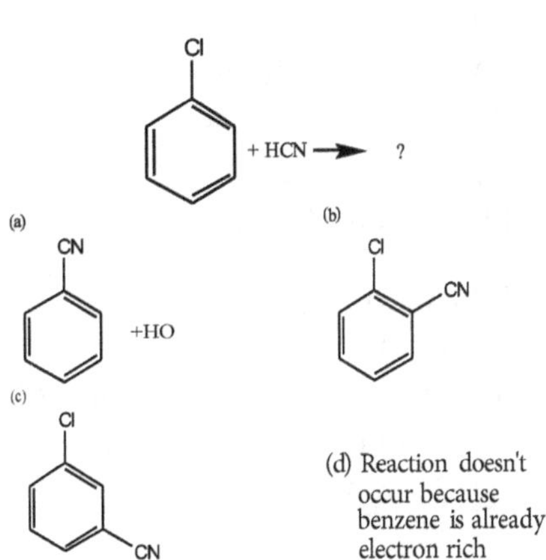

What are X & Y?
    (a) $KMnO_4$; $NaNO_2$, HCl, $0°$ C- $10°$ C
    (b) H_2/Ni; $NaNO_2$, HCl, $0°$ C- $10°$ C
    (c) H_2/Ni; N_2,HCl
    (d) $K_2Cr_2O_1$; N_2,HCl

122.

1,3,5-trimethyl benzene is
    (a) Mesitylene   (b) m-Xylene
    (c) Cresol   (d) Catechol

123.

(d) Reaction doesn't occur because benzene is already electron rich

124.

= ?
    (a) 1,3-Cyclohaxadiene
    (b) Cyclohexane
    (c) Benzene analogue
    (d) Adamantane

125. The structure in the above question is present in which of the following class of drugs?
    (a) Anticancer
    (b) Antiviral
    (c) Antiulcer
    (d) Anti-Parkinson's drugs

126.

$= ?$

(a) 1,4-oxazine
(b) 1,3-dioxetane
(c) 1,4-dioxane
(d) Tetrahydrofuran

127. Ethers are
(a) Aprotic solvents
(b) Protic solvent
(c) Polar solvent
(d) Aprotic & polar solvent

128. Which of the following are used as phase-transfer catalysts?
(a) Alcohols   (b) Ethers
(c) Aromatic hydrocarbon
(d) Crown ethers

129. Which of the following antibiotics contain crown ether structure in it?
(a) Cefaclor, ampicillin
(b) Amoxicillin, cefalexin
(c) Chlortetracycline, aminoglycosides
(d) Gramicidin, valinomycin

130.

$H_3C - MgBr + $ [epoxide] $\xrightarrow{} \xrightarrow[H_2O]{H^+} ?$

(a) Propanol   (b) Butanol
(c) Propanal   (d) Methanol

131. Which of the following is a cumulated diene (allene)?
(a) 1,4-Pentadiene b) 1,2-Butadiene
(c) 1,3-Butadiene   d) I-Butene

132. 1,3-Pentadiene is a
(a) Conjugated diene
(b) Allene
(c) Non-conjugated diene
(d) Aromatic hydrocarbon

133. The true statements of conjugated dienes when they are compared with simple alkenes
(P) They are more stable
(Q) They are the preferred products of elimination
(R) They undergo 1,4-addition, both electrophilic & free radical
(S) Toward free-radical addition, they are more reactive
(a) Only P, S
(b) Only Q,S
(c) Only R
(d) All P, Q, R& S

134. Which of the following molecule undergo 1,4-electrophilic addition reactions
(a) 1,3-Pentadiene
(b) 1,4-Pentadiene
(c) 1,2-Pentadiene
(d) 3-Pentene

135.

$H_2C= \underset{H}{C} - \underset{H}{C} = CH_2 + HCl ?$

(a) Only 2-Chloro-3-butene
(b) Only 1-Chloro-2-butene
(c) Both a & b
(d) 1-Chlorobutene

136.

$$H_2C=\underset{H}{C}-\underset{H}{C}=CH_2 \quad + \quad HBr \quad \cdots\cdots \rightarrow \quad H_3C-\underset{Br}{\overset{H}{C}}-C=CH_2$$

Br   1,2-addition product

$$+$$

$$H_3C- \quad \underset{H}{C}=C-\underset{H}{C}^{H2}-Br$$

1,4-addition product

In this reaction 1,4-addition product is the major one because of the formation of

(a) $3°$ carbocation
(b) $2°$ carbocation
(c) $1°$ carbocation
(d)   Allylic cation

137. In the above reaction at $-80°C$ (at lower temperature) which addition product is the major one?
(a)   1,2-addition
(b)   1,4-addition
(c)   Both will be formed in equal amount
(d)   No product is going to form at $-80°C$

138. IUPAC name of isoprene is
(a)   1,3-Butadiene
(b)   2-Methyl-1,3-butadiene
(c)   2-Methyl butane
(d)   2-Methyl-1-butene

139. In the *vulcanization* of rubber formation of which of the following bridges makes the rubber harder & stronger?
(a)   Nitrogen bridges
(b)   Oxygen bridges
(c)   Sulphur bridges
(d)   Extra carbon bridges

140. Natural rubber has .... configuration at (nearly at) every double bond

(a)   Cis
(b)   Trans
(c)   Cis or Trans that depends on the chain length
(d)   No configuration, rubber is a saturated compound

141. The hybridization state of 'oxygen' in ethers is
(a)   Sp3
(b) Sp^2
(c)   Sp
(d) Sp^3d

142.

$$H_3C- \quad -\overset{H2}{C}-C^{H2}-O-CH_3$$

Name of this ether is
(a)   1-Methoxypropane
(b)   Propoxy methane
(c)   Propylmethylether
(d)   Dipropyl ether

143. Reaction mechanism that is involved in Williamson's synthesis
(a)   Electrophilic substitution
(b)   Free radical addition
(c)   Nucleophilic substitution
(d)   Nucleophilic addition

144. Which of the following molecule is prepared by Williamson's synthesis?

(a)
    $H3C-\underset{H}{C}=CH2$

(b)
    $H3C-\overset{H2}{C}-O-CH3$

(c)
    $H3C-\overset{H2}{C}-\overset{H2}{c}-OH$

(d)
    CH
    O

145. The tendency of alkyl halides to undergo elimination reaction is
(a) $1^° > 2^° > 3^°$ (b) $2^° > 3^° > 1^°$
(c) $3^° > 2^° > 1^°$ (d) $1^° > 3^° > 2^°$

146. Which of the following alkyl halide doesn't undergo nucleophilic substitution reaction with sodium ethoxide to form an ether instead of it, it undergoes elimination reaction to form an alkene?

(a)
    $C-C-\overset{H_2}{C}-\overset{H_2}{C}I$

(b)
    $C-C-\overset{CH_3}{\underset{a}{C}}H3$

(c)
    $HC-\overset{H}{\underset{a}{C}}-CH$
    3   3

(c)
    $HC-\overset{H}{\underset{a}{C}}-CH$
    3   3

147. Which of the following ether undergoes SN_1 reaction with alkyl halides **R-X?**

(a)
    $I-'3C-\overset{li}{C}-O-CH\_i$

(b)
    $H3C-\overset{lil}{C}-O-C\overset{H2}{}-CH3$

(c)
    $H-O-CH3$

(d)
    $H-\overset{CH_3}{\underset{CH3}{C}}-O-CH3$

148. Which of the following statement/s is/are correct?
(P) R-OH group is a weak base & good leaving group
(Q) R-OH group is a strong base & poor leaving group
(R) R-0- ion is a strong base & poor leaving group
(S) R-0- ion is a weak base & good leaving group
(a) Q, S
(b) **P,R**
(c) P,Q
(d) Only R is correct

149.

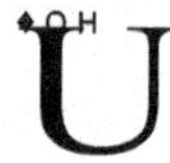

O-Hydroxy toluene

The common name of molecule is
(a) Catechol
(b) Resorcinol
(c) Hydroquinone
(d) O-Cresol

150. Picric acid is
(a) 2,3,4-Trinitrophenol
(b) 2,6-Dinitrophenol
(c) 2,4,6-Trinitrophenol
(d) 3,4,5-Trinitrophenol

151. Phenols are more acidic than alcohols. This is due to one of the following reasons. Identify that.
  (a) Alkoxide ions are better stabilized by the electron releasing alkyl groups
  (b) Resonance stabilizes both phenols and phenoxide ions to the same extant
  (c) Phenols are better stabilized than the phenoxide ions while reverse is true for alcohols and alkoxides
  (d) Phenoxide ions are much better stabilized than the alkoxide ions

152.

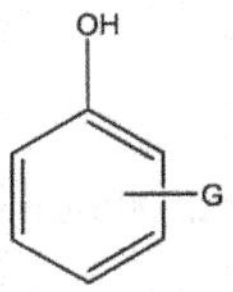

Which of the following group increases the acidity of phenols?
  (a) -NH2   (b) -OH
  (c) -CH3   (d) -CN

153. Which of the following is correct?
  (a) Phenols are stronger acids than alcohols
  (b) Alcohols are stronger acids than phenols
  (c) Alcohols are stronger bases than phenols
  (d) Phenols are stronger bases than alcohols

154. In which of the following reaction 'acylonium ion', is the electrophile?

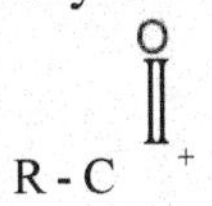

$$R-C$$

  (a) Chichibabin reaction
  (b) Oppenear oxidation
  (c) Curtis reaction
  (d) Fries reaction

155.

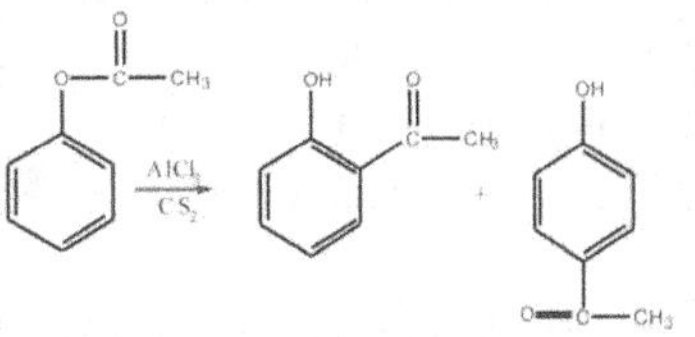

  (a) Kolbe's reaction
  (b) Reimer-Tiemann reaction
  (c) Fries rearrangement
  (d) Philip's condensation

156. Which of the following reaction is used for the synthesis of phenolic ketones?
  (a) Kolbe's reaction
  (b) Reimer-Tiemann reaction
  (c) Fries rearrangement
  (d) Philip's condensation

157. Which of the following reaction is used for the synthesis of phenolic acids (ex: salicylic acid)?
  (a) Kolbe's reaction
  (b) Reimer-Tiemann reaction
  (c) Fries rearrangement
  (d) Philip's condensation

158. CO_2 is used as one of the substrate in which of the following reaction?
  (a) Kolbe's reaction
  (b) Reimer-Tiemann reaction
  (c) Fries rearrangement
  (d) Philip's condensation

159.

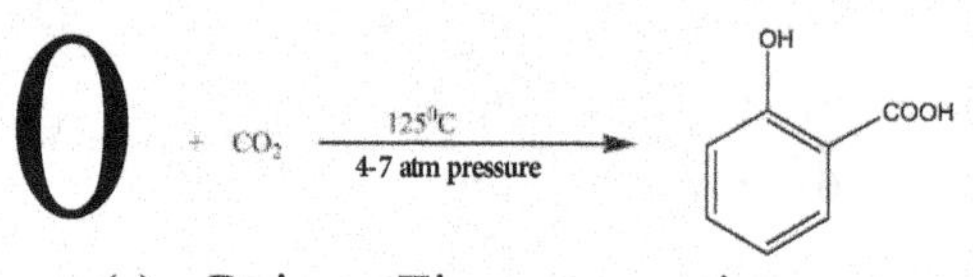

(a) Reimer-Tiemannreaction
(b) Kolbe's reaction
(c) Vilsmeier-Haack reaction
(d) Cannizzaro reaction

160. Which of the following reaction is used for the synthesis of 'phenolic aldehydes' (salicyladehyde)?
(a) Kolbe's reaction
(b) Reimer-Tiemann reaction
(c) Fries rearrangement
(d) Philip's condensation

161. In which of the following reaction Dichlorocarbene (:CClz) is the electrophile?
(a) Kolbe's reaction
(b) Reimer-Tiemann reaction
(c) Fries rearrangement
(d) Philip's condensation

162. Number of electrons present in the valancy shell of dichlorocarbene (CClz) which is the electrophile in the synthesis of 'phenolic aldehydes' (Reimer-Tiemann reaction).
(a) 6　　　　　(b) 8
(c) 4　　　　　(d) 2

163. The isomerism in which different arrangements of atoms that can be converted into one another by rotation about single bonds is
(a) Configurational isomerism
(b) Entgegen
(c) Zussamen
(d) Conformational isomerism

164. The dihedral angle in anti or staggered conformation of n-butane is
(a) 90°　　　　(b) 60°
(c) 45°　　　　(d) 180°

165. Structurally which of the following pair is not correct?
(a) Staggered-Anti
(b) Eclipsed-Gauche
(c) *Cis-Trans*
(d) All the above

166. The stereoisomer's which are non-superimposable, mirror images of each other are called as
(a) Conformers
(b) Diastereomers
(c) Enantiomers
(d) Isomers

167. Which of the following statement/s is/are correct?
(P) Enantiomers have same physical properties
(Q) Diastereomers have same physical properties
(R) Racemic mixture consists of equal amounts of enantiomers
(S) The direction of rotation of plane polarized light is different for enantiomers
(a) P, R & S　　　　(b) Only Q
(c) P, Q & R　　　　(d) R & S

168. The isomers in which compounds have same MF but differ in their arrangement of atoms are called
(a) Conformational isomers
(b) *Cis-Trans*
(c) E-Z
(d) Configurational isomers

169. Of the following groups in the R/S system of nomenclature highest priority goes to
     (a) -CH2OH
     (b) –CHO
     (c) -CH3
     (d) $-C_2H_5$

170. Muscle contraction results in the formation of (+)-lactic acid. The number of possible stereoisomer's of that (+)-lactic acid are?
     (a) 4
     (b) 8
     (c) 10
     (d) 2

171. Calcite a substance which is used as a polaroid, is?
     (a) A particular crystalline form of CaCO3
     (b) A particular crystalline form of CaO
     (c) A particular crystalline form of CaSO4
     (d) A particular crystalline form of NaCl

172. Nicol prism which is used as a Polaroid is used to convert
     (a) Plane polarized light into ordinary light
     (b) Separation of racemic mixture
     (c) Identification of enantiomers
     (d) Ordinary light into plane polarized light

173. Match the following
     (P) d   (Q) l
     (R) D   (S) L
     (1) -OH group at the penultimate carbon is on the right side
     (2) Rotate the plane polarized light to the right
     (3) Rotate the plane polarized light to the left
     (4) -OH group at the penultimate carbon is on the left side
     (a) P-2, Q-3, R-1, S-4
     (b) P-3, Q-2, R-1, S-4
     (c) P-4, Q-2, R-3, S-1
     (d) P-4, Q-3, R-2, S-1

174. Number of stereoisomers that are possible in 2-methyl-1-butanol.
     (a) 4
     (b) 8
     (c) 2
     (d) 6

175. Which of the following molecule is achiral
     (a) Lactic acid
     (b) 2-Methyl-1-butanol
     (c) 2-Chlorobutane
     (d) 2,3-dichlorobutane

176. Which of the following molecule is a *mesa* compound?
     (a) Lactic acid
     (b) 2-Methyl-1-butanol
     (c) 2-Chlorobutane
     (d) 2,3-dichlorobutane

177. Number of chiral centers in 2-methyl-1-butanol?
     (a) 2
     (b) 1
     (c) 3
     (d) O

178. Match the following
     (P) Manic acid
     (Q) Malonic acid
     (R) Succinic acid
     (S) Maleic acid

(I) 4C containing saturated dicarboxylic acid

(2) 2-hydroxy succinic acid

(3) 4C containing unsaturated dicarboxylic acid (cis-form)

(4) 3C containing saturated dicarboxylic acid

(a) P-4, Q-2, R-1, S-3

(b) P-2, Q-1, R-3, S-2

(c) P-3, Q-4, R-2, S-I

(d) P-2, Q-4, R-1, S-3

179. The reactions which produce one diastereoisomer or diastereoisomeric dl pair of a given structure in considerable predominance over all other possible diastereoisomers of the same structure are called as

(a) Stereoselective

(b) Stereospecific

(c) Chemoselective

(d) Regioselective

180. Which of the following compounds show *cis-trans* isomerism?

(a) Timethylamine

(b) Propene

(c) Dimethylamine

(d) 2-Butene

181. $-CH_2NO_2$, $-NO_2$, $-C$ triple bond CH, & $-C$ triple bond N.
These are the groups around a chiral center. According to priorities rules highest priority goes to?

(a) $-CH_2NO_2$

(b) $-NO_2$

(c) $-C$ triple bond CH

(d) $-C$ triple bond N

182. Which of the following solvents is not suitable for determining the specific rotation of a chiral unknown?

(a) Water

(b) Methyl alcohol

(c) 2-Butanol

(d) Diethyl ether

183. A molecule is said to be chiral

(a) If it contains plane of symmetry

(b) If it contains center of symmetry

(c) If it cannot be superimposed on its mirror image

(d) If it can be superimposed on its mirror image.

184. Which of the following statements is false regarding chiral compounds?

(a) Rotate the plane of polarized light

(b) Have *cis-trans* isomers

(c) Exist as enantiomers

(d) Can be detected with a polaimeter

185. Which of the following compounds will be optically active?

(a) Propanoic acid

(b) 3-Chloropropanoic acid

(c) 2- Chloropropanoic acid

(d) 3-Chloropropene

186. Which of the following compounds will be optically active?

(a) Succinic acid

(b) Meso-Tartaric acid

(c) Lactic acid

(d) Chloroacetic acid

187. Optical isomers that are not mirror images are called
    (a) Diastereomers
    (b) Enantiomers
    (c) Metamers
    (d) *Mesa* compounds

188. Which of the following statements is false regarding enantiomers?
    (a) Rotate plane-polarized light
    (b) Are superimposable mirror images
    (c) Are nonsuperimposable mirror images
    (d) Have the same melting point

189. A *mesa* compound:
    (a) Is an a chiral molecule which contains chiral carbons
    (b) Contains a plane of symmetry or a center of symmetry
    (c) Is optically inactive
    (d) Is characterized by all of the above

190. Which of the following represents a racemic mixture?
    (a) 75% (R)-2-butanol, 25% (S)-2-butanol
    (b) 25% (R)-2-butanol, 75% (S)-2-butanol
    (c) 50% (R)-2-butanol, 50% (S)-2-butanol
    (d) None of the above

191. Consider (R) - and (S)-2-butanol. Which physical property distinguishes the two compounds?
    (a) Melting point
    (b) Solubility in common solvents
    (c) Rotation of plane-polarized light
    (d) Infrared spectrum

192. In the R/S system of nomenclature - NH2, -C2H5, -CH3 & -H are atoms/groups. Second priority goes to?
    (a) $-NH_2$
    (b) $-C_2H_5$
    (c) $-CH_3$
    (d) $-H$

193. Penicillium glaucum is used for?
    (a) Synthesis of steroids
    (b) Interconvertion of functional groups
    (c) Production of enzymes that can cleave the molecules
    (d) For the resolution of racemic mixture of tartaric acid in which it selectively consumes the (+)-form of tartaric acid.

194. The stereoisomers which are nonsuperimposable, not mirror images of each other & which differ in their physical properties are called as
    (a) Diastereomers
    (b) Enantiomers
    (c) Metamers
    (d) *Mesa* compounds

195. The relative configuration of the below molecule is D- because

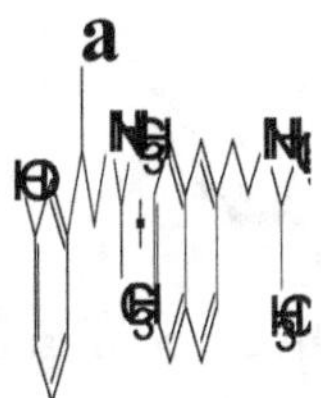

(a) -OH group at the 4th C is on the right side.

(b) -OH group at the 3rd C is on the left side.

(c) -OH group at the 2nd C is on the right side.

(d) -OH group at the 5th C is on the right side.

196.

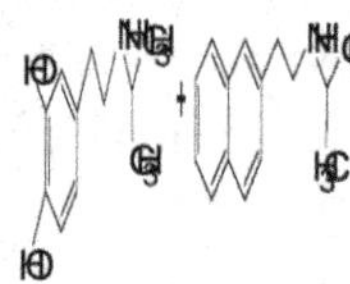

The absolute configuration of above molecule is

(a) R

(b) S

(c) D

(d) L

197.

The absolute configuration of above molecule is

(a) R

(b) S

(c) D

(d) L

198.

c6

The relative configuration of the above molecule is

(a) D

(b) R

(c) S

(d) L

199.

In the above structure in the designation of **R & S** nomenclature 2nd highest priority goes to

(a) Isopropyl group

(b) -NH2

(c) Vinyl

(d) Hydrogen

200.

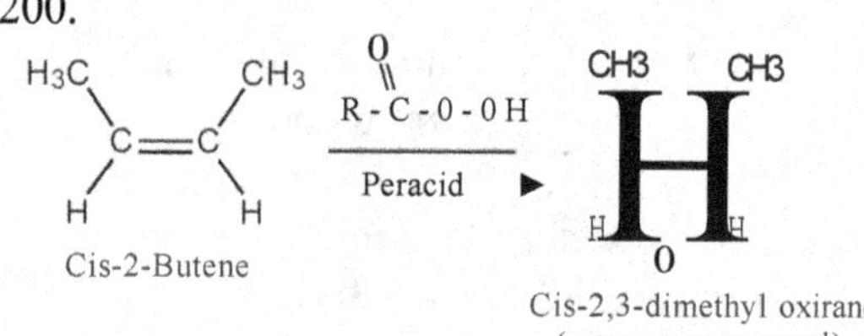

The above reaction is a

(a) Stereoselective

(b) Stereospecific

(c) Chemoselective

(d) Regioselective

201. The reactions which produces one diastereoisomer (or diastereoisomeric dl pair) of a given structure in considerable predominance over all the other possible diastereoisomers of the same structure are called as

(a) Stereoselective

(b) Stereospecific

(c) Chemoselective

(d) Regioselective

202.

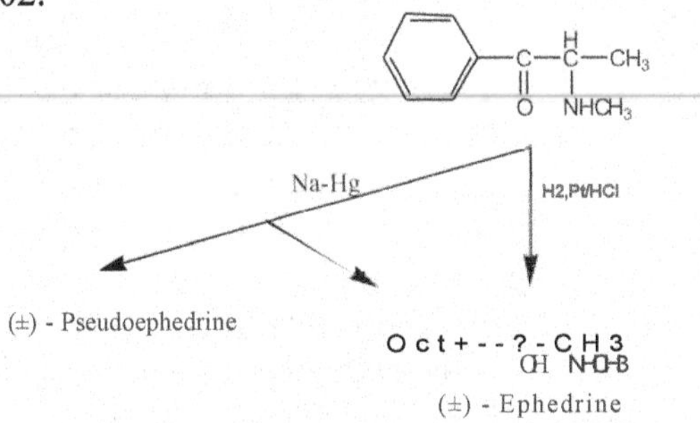

Na-Hg

H2,Pt/HCl

(±) - Pseudoephedrine

Oct +--?- CH3
CH NHCH3

(±) - Ephedrine

The reduction by Pt/HCl to produce only(±) - ephedrine is called as
(a) Chemoselective
(b) Stereospecific
(c) Regioselective
(d) Stereoselective

203. Which of the following is a newman projection of ethane

(a)

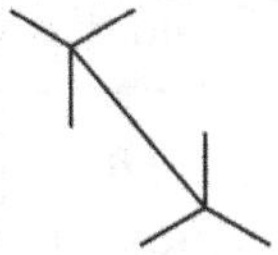

(b)

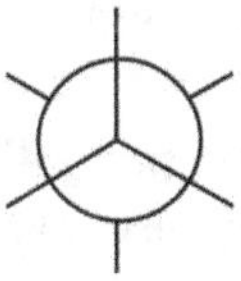

(c) C_2H_6

(d)

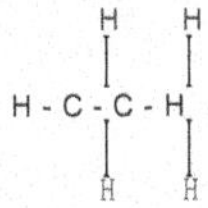

H - C - C - H

204. Which of the following statement/s is/are correct?
   (a) The energy of the electrons in an orbit remains unchanged, as long as the electrons remains in that orbit

(b) Energy is absorbed when an electron moves from a lower stationary state to a higher stationary state
(c) Energy is emitted when an electron moves from a higher stationary state to a lower stationary state
d) All the above

205. Bohr proposed that the angular momentum of an electron is quantized. Which of the following is the correct relationship?
   (a) fileVr = n.h/2lt
   (b) fileVr = h/ nx2n
   (c) fileVr = 2n
   (d) fileVr = nh

206. Shapes of atomic orbital's help to determine the chemical behavior of atoms. Which of the following is the correct decreasing order of energy of orbitals?
   (a) 1s>2s>2p   (b) 2s>1s>2p
   (c) 2p>2s>1s   (d) 2p>1s>2s

207. Electrons have which of the following nature/s?
   (a) Particle nature (b) Wave nature
   (c) Both a & b   (d) None

208. In the propagation of a wave, the place where the amplitude is zero is called?
   (a) Nodal plane
   (b) Node
   (c) Crust
   (d) Trough

209. Which of the following molecules have covalent bonds?
    (a) H2, HCl, NH3
    (b) H2, Ch, C
    (c) HCl, NaCl, KCl
    (d) NaCl, HCl, Br2

210. Which of the following molecule has linear shape (bond angle 180°)?
    (a) BF3   (b) CCl4
    (c) NH3   (d) BeCh

211. Bond angle in methane molecule is?
    (a) 180°   (b) 109°5'
    (c) 120°   (d) 90°

212. According to Lewis theory of acids & bases, an acid is a substance
    (a) Which donates a pair of electrons
    (b) Which donates a proton
    (c) Which accepts a proton
    (d) Which accepts a pair of electrons.

213. Which of the following is more basic?
    (a) Ammonia   (b) 1° amine
    (c) 2° amine   (d) 3° amine

214. 3° amines even though contains 3 alkyl groups it is less basic than 2° amines & 1° amines. Why?
    (a) Alkyl groups decreases the electron density on the N atom
    (b) Alkyl groups increases the electron density on the N atom
    (c) Alkyl groups causes the steric hindrance due to which electrons are not easily available
    (d) Alkyl groups decreases the electronegativity of N atom

215. Which of the following statement is correct?
    (a) A bonding orbital is more stable than the component atomic orbital
    (b) An antibonding orbital is more stable than the component atomic orbital
    (c) A bonding orbital is less stable than the component atomic orbital
    (d) A bonding orbital is less stable than an antibonding orbital

216. Which of the following statement is correct?
    (a) Heterolytic bond dissociation energy of a molecule is greater than homolytic bond Dissociation energy
    (b) Heterolytic bond dissociation energy of a molecule is less than homolytic bond dissociation energy
    (c) Heterolytic bond dissociation energy of a molecule is equal to homolytic bond dissociation energy
    (d) Heterolytic bond dissociation energy and homolytic bond dissociation energy of a molecule depends on the temperature and pressure.

217. Polarity of a molecule depends upon
    (a) Atomic number of atoms
    (b) Atomic weight of atoms
    (c) Valency of atoms
    (d) Electronegativity of atoms

218. In which of the molecule dipole moment is equal to 0
    (a) Water
    (b) Ammonia

    (c) Methyl chloride

    (d) Carbon tetrachloride

    (c) Free radical

    (d) None

219. Which of the following statement is correct?
    (i)   All electron pair acceptors are acids
    (ii) All electron pair donors are acids
    (iii) An acid is a substance that gives up a proton
    (iv) An acid is a substance that accepts a proton
    (a) i and ii   (b) ii and iii
    (c) iii and iv   (d) i and iii

220. The homolytic bond dissociation energy of which of the following radical is least
    (a) $3°$ (b) 2^0
    (c) $1°$ (d) Methyl

221. An organic ion with a pair of available electrons and a negative charge on the central carbon atom is called
    (a) Carbanion   (b) Carbocation
    (c) Carboniumion (d) Carbene

222. Carbanions are more stable, when
    (a) The presence of adjacent electron releasing groups
    (b) The presence of adjacent functional groups
    (c) The presence of adjacent electron withdrawing groups
    (d) None

223. Carbanion behaves as
    (a) Potent electrophile
    (b) Potent nucleophile

224.

$$H_3C-CHO \ + \ OH. \ \xrightarrow{-H_2O}$$

$$A \ + \ H_3C-CHO \ \longrightarrow$$

$$H_3C \underset{O}{\overset{CHO}{\diagup}} \xrightarrow[H_2O]{H^+} B.$$

    (a) Carbocation + aldol
    (b) Carbanion + aldol
    (c) Carbocation + alcohol
    (d) Carbanion + alcohol

225. What is the intermediate occurs in perkin's reaction
    (a) Carbenes
    (b) Carbocations
    (c) Carbanions
    (s) Carbonium ion

226. Which reactive intermediate is participates in nucleophilic substitution reaction
    (a) Carbonium ion
    (b) Carbene
    (c) Carbocation
    (d) Carbanion

227. Carbocation is more stable,
    (a) Due to electron releasing substituent
    (b) Due to electron withdrawing substituent
    (c) Due to adjacent functional groups
    (d) None

228.

$$H_3C—\overset{\overset{H_3C}{|}}{\underset{\underset{CH_3}{|}}{C}}—\overset{CH_2}{\underset{H}{C}}—H \longrightarrow A + B$$

(a) A= 3-iodo-2,2-dimethyl butane,
    B= 3-iodo-2,3-dimethyl butane
(b) A= 2-iodo-3,3-dimethyl butane,
    B= 3-iodo-2,3-dimethyl butane
(c) A= 3-iodo-2,2-dimethyl butane,
    B= 2-iodo-3,3-dimethyl butane
(d) A= 2-iodo-3,3-dimethyl butane,
    B= 2-iodo-3,3-dimethyl butane

229. Which reactive intermediates are produced by heterolysis of a covalent bond
(a) Carbonium ion
(b) Carbine
(c) Carbocation
(d) Nitrene

230. The relative stabilities of carbocation
(a) $3^\circ > 2^\circ > 1^\circ >$ methyl cation
(b) $3^\circ > 2^\circ > 1^\circ <$ methyl cation
(c) $3^\circ < 2^\circ < 1^\circ <$ methyl cation
(d) $3^\circ < 2^\circ > 1^\circ >$ methyl cation

231. The decreasing order of stability of alkyl carbocation
(a) $CH_3 < 1^0 < 2^\circ < 3^\circ$
(b) $CH_3 > 1^\circ > 2^\circ > 3^\circ$
(c) $CH_3 < 1^\circ < 2^\circ < 3^\circ$
(d) $CH_3 < 1^\circ < 2^\circ > 3^\circ$

232. Diazomethane on thermal or photochemical decomposition
(a) Methyl group+ Nitrogen
(b) Methane + Nitrogen
(c) Methylene group + Nitrogen
(d) None

233. The neutral highly reactive intermediates
(a) Carbenes
(b) Carbocations
(c) Carbanions
(d) Free radicals

234. Highly reactive intermediate of nitrenes are also called as
(a) Azides
(b) Azenes
(c) Azocompounds
(d) None

235. Which of the below reactive intermediate is formed in curtius rearrangement
(a) Carbene   (b) Carbocation
(c) Carbanions   (d) Nitrene

236. Pericyclic reactions includes
(a) Cycloaddition reactions
(b) Electrocyclic reactions
(c) Sigmatropic reactions
(d) All the above

237. Diel's Alder reaction is -------type of pericyclic reaction
(a) Electrocyclic reactions
(b) Sigmatropic reactions
(c) Cycloaddition reactions
(d) All the above

238. Two unshared molecules combine to form a cyclic compound with lt electron being used to form new a bond is known as
(a) Sigmatropic reaction
(b) Cycloaddition reaction
(c) Electrolytic reaction
(d) None

239. Which reaction involves either the formation of a ring, with the generation of a new a bond and the consumption of n-bond
    (a) Electrolytic reaction
    (b) Cycloaddition reactions
    (c) Sigmatropic reactions
    (d) None

240. An atom or group in a lt electron system migrates with the a bond without in the number of or a bond or n-bonds are called
    (a) Electrolytic reaction
    (b) Cycloaddition reactions
    (c) Sigmatropic reactions
    (d) None

241. The arrangement of substituent on the benzene ring is often referred as
    (a) Orientation
    (b) Isomersation
    (c) Epimerisation
    (d) None

242. The substituent which cause the compound C_6H_5-S to undergo second substitution faster than benzene are called the
    (a) Activating Substituent
    (b) Deactivating Substituent
    (c) Substituent with less activity
    (d) None

243. The alkyl groups attached to a conjugate system are known to exhibit a special type of resonance called
    (a) Hyper conjugation
    (b) Mesomeric effect
    (c) Inductive effect
    (d) None

244. The relative ability of alkyl groups to be involved in hyperconjugation in the order
    (a) Methyl> 1° >2 °>3 °
    (b) Methyl <1° <2 °<3 °
    (c) Methyl <1° >2 °>3 °
    (d) Methyl> 1° >2 °<3 °

245. When methylene is generated in the presence of alkenes, there are formation of
    (a) Isobutane
    (b) Cyclopropane
    (c) Cyclobutane
    (d) None

246. Which of the following penicillin contains isoxazole group
    (a) Ampicillin   (b) Cloxacillin
    (c) Naficillin   (d) Ticarcillin

247. In the nomenclature of penicillins for example [3.2.0] indicates
    (a) Peripheral numbering
    (b) Numbering of heteroatoms
    (c) Number of atoms in each bridge
    (d) None of the above

248. Which of the following penicillin will have an intermediate spectrum of activity
    (a) Ampicillin   (b) Oxacillin
    (c) Naficillin   (d) Piperacillin

249. Which of the following group has to be introduced at the alpha position in the acylamino side chain of penicillin in order to increase the oral bioavailability
    (a) Electron releasing
    (b) Electron withdrawing
    (c) Electron donating
    (d) Any of the above

250. Which of the following penicillin contains imidazolidine-2-one group in its side chain at 6th position
(a) Piperacillin
(b) Penicillin-G
(c) Amoxacillin
(d) Mezlocillin

251. Carbenicillin is a
(a) Narrow spectrum penicillin
(b) Intermediate spectrum penicillin
(c) Broad spectrum penicillin
(d) B-lactamase resistant penicillin

252. Ortho substitution or substitution by bulky groups in the side chain at the 6th position of penicillins
(a) Decreases B-lactamase resistant
(b) Decreases oral stability
(c) Increases metabolism
(d) Increases B-lactamase resistant

253. Cyclacillin acts by
(a) Inhibiting protein synthesis
(b) Inhibiting cell wall synthesis
(c) Inhibiting bacterial entry into the body
(d) Inhibiting bacterial metabolism

254. Which of the following is the common feature of both Amoxacillin and Cefixime
(a) Side chain at the 6th position
(b) Mechanism of action
(c) Presence of B-lactam ring
(d) Both b and c

255. All naturally occurring penicillins are
(a) Strongly dextro-rotatory
(b) Strongly leavo-rotatory
(c) Racemic mixtures
(d) Optically inactive

256. Which of the following is a Class-I B-lactamase inhibitor
(a) Meropenem
(b) Imipenem
(c) Biapenem
(d) Tazobactam

257. Which of the following B-lactamase inhibitor contains 1,2,3-Triazole ring
(a) Biapenem
(b) Clavulanic acid
(c) Tazobactam
(d) Sulbactam

258. Which of the following B-lactamase inhibitor contains 2-hydroxy ethylidene moiety at C-2
(a) Biapenem
(b) Clavulanic acid
(c) Tazobactam
(d) Sulbactam

259. 1, 1-dioxo penicillanic acid is
(a) Thienemycin
(b) K^{+} Clavulanate
(c) Tazobactam
(d) Sulbactam

260. Which of the following Cephalosporin does not contain a Sulphur atom
(a) Cephradin
(b) Cefepime
(c) Loracabef
(d) Cefexim

261. Methyl pyrrolidine containing Cephalosporin is
(a) Cephradin
(b) Cefepime
(c) Loracabef
(d) Cefexim

262. Cefepime belongs to
(a) 1st generation
(b) 2nd generation
(c) 3rd generation
(d) 4th generation

263. Which of the following does not contain a Phenylglycyl group in the side chain at 7th position
    (a) Cefuroxime   (b) Cephradine
    (c) Cefaclor   (**d**) Cefadroxil

264. Cefixime belongs to which generation
    (a) lst   (b) 2nd
    (c) 3rd (d) 4th

265. Cephalosporins which contain a Phenylglycyl substituent are
    (a) Parenterally active
    (**b**) Subcutaneously active
    (c) Orally active
    (d) Both parenterally and orally active

266. Antibiotics which are derived from amino acids are
    (a) Tetracyclines   (b) Penicillins
    (c) Cephalosporins (d) Both b & c

267. Sulphur containing antibiotics are
    (a) Amphotericin & nystatin
    (**b**) Chloramphenicol
    (c) Lincomycin & clindamycin (cleomycin)
    (d) Tetracyclins

268. The bicyclic system of penicillins contains a -lactam ring fused with ……..
    (a) Dihydrothiazine
    (**b**) Thiazolidine
    (c) Imidazolidine
    (d) Pyrrolidine

269. In the nomenclature of penicillins the unsubstituted bicyclic system including carbonyl amide group ls called as
    (a) Penicillanic acid

    (b) Penicillin
    (c) Cepham
    (d) Penam

270. Penicillin   D-penicillamine. X= ?
    (a) Cold dil.HNO3
    (b) Hot dil.mineral acid
    (c) -lactamase
    (**d**) Acid catalysed rearrangement

271. The following are the statements regarding procaine & benzathine salts of benzyl penicillin. Which of the following statements are incorrect?
    (P) They are water soluble
    (Q) They are water insoluble
    (R) Used for repository purposes
    (S) Used when long term blood levels of benzyl penicillin are required
    (a) Only P   (b) Q, R & S
    (c) R & S   (d) P & S

272. The combination of administration of which of the following with penicillins prolongs the tl2 of penicillins by competing effectively for excretion
    (a) Tolbutamide   (b) Propranolol
    (c) Probucol   (d) Probenicid

273. One of the following groups is present in a cephalosporin which is the only cephalosporin which is used both orally & peranterally
    (a) 1,3,4-Triazole
    (b) a-Amino benzyl
    (c) Cyclohexadiene
    (d) Furyl

274. Penicillin ring system is derived from two of the following amino acids:
(P) Alanine & methionine
(Q) Cysteine & valine
(R) Glycine & cysteine
(S) Methinine & leucine
Choose the correct pair.
(a) P
(b) Q
(c) R
(d) S

275. 6-Amino penicillanic acid contains?
(a) A 1° amino group
(b) A 2° amino group
(c) A 3° amino group
(d) A 4° amino group

276. When penicillins are taken orally they will have poor oral absorption because penicillins are converted into .... in presence of acid of stomach.
(a) Penicillenic acid
(b) D-penicillamine
(c) Penicilloic acid
(d) Penillic acid

277. Assertion[A]: Introduction of methoxy, ethoxy groups into the side chain of 6-APA increases the P-lactamase resistance. Reason[R]: As the steric hindrance increases in the side chain resistance to P-lactamase also increases.
(a) Only A is correct
(b) Only R is correct
(c) Both A & R are correct but R is not correct explanation of A.
(d) Both A & R are correct and R is the correct explanation of A.

278. Which of the following enzyme/s are referred to as 'suicide substrates'?
(a) Oxidoreductases
(b) Transferases
(c) P-lactamases
(d) Hydrolases

279. Which of the following P-lactamase inhibitors contains a sulfone group?
(a) K^+ Clavulanate, Tazobactam
(b) Tazobactam, Sulbactam
(c) Sulbactam, Imipenem
(d) Meropenem, Biapenem

280. Thienamycin a class-II P-lactamase inhibitor (belongs to carbapenems) isolated from?
(a) Streptomyces cattleya
(b) Streptomyces clavuligeris
(c) Penicillium glaucum
(d) Penicillium chrysogenum

281. A-CH=NH group containing P-lactamase inhibitor is?
(a) Tazobactam   (b) Ertapenem
(c) Thienamycin   (d) Imipenem

282. The concomitant administration of Imipene with which of the following antibiotic results in synergistic antibacterial activity *in vivo*.
(a) Aminoglycosides
(b) Tetracyclins
(c) Macrolides
(d) Rifampicin

283. A bicyclic system containing P-lactamase inhibitor is?
(a) Ertapenem   (b) Sulbactam
(c) Meropenem   (d) Biapenem

284. The 5 membered ring system that is present at C-3 position im cephalosporins is
     (a) 1,2,3,4-tetrazole
     (b) 1,2,3,5- tetrazole
     (c) 1,2-diazole
     (d) 1,3-diazole

285. Which of the following statement/s is/are correct?
     (P) Cephalosporins which contain a phenylglycyl substituent in the side chain at C-7 are orally active
     (Q) Cephalosporins which contain a phenylglycyl substituent in the side chain at C-7 are orally inactive
     (R) Cephalosporins which contain an acetyloxy group in the side chain at C-3 are orally active
     (S) Cephalosporins which contain an acetyloxy group in the side chain at C-3 are orally inactive
     (a) P, R
     (b) Q, R
     (c) P, S
     (d) None of the above

286. Which of the following statement/s is/are correct?
     (a) In the case of cefixime E-isomer has more P-lactamase resistant than Z-isomer
     (b) In the case of cefixime Z-isomer has more P-lactamase resistant than E-isomer
     (c) Cephalosporins with 'S' at 1st position are more P-lactamase resistant than with 'O' at 1st position
     (d) Cephalosporins with a bulkier substituent in the side chain at C-7 are less P-lactamase resistant

287. Which of the following statement is correct regarding Cephamycins?
     (a) They contain ^{2}-cephem
     (b) They contain 'O' atom at 1st position
     (c) They do not contain -COOR at 4th position
     (d) They contain a-OCH_3 at i ^{h} position

288. Cephalosporins are potent antibacterials than penicillins, against potent species of bacteria because of which of the following?
     (a) They are more resistance to inactivation by P-lactamases
     (b) They have more permeability into bacterial cells
     (c) They have intrinsic activity against bacterial enzymes involved in cell wall synthesis and cross-linking
     (d) All the above

289. Cefoperazone contains
     (a) Pyridazine   (b) Pyrimidine
     (c) Piperazine   (d) Pyrazole

290. Cephalosporin $\xrightarrow{\text{-lactamases}}$?
     (a) Cephalosporoic acid
     (b) Desacetyl cephalosporin
     (c) Desacetyl cephalosporin lactone
     (d) 7-amino cephalosporanic acid

291. -lactam ring is
  (a) Azetidine-3-one
  (b) Azetidine-2-one
  (c) Oxetidine-3-one
  (d) Oxetidine-2-one

292.

$$R - C -) = \overset{H}{\underset{}{r}}$$

COOH

In the above molecule the weakest bond is the bond that is present between which atoms
  (a) 4,5
  (b) 1,2
  (c) 4, 7
  (d) 3,4

293. Which of the following tetracycline contains a methylidene group
  (a) Doxycycline
  (b) Minocycline
  (c) Methacycline
  (d) Demeclocycline

294. Which ring of the tetracycline molecule is completely unsaturated
  (a) C
  (b) A
  (c) D
  (d) B

295. In tetracycline molecule epimerization occurs at
  (a) C-4
  (b) C-5
  (c) C-2
  (d) C-6

296. Which of the following group is present at C-2 in tetracycline molecule?
  (a) Acid
  (b) Ester
  (c) Alcohol
  (d) Amide

297. The group that is present at the 4th m the tetracycline molecule is
  (a) -dimethylamino
  (b) -diethylamino
  (c) a-diethylamino
  (d) a-dimethylamino

298. How many acidity constants are there in a tetracycline molecule?
  (a) 3
  (b) 4
  (c) 5
  (d) 1

299. At physiological pH tetracyclines exists as
  (a) Acid compounds
  (b) Amphoteric compounds
  (c) Basic compounds
  (d) None of the above

300. Which of the following antibiotic forms complexe with milk?
  (a) Erythromycin
  (b) Ampicillin
  (c) Cefixime
  (d) Minocycline

301. Tetracyclines treat the bacterial infections by
  (a) Inhibiting peptidoglycon synthesis by preventing cross linking
  (b) Inhibiting bacterial growth by forming complexes
  (c) Inhibiting the release of carrier
  (d) Inhibiting protein synthesis

302. Which of the following tetracycline contains a glycyl substituent?
  (a) Tigecycline
  (b) Minocycline
  (c) Doxycycline
  (d) All of the above

303. Which of the following antibiotic is bactereostatic but not bactericidal
   (a) Ciproflaxacin   (b) Ampicillin
   (c) Cefixime   (d) Minocycline

304. Tetracyclins are painful on IM injection. This is because of the formation of insoluble calcium complexes. To overcome this, the preparations must contain
   (a) Ethyleneglycol
   (b) Propyleneglycol
   (c) Ethylenediaminetetraacetic acid
   (d) Both b and c

305. Tetracyclines are characterized by having a
   (a) Partially reduced naphthalene
   (b) Completely reduced naphthacene
   (c) Partially reduced naphthacene
   (d) Completely reduced naphthalene

306. Which of the following antibiotic competes with tRNA for the A site
   (a) Erythromycin
   (b) Ampicillin
   (c) Cefixime
   (d) Chlortetracycline

307. Which of the following antibiotics contain a -lactam ring?
   (a) Ampicillin, cefepime, azithromycin
   (b) Ampicillin, cefepime, doxicycline
   (c) Ampicillin, cefepime only
   (d) Ampicillin, cefepime, tigemonam, sulphazecin, aztreonam

308. Which of the following antibiotic does not contain a bicyclic system in its structure?
   (a) Piperacillin

(b) Cephamandole
(c) Aztreonam
(d) Mezlocillin

309. Which of the following monobactam antibiotic contains a Glutamoyl group?
   (a) Aztreonam   (b) Sulphazecin
   (c) Tigemonam   (d) Tigecycline

310. Which of the following antibiotic prevents the movement of ribosome from one codon to another (Translocation process)
   (a) Clarithromycin
   (b) Vancomycin
   (c) Bacitracin
   (d) Cefazoline

311. Which of the following antibiotics contain a lactone ring?
   (a) Dirithromycin, telithromycin, azithromycin
   (b) Dirithromycin, telithromycin, cefotetan
   (c) Naficillin, cefmetazole, azithromycin
   (d) Carbenicillin, ticarcillin, dirithromycin

312. Gentamicin contains
   (a) Streptadine
   (b) 2-deoxystreptamin
   (c) Spectinamine
   (d) Both a and b

313. The tetracycline with 'methylidine' group is
   (a) Oxytetracycline
   (b) Demeclocycline
   (c) Methacycline
   (d) Doxycycline

314. The tetracycline with a 'dimethyl amino group' at C-7 is
    (a) Demeclocycline
    (b) Methacycline
    (c) Doxycycline
    (d) Minocycline

315. The group that is present in the side chain at C-9 of 'tigecycline' is
    (a) Isopropyl   (b) 3°-Butyl
    (c) Isopentyl   (d) n-Hexyl

316. During the action of tetracyclines on bacteria, the binding of tetracyclines at the ribosomal binding site require .... ions
    (a) Mg^{+2} (b) Ca^{+2}
    (c) Na^{+} (d) K^{+}

317. In the SAR of tetracyclines only slight modifications can be done on which of the following ring without dramatic loss of antibacterial potency
    (a) A ring   (b) B ring
    (c) C ring   (d) D ring

318. When tetracyclines are combined with which of the following they form water insoluble salts
    (a) HCl
    (b) NaOH
    (c) Fe^{+2}
    (d) All the above

319. The number of acidity constants in tetracycline molecule is
    (a) 1   (b) 3
    (c) 2   (d) 4

320. In the tetracycline molecule the acidity constant PKa_1 is formed by the combination of groups that are present on which of the following atoms
    (a) 4, 4a   (b) 10, 11, 12
    (c) 5,6,7   (d) 1,2,3

321. In the tetracycline molecule the acidity constant PKa_3 is formed by the combination of groups that are present on which of the following atoms
    (a) 4, 4a   (b) 10, 11, 12
    (c) 5,6,7   (d) 1,2,3

322. In the tetracycline molecule the acidity constant PKa_2 is formed by the combination of groups that are present on which of the following atoms
    (a) 4, 4a   (b) 10, 11, 12
    (c) 5,6,7   (d) 1,2,3

323. Which of the following tetracycline is obtained from Streptomyces rimosus?
    (a) Doxycycline
    (b) Methacycline
    (c) Terramycin (oxytetracycline)
    (d) Minocycline

324. Which of the following is an 'amphoteric' molecule?
    (a) Azlocillin
    (b) Minocycline
    (c) Azithromycine
    (d) Cefepime

325. Following are some drug derivatives used to increase/decreases the water solubility of the parent drugs:
    (P) Rolitetracycline
    (Q) Erythromycin lactobionate
    (R) Chloramphenicol succinate
    (S) Erythromycin stearate

Choose the correct combination of statements.

(a) Q & R are used to increases water solubility while P & S are used to decrease it

(b) P, Q & R are used to increases water solubility while S is used to decrease it

(c) Q, S & R are used to increases water solubility while P is used to decrease it

(d) Q & S are used to increases water solubility while P & Q are used to decrease it

326. The heterocyclic ring that is present in 'Rolitetracycline' is
(a) Pyrazolidine
(b) Imidazolidine
(c) THF
(d) Pyrrolidine

327. Macrolides are the 14 membered lactone ring containing antibiotics. The macrolide with 16 membered lactone ring is
(a) Tylosin
(b) Telithromycin
(c) Clarithromycin
(d) Oleandomycin

328. Which of the following statements are correct regarding macrolide antibiotics?
(P) Salt formation with glucoheptonic & lactobionic acid increases water solubility

(Q) Salt formation with lauryl sulfate & stearic acid decreases water solubility

(R) Salt formation with lauryl sulfate & stearic acid increases water solubility

(S) Salt formation with gluco-heptonic & lactobionic acid decreases water solubility

(a) R & S   (b) Q & S
(c) P & Q   (d) Only P

329. The 14 membered ring macrolides are biosynthesiszed from which of the following?
(a) Propanoic acid units
(b) Butanoic acid units
(c) Ethanoic acid units
(d) Pentanoic acid units

330. The sugars *cladinose* & *desosamine* are present in which of the following antibiotics
(a) Chloramphenicol
(b) Aminoglycosides
(c) Polypeptide antibiotics
(d) Macrolides

331.

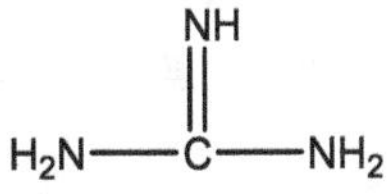

The above group containing aminoglycoside is
(a) Gentamicin
(b) Streptomycin
(c) Spectinomycin
(d) Tobramycin

332. When gentamicin or other aminoglycosides are combined with which of the following in the same solution or given to a patient at a time, then both will be inhibited (inactive)
     (a) Ticarcillin
     (b) Cefixime
     (c) Both a & b
     (d) Azithromycin

333. The aminoglycoside which is obtained from *Micromonospora purpurea* is
     (a) Streptomycin
     (b) Spectinomycin
     (c) Gentamicin
     (d) Kanamycin

334. The penetration of aminoglycosides through the cell membrane of the bacterium depends partly on oxygen-dependent active transport by a polyamine earrier system. This transport system is blocked by ......
     (a) Dirithromycin
     (b) Chloramphenicol
     (c) Vancomycin
     (d) Carbenicillin

335. The stereochemistry of aminoacids that are present in the polypeptide antibiotics which are produced by bacteria is
     (a) D
     (b) L
     (c) Both a & b
     (d) Amino acids are achiral

336. The antibiotics which have a pendant fatty acid chain in their structure are
     (a) Macrolides
     (b) Penicillins
     (c) Aminoglycosides
     (d) Polypeptide antibiotics

337. The antibiotic which inhibits the release of carrier from the building block unit of peptidoglycon layer during the formation of peptidoglycon layer outside the cell membrane
     (a) Bacitracin
     (b) Streptomycin
     (c) Dirithromycin
     (d) Vancomycin

338. The antibiotic which interferes with the regeneration of the lipid carrier by blocking its dephosphorylation during the formation of peptidoglycon layer
     (a) Bacitracin
     (b) Streptomycin
     (c) Dirithromycin
     (d) Vancomycin

339. The antibiotic which contain an ester functional group in its structure is
     (a) Cefixime
     (b) Ampicillin
     (c) Clarithromycin
     (d) Vancomycin

340. Naphthyridine is
     (a) 1,8-diaza-naphthalene
     (b) 1,2-diaza-naphthalene
     (c) 1,3-diaza-naphthalene
     (d) 2,3-diaza-naphthalene

341. Cinnoline is
     (a) 1,8-diaza-naphthalene
     (b) 1,2-diaza-naphthalene
     (c) 1,3-diaza-naphthalene
     (d) 2,3-diaza-naphthalene

342. The heterocyclic ring that is present in nalidixic acid a fluroquinolone is
(a) Naphthyridine (b) Cinnoline
(c) Phthalazine (d) Quinazoline

343. Quinolone antimicrobials are .... substances
(a) Biosynthetic
(b) Synthetic
(c) Semisynthetic
(d) Naturally obtained

344. The antibiotics which possess in common an N-1-alkylated-3-carboxy pyridine-4-one are
(a) Penicillins
(b) Tetracyclines
(c) Fluroquinolones
(d) Macrolides

345. The group that is present at 3rd position in the structure of ofloxacin (racemic) is
(a) Keto (b) Fluoro
(c) Methyl (d) Carboxy

346. In the basic nucleus of fluroquinolones addition of fluoro group at which position greatly increases the biological activity
(a) 2nd (b) 5th
(c) 6th (d) 7th

347. The group that is present at C-7 in most of the fluoroquinolones is
(a) Pyrimidine (b) Piperazine
(c) Pyrazine (d) Pyrazole

348. Which of the following fluoroquinolones contain a 3rd ring in its basic nucleus?
(a) Levofloxacin (b) Ofloxacin

(c) Sparfloxacin (d) Both a & b

349. The heterocyclic ring that is present in Cinoxacin a fluroquinolone is
(a) Naphthyridine (b) Cinnoline
(c) Phthalazine (d) Quinazoline

350. Which of the following fluoroquinolones contain a morpholine ring in its basic nucleus?
(a) Levofloxacin (b) Ofloxacin
(c) Both a & b (d) Sparfloxacin

351. An imine group containing fluoroquinolone is
(a) Norfloxacin
(b) Moxifloxacin
(c) Gatifloxacin
(d) Gemifloxacin

352. Which of the following is a prodrug of trovafloxacin a fluoroquinolone?
(a) Alatrovafloxacin
(b) Moxifloxacin
(c) Gatifloxacin
(d) Gemifloxacin

353. Topoisomerase II or DNA gyrase is an enzyme that produces a negative supercoil (unwinding) in DNA & thus permits transcription or replication. The antibiotic which inhibits DNA gyrase enzyme is
(a) Cefixime
(b) Ampicillin
(c) Clarithromycin
(d) Moxifloxacin

354. In fluoroquinolone antibiotics the group that is present at 4th position is
(a) Hydroxy (b) Amino
(c) Keto (d) Mercapto

355. The groups those are present at which positions in the fluoroquinolone structure are involved in binding to the DNA/DNA-gyrase enzyme system
(a) 6th & 7th
(b) 3rd & 4th
(c) $?^{th}$ & 8th
(d) 1st & 2nd

356. In the basic structure of fluoroquinolones substitution by fluorine at which position increases antimicrobial activity by increasing the lipophilicity of the molecule (increasing the drugs penetration through the bacterial cell wall)
(a) 7th
(b) 6th
(c) 2nd
(d) 5th

357. The basic structure of fluoro-quinolones contain a fluorine atom at 6th position, an additional fluoro group at ...... position improves drug absorption & t1/2 but may increases drug-induced photosensitivity
(a) 8th
(b) 6th
(c) 2nd
(d) 5th

358. The piperazinyl group that is present at which position in the basic nucleus of fluoroquinolones increases binding to CNS GABA receptors, which accounts for CNS side effects
(a) 7th
(b) 6th
(c) 2nd
(d) 5th

359. In the structure of Ofloxacin a chiral (asymmetric) center is present at which position
(a) 2nd
(b) 3rd
(c) 4th
(d) 1st

360. In the SAR of fluoroquinolones a fluorine atom at which position produces the highest incidence of photosensitivity via singlet oxygen & radical induction
(a) 8th
(b) 6th
(c) 2nd
(d) 5th

361. In the SAR of fluoroquinolones a fluorine atom at 8th position produces the highest incidence of photosensitivity via singlet oxygen & radical induction, introduction of which of the following group at the same 8th position by replacing F atom decreases photosensitivity
(a) -OH
(b) -NH2
(c) -OCH3
(d) -CH3

362. When fluoroquinolones are combined with polyvalent metal ions such as Ca+2, Mg+2 chelation occurs between metal & groups that are present at which positions in basic structure
(a) 6th & 7th
(b) 3rd & 4th
(C) 7th & 8th
(d) 1st & 2nd

363. Which of the following anticancer drug contains aziridine nucleus
(a) Thiotepa
(b) Cyclophosphamide
(c) Busulfhan
(d) All the above

364. Bis- -haloalkylamines are commonly called as
(a) Taxanes
(b) Mustines
(c) Podophyllotoxins
(d) Nitrogen mustards

365. The position of guanine that is attacked by bifunctional alkylating agents is
   (a) 1st
   (b) 3rd
   (c) 2nd
   (d) 7th

366. The presence of which of the following group on the nitrogen atom of nitrogen mustards decreases the risk of serious side effects
   (a) Aromatic
   (b) Aliphatic
   (c) Both
   (d) None

367. Steroidal nucleus containing Anticancer Agent is
   (a) Carmustin
   (b) Estromustin phosphate sodium
   (c) Comptothecin
   (d) Methotrexate

368. Which of the following Is a nitrosourea?
   (a) Cisplatin
   (b) Doxorubicin
   (c) Lomustine
   (d) Procarbazine

369. The cytotoxic metabolite that Is formed from the metabolism of cyclophosphamide is
   (a) Propanaldehyde
   (b) Propenaldehyde
   (c) 2-Propenol
   (d) Propanone

370. The acrolein that is formed from the anticancer drug cyclophosphamide causes
   (a) Renal Damage
   (b) Cardiac damage
   (c) Hemorrhagic cystitis
   (d) Cataracts

371. Which of the following is an organometallic anticancer drug?
   (a) Altretamine
   (b) Carboplatin
   (c) Fluorouracil
   (d) Paclitaxel

372. Oxetane ring containing compound is
   (a) Teniposide
   (b) Vinblastin
   (c) Docetaxel
   (d) Topotecan

373. Mechanism of action of doxorubicin Is
   (a) Mitotic spindle formation inhibition
   (b) DNA alkylation
   (c) DNA intercalation
   (d) Inhibition of dihydrofolate reductase

374. The heterocyclic ring that is present in methotrexate is
   (a) Quinoline
   (b) Quanazoline
   (c) Pteridine
   (d) Pynolidine

375. Of the following which Is a topoisomerase 2 inhibitor
   (a) Paclitaxel
   (b) Vinca alkaloids
   (c) Topotecan
   (d) Teniposide

376. Of the following anticancer drugs which causes demethylation of DNA
   (a) Azacitidine
   (b) Dacarbazine
   (c) Flurouracil
   (d) Camptothecin

377. Tricyclic system is present in _____ drug
    (a) Acyclovir
    (b) Rimantadine
    (c) Zidorudine
    (d) IFN-y

378. Which of the following is a protease inhibitor
    (a) Didanosine   (b) Amprenavir
    (c) Amantadine   (d) Zidorudine

379. Of the following interferons which is termed as "immune interferon".
    (a) IFN-a   (b) IFN-
    (c) IFN-y   (d) Both a & c

380. 'Azido' group containing Nucleoside reverse transcriptase inhibitor is
    (a) Abacavir   (b) Starudine
    (c) Lamivudine   (d) Zidovudine

381. Nevirapine and efavirenz are
    (a) Protease inhibitors
    (b) Non-nucleoside reverse transcriptase inhibitors
    (c) Nucleoside reverse transcriptase inhibitors
    (d) DNA polymerase inhibitors

382. Undecylenic acid is a
    (a) Bactereostatic
    (b) Antimalarials
    (c) Fungistatic
    (d) Antihelmenthetic

383. Lorazepam is a
    (a) Benzo (f)-1,4-diazepine
    (b) Benzo (f)-1,4-thiazepine
    (c) Benzo (f)-1,3-diazepine
    (d) Benzo (e)-1,4-diazepine

384. The heterocyclic ring that is present in Alprazolam
    (a) 1,2,3-triazole
    (b) 1,3,4-triazole
    (c) 1,2,4-triazole
    (d) None of the above

385. In the benzodiazepine nucleus an electronegative substituent is present at which position
    (a) 6th (b) 9th
    (C) 8th (d) 7th

386. Midazolam
    (a) Closes er channel
    (b) Opens Na^+ channel
    (C) Opens er channel
    (d) Closes Ca+zchannel

387. Barbituric acid is
    (a) Pyrimidine-2,4,5-trione
    (b) Pyrimidine-2,6-dione
    (c) Pyrimidine-2,5,6-trione
    (d) Pyrimidone-2,4,6-trione

388. Which of the following is an ultra short acting barbiturate?
    (a) Amobarbital
    (b) Pentobartial
    (c) Thiamylal
    (d) Mephobarbital

389. If both the hydrogens at 5th position of barbituric acid are not replaced, then it leads to
    (a) Lactonization
    (b) Cleavage of molecule
    (c) Tautomerization
    (d) Ring expansion

390. Which of the following statements are correct regarding barbituric acids?

    (i) 1,3-disubstituted barbituric acids are active

    (ii) 5- monosubstitued barbituric acids are active

    (iii) 5,5- disubstitued-2-thiobarbituric acids are active

    (iv) 1,5,5- trisubstituted barbituric acids are active

(a) i, iii   (b) ii, iii

(c) iii, Iv   (d) I,Iv

391. In the structure of barbituric acid replacement of oxygen by sulfur at which position increases activity

(a) 4th (b) 2nd & 6th

(c) 2nd & 4th (d) 2nd

392. Chloral is

(a) Dichloroacetaldehyde

(b) Trichloroacetic acid

(c) Dichloroacetic acid

(d) Trichloroacetaldehyde

393. Meprobamate is a hypnotic and sedative which contains

a) 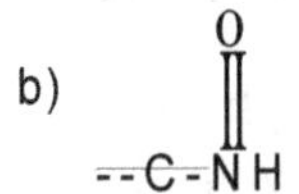   b) 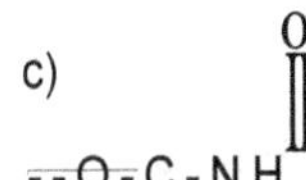   c) 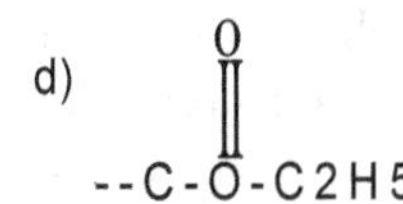   d)

(a) 3rd (b) 2nd

(C) 4th (d) 1st

394. Modifications of which antitubercular drug leads to the production of antidepresent drugs

(a) Ethambutol

(b) Pyrazinamide

(c) Isoniazid

(d) Rifampin

395. Which of the following is a selective MAO-B inhibitor?

(a) Moclobemide

(b) Deprenyl(Selegiline)

(c) Tranylcypromine

(d) Imipramine

396. Which of the following contains dibenzocycloheptane nucleus?

(a) Clomipramine   (b) Maprotiline

(c) Fluroxamine   (d) Nortriptyline

397. In Clomipramine 'Chlorine' is present at which position

398. The bridge that is present between ring nitrogen and the basic amino nitrogen in the tricyclic antidepressants is

(a) Ethylene   (b) Butylene

(c) Propylene   (d) Methylene

399. Sertraline and Citalopram are

(a) TCAs

(b) MAO inhibitors

(c) 5-HT$_{1A}$ agonist

(d) SSRis

400. 5HT$_{1A}$ agonist 'Buspirone' contains

(a) Bicyclic system

(b) Tricyclic system

(c) Spiro system

(d) Tetracyclic system

401. Mirtazepine and Mianserin which contains Benzo[e]-pyrido[b]-azepine ring are
    (a) Pl -agonists
    (b) arantagonists
    (c) Both a & b
    (d) aragonists

402. Imidazolidine-2,4-dione ring containing compound is
    (a) Phensuximide
    (b) Dimethoadione
    (c) Ethotoin
    (d) Phenobarbital

403. Match the following
    (P) Methsuximide
        1. Blocks T-type Ca^+z channels
    (Q) Phenytoin
        2. Blocks Na^+ channels
    (R) Valproic acid
        3. GABA-T inhibitor
    (S) Tiagabine
        4. GABA reuptake inhibitor
    (a) P-4' Q-3' R-2' S-1
    (b) P-1' Q-2' R-3' S-4
    (c) P-2' Q-3' R-1' S-4
    (d) P-2' Q-3' R-4' S-1

404. Which of the following is an iminostilbene?
    (a) Oxcarbazepine
    (b) Diazepam
    (c) Vigabatrin
    (d) Felbamate

405. Which of the following drugs contains 'ethenyl' group
    (a) Vigabatrin, etchlorvynol
    (b) Carbamazepine, vigabatrin
    (c) Ethchlorvynol, valproic acid

    (d) Valproic acid, vigabatrin

406. Which of the following is used for the screening of potential anticonvulsant drugs in experimental animals?
    (a) Caffeine
    (b) Amphetamine
    (c) Pentylenetetrazole
    (d) Sibutramine

407. 1,3-dimethylxanthine is
    (a) Caffeine
    (b) Theophylline
    (c) Theobromine
    (d) Picrotoxin

408. Methylxanthines acts as diuretics by
    (a) Vasodilation of the afferent glomercular arteriole
    (b) Vasodilation of the efferent glomercular arteriole
    (c) Vasoconstriction of efferent glomercular arteriole
    (d) Vasoconstriction of afferent glomercular arteriole

409. Branching with smaller alkyl groups at …….. position of P-phenylethylamine increases central sympathomimetic activity
    (a) P-to amino group
    (b) On the phenyl ring
    (c) On the amino group
    (d) a-to amino group

410. Triflupromazine contains
    (a) Benzo[b]-thiazine
    (b) Benzo[b]-thiazole
    (c) Benzimidazole
    (d) Phenothiazine

411. Thioridazine acts by blocking
   (a) D r receptors   (b) Bl-receptor
   (c) a l- receptors (d) B₃-receptors

412. Droperidol chemically is a
   (a) Iminostilbene
   (b) Phenothiazine
   (c) Succinimide
   (d) Fluorobutyrophenone

413. Maximum potency of antipsychotic activity is observed when substituents are present at which at position on phenothiazine ring
   (a) 1st (b) 3rd
   (c) 4th   (d) 2nd

414. The tautomerism that will see in barbiturates
   (a) Keto-enol
   (b) Amine-imine
   (c) Lactam-lactim
   (d) Both a & c

415. If in the synthesis of a compound, a, B-unsaturated esters are going to be formed means, then name of that reaction is called as
   (a) Michael addition
   (b) Polonovsky rearrangement
   (c) Aldol condensation
   (d) Knoevanagel reaction

416. Aminophylline is a combination of
   (a) Theophylline + ethylenediamine
   (b) Caffeine + ethylenediamine
   (c) Theobromine + ethylenediamine
   (d) Caffeine + theobromine

417. 'Formaldehyde' is used in which of the following reaction
   (a) Aldol condensation
   (b) Michael addition
   (c) Mannich reaction
   (d) Knoevanagel reaction

418. 'Spiro glutaric anhydride' is used in the synthesis of
   (a) Carbamazepine
   (b) Buspirone
   (c) Phenobarbital
   (d) Phensuximide

419. Butabarbital is
   (a) Basic   (b) Neutral
   (c) Amphoteric   (d) Acidic

420. Clomipramine contains
   (a) Dibenzocycloheptane ring
   (b) Benzo [b-1,5]- thiazepine
   (c) Benzo[e]-1,2,4-thiadiazine-1, 1-dioxide
   (d) Dibenzazepine

421. $R\text{-}CHrCN$ + Ethyl propenoate ---------
   ----> x Name of this kind of reaction is
   (a) Mannich reaction
   (b) Cannizzaro reaction
   (c) Kolbe's reaction
   (d) Michael addition

422.

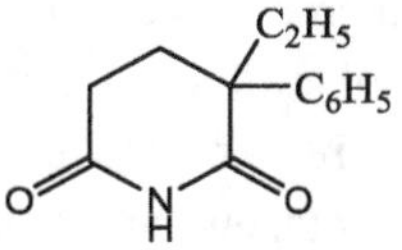

This is a hypnotic & sedative, what is this drug
   (a) Secobarbital   (b) Diazepam
   (c) Meprobamate   (d) Glutethimide

423. Zaleplon, zopiclone & zolpidem are
(a) Barbiturates
(b) Benzodiazepines
(c) Carbamates
(d) Non barbiturates & non benzodiazepines with CNS depressant
activity

424.

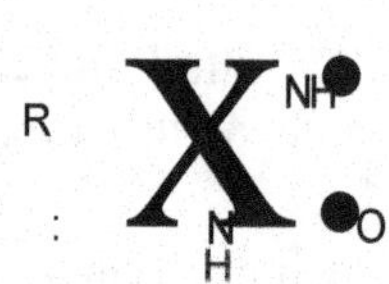

The type of tautomerism that is present in the above molecule is
(a) Lactam-lactim
(b) Keto-enol
(c) Both a & b
(d) Amine-imine

425.

Which of the following statement is correct regarding the SAR of above molecule?
(a) Substitution at both N1 & N3 decreases activity
(b) Substitution at both N_1 & N3 increases activity
(c) Replacement of all the 3 oxygen atoms by sulfur atoms increases activity
(d) Mono substitution at C-5 increases activity

426.

This is a metabolite of diazepam, prazepam, halazepam & clorazepate, during the further metabolism of this drug hydroxylation occurs at
(a) 3rd position
(b) 6th position
(c) 4th position
(d) On phenyl ring at C-5

427.

Name of this reaction is
(a) Friedel-Crafts reaction
(b) Polonovsky rearrangement
(c) Wagner-meerwien rearrangement
(d) Reimer-Tiemann reaction

428.

Name of this reaction is
(a) Friedel-Crafts reaction
(b) Polonovsky rearrangement
(c) Wagner-meerwien rearrangement
(d) Reimer-Tiemann reaction

429. Which of the following statement is correct regarding the SAR of benzodiazepines?
   (a) Saturation of 4,5 double increases activity
   (b) Substitution at meta & para positions of C-5 phenyl ring increases activity
   (c) Saturation of 4,5 double decreases activity
   (d) Substitution at 6,8,9 positions increases activity

430.

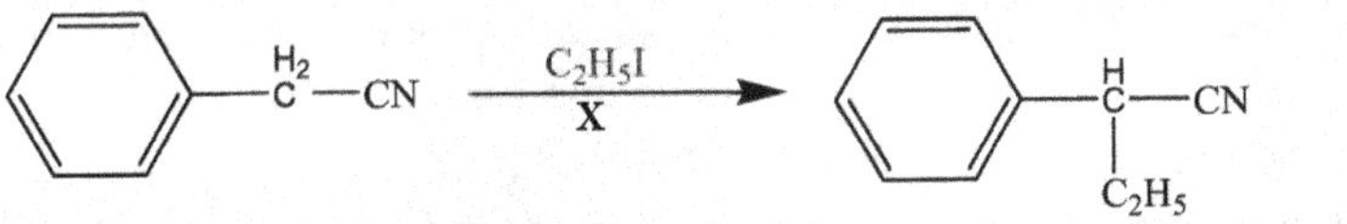

In the above reaction what is X
   (a) Conc.HCl   (b) Heat   (c) Water   (d) NaNH2

431. A person in a suicide attempt consumed over dose of benzodiazepines, which of the following drug is given to that person
   (a) Tiagabin   (b) Flumazenil
   (c) Acetaminophen (d) Nifedipine

432. When chloral hydrate is taken, it is very quickly converted to one of the following, which is responsible for almost all of the hypnotic effect of chloral hydrate
   (a) 2,2-dichloroethanol
   (b) 2,2,2-trichloroethanol
   (c) 1,1,2-trichloroethanol
   (d) 1,1-dichloroethanol

433. The term saponification is related to one of the following
   (a) Dil.HCl   (b) Conc)H2SO4
   (c) KOH   (d) Na2SO4

434. $3\ CH_3CHO \xrightarrow[-3\ H_2O]{H_2SO_4}$?

a) 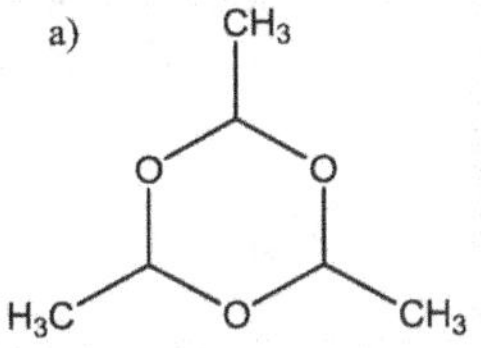 (a)

(b)

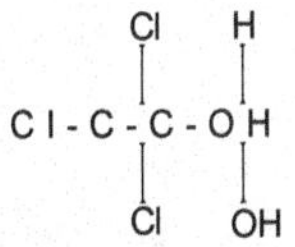

(c) Ethchlorvynol
(d) Meprobamate

435.

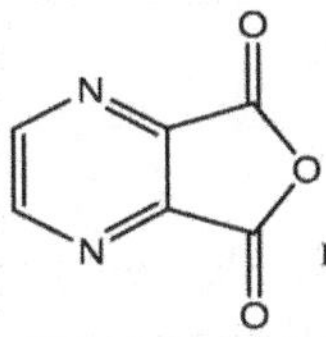

Furo[3,4-b]pyrazine-5,7-dione

It is the starting material of
   (a) Zolpidem
   (b) Zopiclone
   (c) Zaleplon
   (d) Buspirone

436.

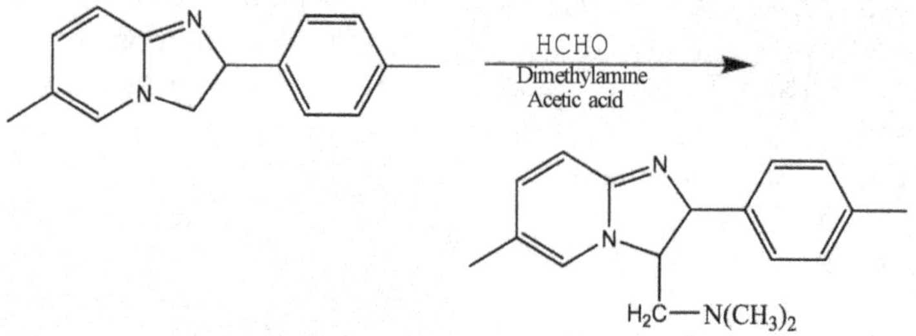

HCHO
Dimethylamine
Acetic acid

$H_2C-N(CH_3)_2$

This is an intermediate reaction in the synthesis of zolpidem this reaction can be called as

(a) Gattermann-koch reaction
(b) Mannich reaction
(c) Benzoin condensation
(d) Kolbe's reaction

437. Trazodone & nefazodone are selective serotonergic reuptake inhibitors & $5HT_{2A}$ antagonists which contain

(a)

(b) (N\N-

(c) o-

(d) CN-

438. The combination of SSRis with one of the following drugs causes "serotonin syndrome" characterized by tremor, hyperthermia & cardiovascular collapse.

(a) Buspirone
(b) Tricyclic antidepressants
(c) MAOis
(d) Phenothiazines

439. Nisoxetine & reboxetine are 'selective NE reuptake inhibitors' which contain a substituent at one of the following positions of benzene ring

(a) Ortho position
(b) Meta position
(c) Para position
(d) Benzene ring is unsubstitued

440. Which of the following statement/s is/are correct regarding the (side chain on the N atom) SAR of "tricyclic antidepressants"?

(P) $3°$ amines are more potent inhibitors of 5HT reuptake
(Q) $2°$ amines are more potent inhibitors of NE reuptake
(R) $3°$ amines are more potent inhibitors of NE reuptake
(S) $2°$ amines are more potent inhibitors of 5HT reuptake

(a) R,S
(b) Q,R
(c) P, S
(d) P, Q

441.

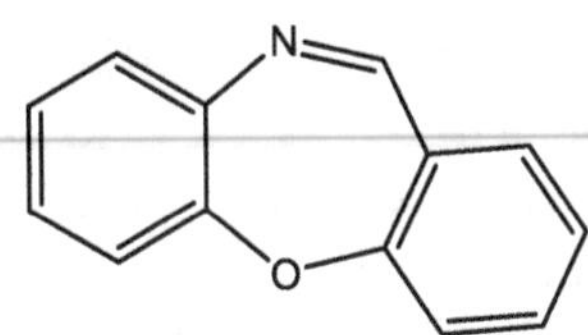

Dibenzo[b,f]-1,4-oxazepine

Which of the following antidepressant contains this basic nucleus in it?
(a) Desipramine   (b) Amoxapine
(c) Maprotiline   (d) Amitriptyline

442.

The above structure is named as ureide & it is present in
(a) Antidepressants
(b) Antiseizures
(c) Antipsychotics
(d) Antitybercular

443.

Which of the following drugs contain the above structures as basic nucleus in them respectively?
(a) Methosuximde, trimethadione
(b) carbamazepine, vigabatrine
(c) Trimethadione, methosuximde
(d) mephenytoin, clonazepam

444. In Oxcarbazepine Oxygen atom is present at .... position
(a) 11th
(b) 2nd
(c) 7th
(d) 10th

445.

H2N - C — H2 __ /I
H2C - COOH

This is an anticonvulsant, what is this drug
(a) Gabapentine
(b) Vigabatrin
(c) Tiagabine
(d) Valproic acid

446.

2-Thienyl

An aniconvulsant which contain above nucleus is
(a) Gabapentin
(b) Vigabatrin
(c) Tiagabine
(d) Valproic acid

447. Which of the following antiepileptic drug is an analogue of 'meprobamate' which is an obsolete anxiolytic drug?
(a) Lamotrigine   (b) Zonisamide
(c) Topiramate   (d) Felbamate

448. Lamotrigine an antiepileptic drug which is
(a) 1,2,4-triazine
(b) 1,2,3-triazine
(c) 1,2,5-triazine
(d) 1,2-diazine

449. 1,3-dimethylxanthine is
(a) Caffeine
(b) Theophylline
(c) Theobromine
(d) Purine

450. Methylxanthines antagonize ………. receptors
(a) D2   (b) M1
(c) A2   (d) Ach

451. Purine is
(a) Imidazolo[4,5-d]pyrimidine
(b) Imidazolo[5,4-d]pyrimidine
(c) Pyrazolo[4,5-d]pyrimidine
(d) Pyrazino[6,5-e] pyrimidine

452. A $3°$ carbon containing central sympathomimetic agent (psychomotor stimulant) is
(a) Amphetamine
(b) Benzphetamine
(c) Phentermine
(d) Fenfluramine

453.

Branching with lower alkyl groups at which position in the above structure increases central activity
(a) a   (b)
(c) Ortho   (d) Meta

454.

Which of the following statement is correct regarding SAR of above compound?
(a) Hydroxylation of the ring or on the -carbon decreases activity
(b) Halogenation of the aromatic ring decreases activity
(c) N-methylation increases activity
(d) All the above

455. One of the following drug increases the rate of synthesis of dopamine & there by acts as an alerting agent
(a) Methylphenidate
(b) Sibutramine
(c) Pemoline
(d) Phendimetrazine

456. In the structure of Chlorpromazine the distance between ring nitrogen & side chain nitrogen is
(a) 3 carbons   (b) 2 carbons
(c) 4 carbons   (d) 1 carbons

457.

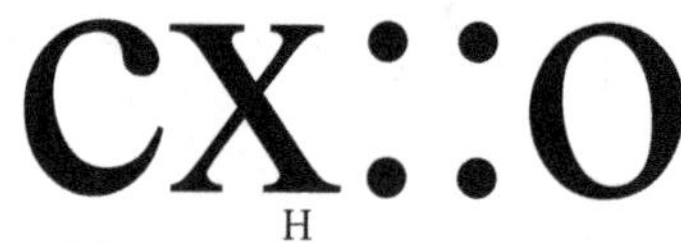

Dibenzo[b,e] 1,4-thiazine

One of the following drugs contains above nucleus
(a) Nortryptilline
(b) Butabarbital
(c) Methamphetamine
(d) Mesoridazine

458. One of the following drugs is an alkyl piperidyl side chain containing phenothiazine
    (a) Promazine
    (b) Perphenazine
    (c) Thioridazine
    (d) Desipramine

459. In Chlorpromazine Chlorine atom is present at ....position
    (a) 2nd
    (b) 3rd
    (C) 1st
    (d) Both 2nd & 3rd

460.

CO)

An antipsychotic with above structure as a basic nucleus is
    (a) Loxapine
    (b) Thiothixene
    (c) Clozapine
    (d) Trifluperazine

461. A dibenzodiazepine antipsychotic is
    (a) Loxapine
    (b) Thiothixene
    (c) Clozapine
    (d) Trifluperazine

462.

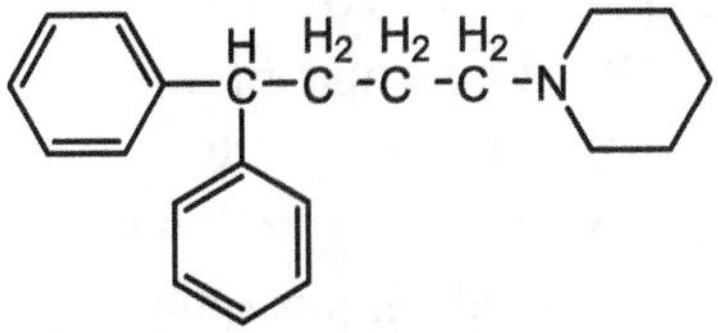

Which of the following antipsychotic drug/s belongs to the class of above structure?
    (a) Pimozide
    (b) Penfluridol
    (c) Loxapine
    (d) Both a & b

463. Morpholine is a
    (a) $1°$ amine   (b) $2°$ amine
    (c) $3°$ amine   (d) $4°$ amine

464. In which of the following disease condition there is a degeneration of dopaminergic neurons in substantia nigra of brain
    (a) Epilepsy
    (b) Schizophrenia
    (c) Parkinson's disease
    (d) Insomnia

465. An antiviral drug which acts as a 'dopamine releaser' used in the treatment of Parkinson's disease is
    (a) Zidovudine   (b) Ganciclovir
    (c) INF-y   (d) Amantadine

466. An antiviral drug which acts as a 'dopamine releaser' used in the treatment of Parkinson's disease contains a
    (a) Spiro system
    (b) Bicyccic system
    (c) Tricyclic system
    (d) Fused system

467.

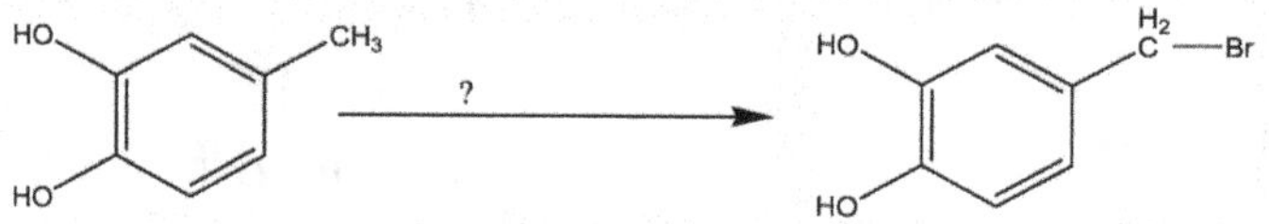

(a) NaBH4   (b)   N-Bromosuccinimde
(c) HBr   (d)   Briwater

468.

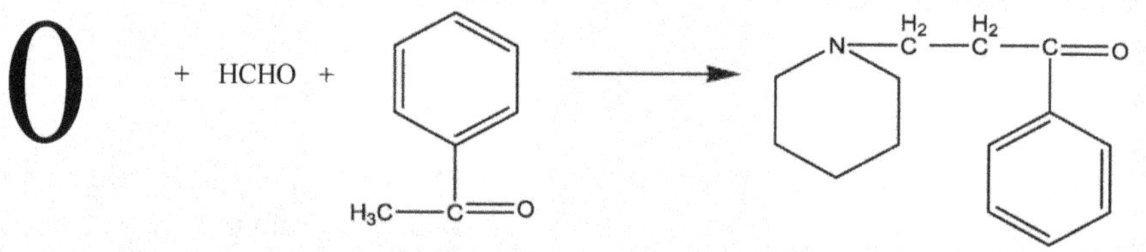

+ HCHO +

(a) Gattermann-koch reaction   (b)   Mannich reaction
(c) Benzoin condensation   (d)   Kolbe's reaction

(d) N-methyl NE

469. Which of the following prevents the storage of neurotransmitters in the vesicles in the presynaptic neurons?
(a) Bosentan   (b) Prazoscin
(c) Tadalafil   (d) Reserpine

470. Which of the following is present in the drugs which acts as selective a_1-antagonists
(a) Benzimidazole (b) Quinoline
(c) Quinazoline   (d) Indole

471. Which of the following contains spiro system?
(a) Guanadrel   (b) Guanethidine
(c) Terazocin   (d) Hydralazine

472. Metabolite of methyldopa, which acts on az-receptors, is
(a) Norepinephrine
(b) a-methyl NE
(c) P-methyl NE

473. The heterocyclic ring system of PDE-5 inhibitors mimic the
(a) Purine ring of cGMP
(b) G-Protien coupled receptors
(c) Guanine of DNA
(d) Amino acids of Angiotensin-I

474. Of the following which is a des-sulfamoyl analogue of benzthiazine diuretics
(a) Minoxidil   (b) Diazoxide
(c) Clonidine   (d) Losartan

475. The heterocyclic rings that are present in the drug minoxidil are
(a) Pyrazine, piperidine
(b) Pyridazine, piperidine
(c) Pyrimidine, pyrrolidine
(d) Pyrimidine, piperidine

476. Which of the following are biphenyl compounds?
    (a) P-blockers
    (b) ACE-inhibitors
    (c) arreceptor antagonists
    (d) AT II receptor antagonists

477. Azacitidine containing antihypertensive drug is
    (a) Prazosin   (b) Hydralazine
    (c) Guanethidine   (d) Minoxidil

478. A selective Pi-blocker is
    (a) Acebutolol   (b) Propranolol
    (c) Pindolol   (d) Carvedilol

479. Carvedilol contains
    (a) Phenothiazine
    (b) Dibenzopyrrole
    (c) Xanthine
    (d) Xanthene

480. Which of the following statement is correct regarding the SAR of P-blockers?
    (a) Aryloxypropanolamines are more potent than Aryloxyethanol-amines
    (b) Aryloxyethanolamines are more potent than Aryloxypropanol-amines
    (c) Replacement of ethereal oxygen by S, CH_2 and NH_3 increases activity
    (d) Substitution on the methylene carbon by alkyl groups increases activity

481. Of the following which can acts as mixed a-and P-antagonist
    (a) Esmolol   (b) Nadolol
    (c) Betaxolol   (d) Labetalol

482. A non-selective P-blocker which is used in the treatment of glaucoma contains
    (a) Pyrimidine
    (b) Thiazole, morpholine
    (c) Morpholine, 1,2,5-thiazole
    (d) Naphthalene

483. Pyrrolidine-2-oic acid is
    (a) Glycine   (b) Alanine
    (c) Tryptophan   (d) Proline

484. A sulfhydryl group containing ACE inhibitor is
    (a) Fosinopril   (b) Quinapril
    (c) Captopril   (d) Ramipril

485. Angiotensin-I is a
    (a) Octapeptide
    (b) Heptapeptide
    (c) Hexapeptide
    (d) Decapeptide

486. In Captopril which group is responsible for the cause of skin rashes and taste disturbances? (Disguesia)
    (a) 2-methyl propionyl
    (b) Mercapto
    (c) -COOR
    (d) Proline

487. Both Arterial & venous vasodilator is
    (a) 1-Hydrazino phthalazine
    (b) Minoxidil
    (c) Disodium pentacyanonitrosyl ferrate
    (d) All the above

488. P-Chloroperbenzoic acid is an
   (a) Reducing agent
   (b) Chelating agent
   (c) Sequiestering agent
   (d) Oxidising agent

489. When guanabenz acts on arreceptors what happens
   (a) Further release of neurotrans-mitter increases
   (b) Further release of neurotransmitter decreases
   (c) No change in the release of neurotransmitter
   (d) Metabolism of neurotransmitter mcreases

490. Clonidine contains
   (a) Pyrazolidine   (b) Pyrrolidine
   (c) Imidazolidine   (d) Oxazolidine

491. A spiro atom containing AT receptor antagonist is
   (a) Losartan   (b) Valsartan
   (c) Telmisartan   (d) Irbesartan

492. 1,4-Dihydropyridines are synthesized by
   (a) Mannich reaction
   (b) Hantzsch reaction
   (c) Cannizzaro reaction
   (d) Kolbe's reaction

493. Which of the following is released from the vascular endothelium of blood vessels?
   (a) Nitrous acid
   (b) Nitrogen dioxide
   (c) Dinitrogen monoxide
   (d) Nitrogen monoxide

494. 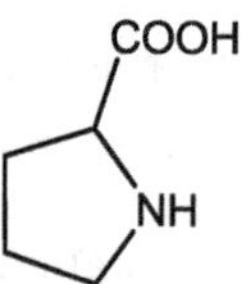

Which of the following class of antihypertensive drugs contains this structure?
   (a) P-blockers
   (b) aragonists
   (c) ACE inhibitors
   (d) ET-receptor antagonists

495. 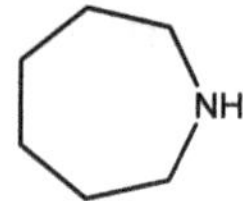

Which of the following ACE inhibitor contains the above nucleus in its structure?
   (a) Lisinopril   (b) Ramipril
   (c) Enalaprilat   (d) Benazepril

496.

An antihypertensive drug which contains the above nucleus acts by
   (a) Causing vasodilation
   (b) Blocking a1-receptors
   (c) By depleting the catecholamines
   (d) Blocking Pl-receptors

497.

An antihypertensive drug which contains this nucleus?

(a) Minoxidil   **(b)** Diazoxide
(c) Clonidine   (d) Losartan

498. Diltiazem an antihypertensive drug which one of the following?

(a)

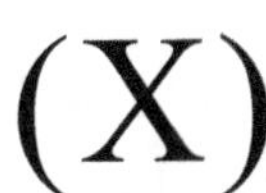

(b)

(X)

(c)

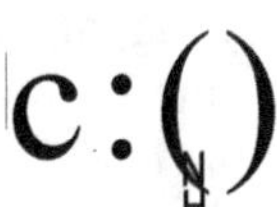

(d)

499. A class I antiarrhythmic which contains the following nucleus?

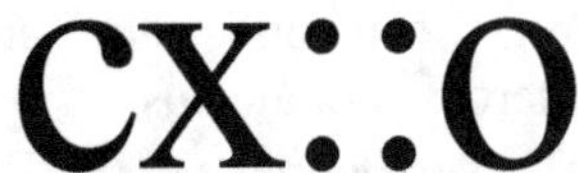

(a) Quinidine

(b) Procainamide
(c) Disopyramide
(d) Moricizine

500. Which of the following class-IA antiarrhythmic agent contains benzo [b]-pyridine basic nucleus?
(a) Procainamide
(b) Quinine
(c) Quinidine
(d) Disopyramide

501. Of the following antiepileptics which is used in the treatment of arrhythmias
(a) Tiagabine
(b) Phenytoin
(c) Phensuximide
(d) Dimethadione

502. Starting material for the synthesis of lidocaine is
(a) m-Xylene
(b) 2-methyl aniline
(c) Aniline
(d) Xylidene

503. Antiarrhythmic agent which contains phenothiazine ring
(a) Propranolol
(b) Nifedipine
(c) Flecainide
(d) Moricizine (Ethmozine)

504. Ca^{+2} channel blockers are
(a) 1,4-dihydropyridines
(b) 1,2-dihydropyridines
(c) 2,3-dihydropyridines
(d) 3,5-dihydropyridines

505. Heterocyclic ring that is present in diltiazem
    (a) Benzo-[b]-azepine
    (b) Benzodiazepine
    (c) Benzothiazepine
    (d) Benzo-[b]-furan

506. Match the following

Drug		Class
(A) Propranolol	(i)	III
(B) Tocainide	(ii)	IB
(C) Amiodarone	(iii)	II
(D) Amlodipine	(iv)	IV

    (a) A-ii' B-i' C-iv' D-iii
    (b) A-ii, B-iii, C-iv, D-i
    (c) A-iii, B-ii, C-iv, D-i
    (d) A-iii, B-ii, C-i, D-iv

507. Vinyl group containing antiarrhythmic is
    (a) Procainamide   (b) Quinidine
    (c) Nifedipine   (d) Diltiazem

508. p-nitrobenzoic acid   p-nitro-benzoylchloride   Procainamide. x= ?
    (a) Phosgene
    (b) Oxalyl chloride
    (c) Thionylchloride
    (d) Ch/ light

509.

$$H_3C-\overset{H_2}{C}-C_6H_5 \ , \ CH_3COCl \xrightarrow{AlCl_3} - 11, c-8' -o--COCH_3$$

Name of this reaction is
    (a) Knoevenogel condensation
    (b) Fries rearrangement
    (c) Beckmann reagement
    (d) Friedel-crafts reaction

510.

CO

One of the following antiarrhythmic drug contains the above basic heterocyclic nucleus
    (a) Mexiletine   (b) Esmolol
    (c) Aprindine   (d) Pilsicainide

511.

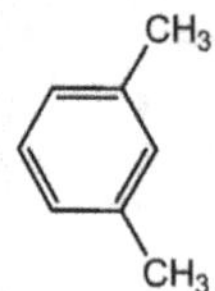

512.

CO

One of the following antiarrhythmic drug contains the above basic heterocyclic nucleus
    (a) Mexiletine   (b) Esmolol
    (c) Aprindine   (d) Pilsicainide

One of the following antiarrhythmic drug contains the above basic heterocyclic nucleus
    (a) Mexiletine   (b) Esmolol
    (c) Aprindine   (d) Pilsicainide

513.

o\

V V

One of the following antiarrhythmic drug contains the above basic

heterocyclic nucleus
(a) Amlodipine
(b) Amiodarone
(c) Lidocaine
(d) Quinidine

514. 2,6-dimethylphenol ls the starting material of
(a) Amiodarone   (b) Amlodipine
(c) Lidocaine   (d) Mexiletine

515.

$Cl-C^{H2}-$

This is used in the synthesis of
(a) Esmolol   (b) Phenytoin
(c) Prazocine   (d) Reserpine

516.

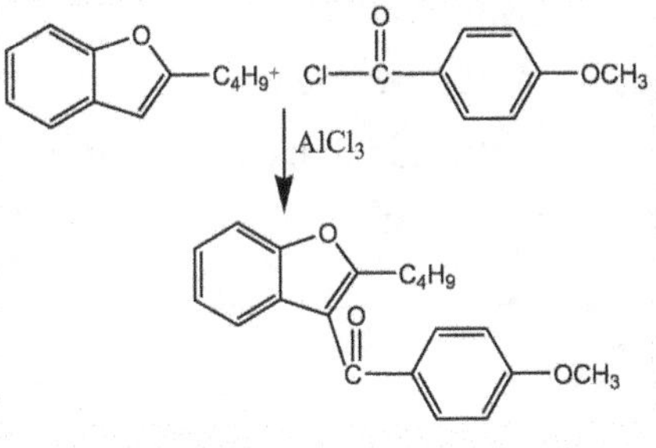

The above reaction is involved in the synthesis of Amiodarone, name of that reaction is?
(a) Knovenogel condensation
(b) Fries rearrangement
(c) Beckmann reagement
(d) Friedel-crafts reaction

517. Which of the following antihyperlipidemic drug is a prodrug?
(a) Lovastatin   (b) Pravastatin
(c) Fluvastatin   (d) Atorvastatin

518. Antih$_{yp}$erlipidemic drug with a decaline ring system is
(a) Probucol   (b) Colestipol
(c) Gemfibrozil   (d) Simvastatin

519.

$$HMG\ CoA \xrightarrow[\text{-re du-ct-as-e}]{\text{HMGCoA}} Mevalonate$$

The enzyme that catalyses the above reaction is inhibited by
(a) Ciprofibrate
(b) Cholestyramine
(c) Niacin
(d) Cerivastatin

520. Statins are
(a) Specific, reversible, competitive HMG CoA reductase inhibitors
(b) Non specific, reversible, competitive HMG CoA reductase inhibitors
(c) Specific, irreversible, competitive HMG CoA reductase inhibitors
(d) Specific, reversible, noncompetitive HMG CoA reductase inhibitors

521. The number of carbon atoms that are present in the dicarboxylic acid unit of HMG CoA reductase enzyme
(a) 4C   (b) SC
(c) 6C   (d) 3C

522. Which of the following is present in the drugs which increases the transcription of the genes for "lipoprotein lipase", apoA1 and apoA5
   (a) Dithiopropylidene
   (b) Decaline
   (c) Fibrate
   (d) Styrene

523. The number of carbon atoms that are present in the spacer group that is present between phenoxy & isobutyric acid groups.
   (a) 1   (b) 2
   (c) 3   (d) 4

524. Vinyl benzene containing antihyperlipidemic drug acts by
   (a) Inhibiting the HMG CoA reductase enzyme
   (b) Enhancing lipoprotein lipase
   (c) Binding to bile acids
   (d) Increasing HDL

525. Cholesterol   Bile acids. What is x?
   (a) HMG CoA reductase
   (b) 7a-hydroxylase
   (c) lipoprotein lipase
   (d) MAO

526. P-Picolic acid is used as ....
   (a) Antihypertensive
   (b) Antiarrhythmic
   (c) Antihyperlipedemic
   (d) Antianginal and coronary vasodilator

527. An antihyperlipedemic which has high lipophilic character with strong antioxidant properties is
   (a) Probucol   (b) Colestipol
   (c) Gemfibrozil   (d) Simvastatin

528. An antihyperlipedemic which reduces both LDL & HDL levels, but does not alter plasma triglycerides is
   (a) Probucol   (b) Colestipol
   (c) Gemfibrozil   (d) Simvastatin

529. Omega-3-marine Triglycerides are used as
   (a) Antihypertensive
   (b) Antiarrhythmic
   (c) Antihyperlipedemic
   (d) Antianginal and coronary vasodilator

530.

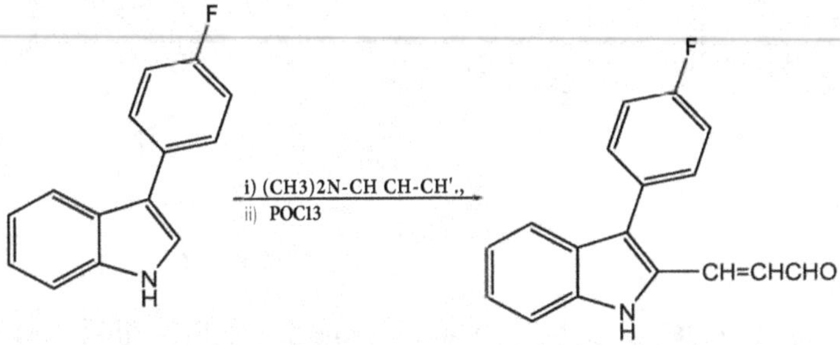

i) (CH3)2N-CH CH-CH'.,
ii) POCl3

This is an intermediate reaction in the synthesis of Fluvastatin. This reaction is called as

(a) HVZ reaction
(b) Mannich reaction
(c) Birch reaction
(d) Vilsmayer reaction

531.

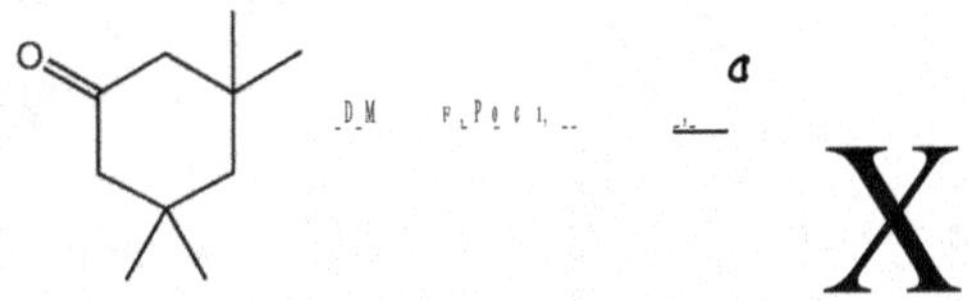

X

This is an intermediate reaction in the synthesis of Dalvastatin. This reaction is called as

(a) HVZ reaction
(b) Mannich reaction
(c) Michael reaction
(d) Vilsmayer reaction

532.

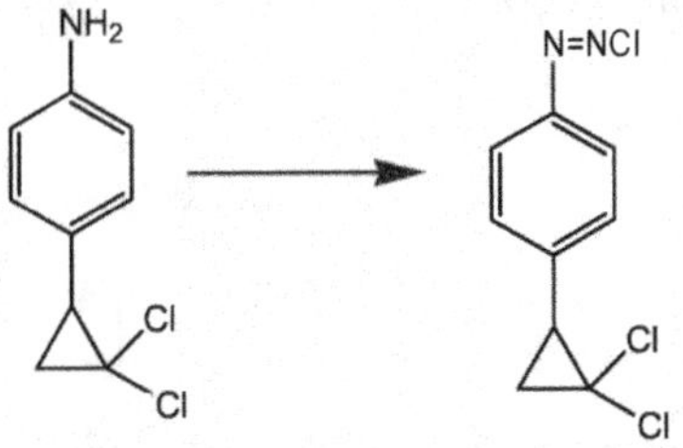

The conversion of starting material into product takes place in presence of?

(a) N2/HCl
(b) N2O/HCl
(c)   NaNO2/HCl
(d)   NaOH

533.

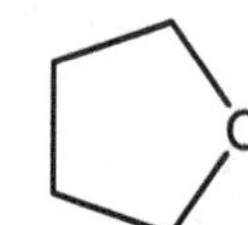

This is an intermediate reaction in the synthesis of Fenofibrate. This reaction is called as
(a) Beckmann rearrangement
(b) Pinacol-pinacolone rearrangement
(c) Clasian rearrangement
(d) Fries rearrangement

534. The starting material for the synthesis of dextro thyroxine
(a) Serine
(b) Alanine
(c) Tyrosine
(d) Phenyl alanine

535.

Tetrahydrofuran

The organic nitrate which contains THF
(a) Glyceryl trinitrate
(b) Amyl nitrite
(c) Tenitramine
(d) Isosorbide dinitrate

536. Which of the following statement/s is or are correct regarding organic nitrates
(P) They are esters of simple organic alcohols or polyols with nitric acid
(Q) They are volatile because of small lipophilic ester character
(R) They are explosive in concentrated form
(S) They are volatile as they contain ester bond
(a) AllP, Q, R & S
(b) Only Q & R
(c) Only Q, R & S
(d) Only P, Q & S

537. Number of carbon atoms in erythrityl tetranitrate
(a) 3
(b) 4
(c) 2
(d) 6

538. Propane-1,2,3-triol is present in which of the following organic nitrate
(a) Erythrityl tetranitrate
(b) Amyl nitrite
(c) Isosorbide dinitrate
(d) Nitroglycerin

539. Nitric oxide is responsible for
    (a) Relaxation of vascular smooth muscle
    (b) Inhibiting platelet aggregation (antithrombotic)
    (c) Inhibiting leucocyte-endothelial interaction (anti-inflammatory)
    (d) All the above

540. When nitroglycerin is taken the unbound group (tissue free) which is present in our body play a key role in the venodilation effect of it?
    (a) -SH
    (b) -NH2
    (c) -OH
    (d) -COOR

541. Molsidomine is an oral nitric oxide donor which is used a an antianginal contains

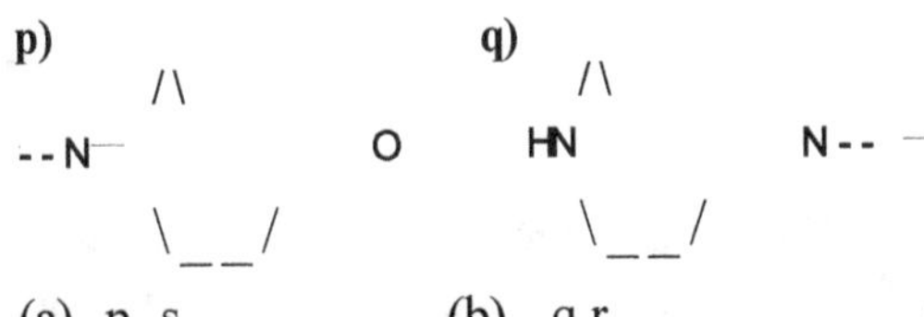

    (a) p, s
    (b) q,r
    (c) p,r
    (d) r,s

542. An anti-anginal which contains piperazine, modulates the metabolism of myocardium by increasing the glucose oxidation & thus generating more ATP per molecule of O_2 consumed is
    (a) Dipyridamole
    (b) Amlodipine
    (c) Amyl nitrite
    (d) Ranolazine

543. A benzylisoquinoline alkaloid which increases the cAMP levels by inhibiting the enzyme PDE
    (a) Morphine
    (b) Ergotamine
    (c) Papaverine
    (d) Brucine

544. D-Glucose is the starting material of which organic nitrate
    (a) Erythrityl tetranitrate
    (b) Amyl nitrite
    (c) Isosorbide dinitrate
    (d) Nitroglycerin

545.

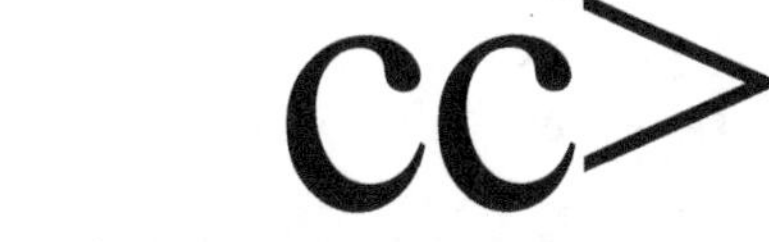

Benzo[c]-1,2,5-oxdiazole
A calcium channel blocker which contains above nucleus is
    (a) Isradipine
    (b) Amlodipine
    (c) Nifedipine
    (d) Nitrendipine

546.

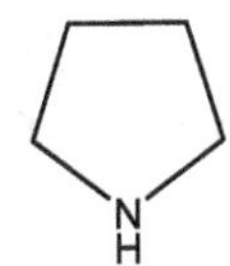

Pyrrolidine is the starting material of which calcium channel blocker?
    (a) Isradipine
    (b) Bepridil
    (c) Nifedipine
    (d) Nitrendipine

547.

The above conversion is an intermediate step in the synthesis of dipyridamole, which will takes place in presence of?

(a) Ch/hu   (b) Ch, red P   (c) PCls   (d) HCl

548. Cardiac glycosides are the drugs which are used in the treatment of CHF contain
(a) Only sugar moiety (glycone)
(b) Only non sugar moiety (aglycone)
(c) Both a & b
(d) None

549. Cardenolides contain
(a) 5-membered a, P-unsaturated lactone
(b) 6-membered a, P-unsaturated lactone
(c) 4-membered a, P-unsaturated lactone
(d) 7-membered a, P-unsaturated lactone

550. In cardiac glycosides the -OH group of .... position of aglycone is involved in the bond formation with sugar moiety
(a) 3 rd   (b) 14th
(c) 16th   (d) 12th

551. Study the following statements about the stereochemistry of steroidal aglycones in cardiac glycosides:
(P) Rings A-Band C-D are *cis* fused while B-C is trans fused
(Q) Rings A-B and C-D are *trans* fused while B-C is cis fused
(R) Rings A-Bare trans fused while B-C and C-D are cis fused
(S) Rings A-Bare cis fused while B-C and C-D are trans fused

Choose the correct statement.
(a) P is true while Q, R & S are false
(b) Q is true while P, R & S are false
(c) R is true while P, Q, & S are false
(d) S is true while P, R & Q are false

552. The glycosidic linkage that is present in cardiac glycosides is
(a) P-1,4   (b) a-1,2
(c) a-1,4   (d) P-1,2

553. Match the following

Cardiac glycoside   Aglycone moiety
(P) Lanatoside A
        1. Digitoxigenin

(Q) Lanatoside B
    2. Gitoxigenin
(R) Lanatoside C
    3. Digoxigenin
(S) G-Strophanthin
    4. Ouabain
(a) P-1' Q-2' R-3' S-4
(b) P-2, Q-4, R-3, S-1
(c) P-4, Q-3, R-2, S-1
(d) P-3, Q-2, R-1, S-4

554. In the cardiac glycosides of *Digitalis lanata,* in the -D-digitoxose sugar acetyl group is present at
(a) 1st position   (b) 4th position
(c) 3rd position   (d) 2nd position

555. Cardiac glycoside present in the seeds of *Strophanthus kombe* contain which sugar moieties
(a) Glucose   (b) Cymarose
(c) Rhamnose   (d) Both a & b

556. Which of the following inhibits the membrane-bound Na^+/K^+-ATPase pump responsible for Na^+/K^+ exchange in cardiac tissue
(a) Nitrendipine
(b) Isosorbide dinitrate
(c) Probucol
(d) Digilanide B

557. Drug with which of the following nucleus possesses cardiac glycosidic activity

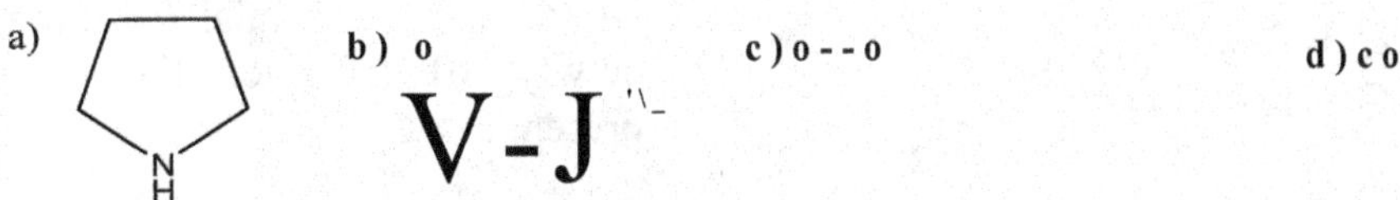

(b) 14-0H group
(c) Carbonyl oxygen of lactone
(d) Ring A

558. Which of the following atom/group of cardiac glycoside is bind to the binding site on Na^+/K^+-ATPase
(a) 3-0H group

559. Inamrinone & Milrinone are the nonglycosidic +ve inotropic agents which inhibits PDE-3 contains

560. Dobutamine a P-agonist which is used in the treatment of CHF that stimulates the synthesis of cAMP contains .... group
    (a) Resorcinol   (b) Catechol
    (c) Hydroquinone (d) 1,2,3-triol

561. Dobutamine a P-agonist which is used in the treatment of CHF is active only by the i.v route because of its rapid first-pass metabolism by
    (a) MAO-A   (b) MAO-B
    (c) COMT   (d) DAO

562. All the diuretics are secreted into the proximal tubule & act from the inside of tubular lumen, on the cells of nephron except one diuretic, that diuretic contains which of the following in its structure.
    (a) 1,3,4-Thiadiazole
    (b) 1,2,4-Benzothiadiazine-1, 1-dioxide
    (c) 5-Sulfamolyl-2-amino benzoic acid
    (d) A spiro system

563. Match the following

    Site of action   Heterocyclic ring present in diuretic
    (P) proximal tubule
        1. Pteridine
    (Q) thick ascending limb of
        2. 1,3,4-Thiadiazole loop of henle
    (R) distal tubule
        3. 5-Sulphamolyl-2-amino benzoic acid
    (S) collecting tubule
        4. 1,2,4-Benzothiadiazine-1,1-dioxide
    (a) P-1, Q-2, R-3, S-4
    (b) P-3, Q-1, R-2, S-4
    (c) P-2, Q-3, R-4, S-1
    (d) P-2, Q-3, R-4, S-i

564. The sulphonamide which exhibited mild diuresis when used for the treatment of bacterial infections
    (a) Sulphamethoxazole
    (b) Sulphisoxazole
    (c) Sulphadiazine
    (d) Sulphanilamide

565. Which of the following diuretic is a derivative of m-disulphamoyl benzene
    (a) Acetazolamide
    (b) Chloraminophenamide
    (c) Furosemide
    (d) Amiloride

566. 1,3,4-Thiadiazole heterocyclic ring containing diuretic is
    (a) Methazolamide
    (b) Benzthiazide
    (c) Xipamide
    (d) Azosemide

567. The sulfamoyl group that is prerequisite for diuretic activity of thiazide diuretics is present at
    (a) 7th (b) 6th
    (c) 3rd **(d) 4th**

568. An activating group such as -Cl, -Br etc that is essential for diuretic acivity of thiazide diuretics is present at

(a) 7th (b) 6th
(c) 3rd (d) 4th

569. Mersalyl (Salyrgan) a substituted 2-acetamido phenoxyacetic acid is a ……….
     (a) Site 1 diuretic
     (b) Site 2 diuretic
     (c) Site 3 diuretic
     (d) Site 4 diuretic

570. A furfuryl group containing diuretic
     (a) Triampterine
     (b) Bumetanide
     (c) Hydrochlorthiazide
     (d) Furosemide

571. Which of the following diuretics belongs to phenoxyacetic acid group
     (a) Triampterine, ethacrynic acid
     (b) Bumetanide, indacrinone
     (c) Azosemide, acetazolamide
     (d) Ethacrynic acid, indacrinone

572. Saturation of = bond b/w 3,4-positions of the benzothiadiazine-1,I-dioxide of thiazide diuretics
     (a) Increases activity
     (b) Decreases activity
     (c) No change in activity
     (d) Can't predict the activity

573. An acrylolyl moiety containing diuretic is
     (a) Indacrinone
     (b) Ethacrynic acid
     (c) Torsemide
     (d) Canrenone

574. A sulfonyl urea moiety containing diuretic is
     (a) Indacrinone
     (b) Ethacrynic acid
     (c) Torsemide
     (d) Canrenone

575. Bumetanide & Piretanide are 5-Sulfamolyl-3-amino benzoic acids, these are
     (a) Site-2: high ceiling/ loop diuretics
     (b) Site-1: carbonic anhydrase inhibitors
     (c) Site-3: thiazide diuretics
     (d) Site-4: potassium sparing diuretics

576. Gitelman's syndrome, a rare monogenetic disorder caused by a class of diuretics which contain one if the following heterocyclic ring system
     (a) 1,3,4-Thiadiazole
     (b) 5-Sulfamolyl-2-amino benzoic acid
     (c) Pteridine
     (d) 1,2,4-Benzothiadiazine-1, 1-dioxide

577. Spironolactone, an aldosterone antagonist (site 4: potassium sparing diuretic) contains
     (a) 5-membered lactone
     (b) 6-membered lactone
     (c) 4-membered lactone
     (d) ?-membered lactone

578. Canrenone, an active aldosterone antagonist, a major metabolite of spironolactone contains
    (a) 5-membered lactone
    (b) 6-membered lactone
    (c) 4-membered lactone
    (d) 7-membered lactone

579. Which of the following statements are true about mannitol an osmotic diuretic
    (a) Pharmacologically inert substance
    (b) Filtered in the glomerulus
    (c) Not reabsorbed by nephron
    (d) All the above

580. Urea + water .   Which of the following diuretic contain X group
    (a) Furosemide
    (b) Dichlorphenamide
    (c) Ethacrynic acid
    (d) Amiloride

581. Spironolactone   canrenone, during this conversion which of the following will takes place
    (a) Saturation of 4,5 double bond
    (b) Formation of 7,8 double bond
    (c) Formation of 6,7 double bond
    (d) Conversion of 5-membered lactone to 6- membered lactone

582. N-acetyl-p-benzoquinoneimine is a metabolite of Furosemide
    (a) Carbamazepine
    (b) Acetaminophen
    (c) Ibuprofen
    (d) phenylbutazone

583. 'Levulinic acid' is the common name of
    (a) Pentanoic acid
    (b) 4-Oxopentanoic acid
    (c) Isobutyric acid
    (d) n-hexanoic acid

584. Saccharine (Benzo[d]-isothiazole-3-one-1,1-dioxide) is the starting material for the synthesis of
    (a) Mefenamic acid
    (b) Oxyphenbutazone
    (c) Ketoprofen
    (d) Oxicams

585. Methylsulfonyl group containing NSAID are
    (a) Rofecoxib, nimesulide
    (b) Nimesulide, meclofenamate sodium
    (c) Rofecoxib, sudoxicam
    (d) Piroxicam, salsalate

586. Name of this reaction is? The products of this reaction are used as Ca^{+2} channel blockers.
     (a) Michael addition
     (b) Mannich condensation
     (c) Polonovski rearrangement
     (d) Aldol condensation

587. 2-Chloromethyloxirane is utilized in the synthesis of
     (a) Diazepam
     (b) Chlorpromazine
     (c) Esmolol
     (d) Valproic acid

588. Acetic anhydride in presence of pyridine is used to determine
     (a) The no. of-COOH groups
     (b) The no. of atoms in a molecule

     (c) Acidity of molecule
     (d) The no. of-OH groups

589. Which of the following combination has not to be given
     (a) Thioridazine+Paracetamol
     (b) Imipramine + Tyramine
     (c) Atendol + Captopril
     (d) Tyramine+Tranylcypromine

590. Synthesis of salicylic acid from phenol in presence of CO_2 and K_2CO_3 is called as
     (a) Fries rearrangement
     (b) Friedel-crafts alkylation
     (c) Kolbe's synthesis
     (d) Knovenogel condensation

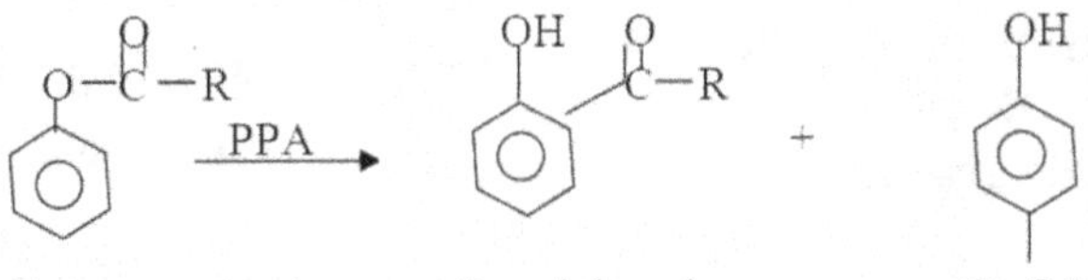

O—C—R
PPA →
Phenylester

OH
C—R
O-acylphenol

+

OH
O= C-R P-acylphenol

591. This rearrangement is called as
     (a) Polonovski rearrangement
     (b) Beckmann's rearrangement
     (c) Michael addition
     (d) Fries rearrangement

592. Which of the following is required for aldol condensation?
     (a) HCl
     (b) Cone. H_2SO_4
     (c) CCl4
     (d) NaOH

593. Which of the following drug acts on the hypothalamic thermoregulatory center?
     (a) Phenacetin (Acetophenetidie)
     (b) Fluoxetine
     (c) Secobarbital
     (d) Fluvastatin

594. Which of the following NSAID contains 2-aminobenzoic acid group
     (a) Meclofenamate sodium
     (b) Sulphinpyrazone
     (c) Sudoxicam
     (d) Ibuprofen

595. E-Z isomerism is shown by
    (a) Diclofenac   (b) Disalcid
    (c) Naproxen   (d) Sulindac

596. The number of carbon-carbon double bonds present in arachidonic acid and prostagland in G_2 are respectively.
    (a) 2,4   (b) 4,0
    (c) 4,2   (d) 0,0

597. The number of carbon atoms that are present in cyclopentanoperhydrophenanthrene are
    (a) 18   (b) 19
    (c) 17   (d) 27

598. Cyclopentanoperhydrophenanthrene is commonly called as
    (a) Androstane   (b) Pregnane
    (c) Cholestane   (d) Sterane

599. Match the following Steroid nucleus Number of carbon atoms
    (P) Progestane (Pregnane)
        1. 21C
    (Q) Androstane
        2. 19C
    (R) Cholestane
        3. 27C
    (S) Estrane
        4. 18C
    (a) P-1, Q-2, R-3, S-4
    (b) P-2, Q-3, R-4, S-1
    (c) P-3, Q-1, R-2, S-4
    (d) P-4, Q-2, R-3, S-1

600. The number of chiral centers in a sterane nucleus are
    (a) 4   (b) 6
    (c) 8   (d) 2

601. Which of the following are chiral centers in a sterane nucleus?
    (aj 6, 11,9,8, 14, 13
    (b) 5, 10, 9, 8, 14, 13
    (c) 4, 13, 14, 10, 11, 12
    (d) 3, 4, 5, 8, 13, 14

602. In the steroidal IUPAC nomenclature, the stereochemistry of the 'H' at which position is always indicated in the name
    (a) 5th (b) 10th
    (c) 9th (d) 13th

603. Which of the following statements are correct regarding the stereochemistry of steroidal drugs
    (P) Steroids with 5a-H configuration will have sex hormone activity
    (Q) Steroids with 5P-H configuration will have sex hormone activity
    (R) Steroids with 5a-H configuration will have cardiac glycoside activity
    (S) Steroids with 5P-H configuration will have cardiac glycoside activity
    (a) P, S
    (b) Q, R
    (c) R, S
    (d) All the above

604. Which of the following statements are correct regarding the stereochemistry of steroidal drugs
    (P) 5a steroids will have A/B *trans* configuration
    (Q) 5p steroids will have A/B *cis* configuration
    (R) 5P steroids will have A/B *trans* configuration

(S) Sa steroids will have A/B *cis* configuration

(a) P,Q
(b) R,S
(c) Q,R
(d) All the above

605.

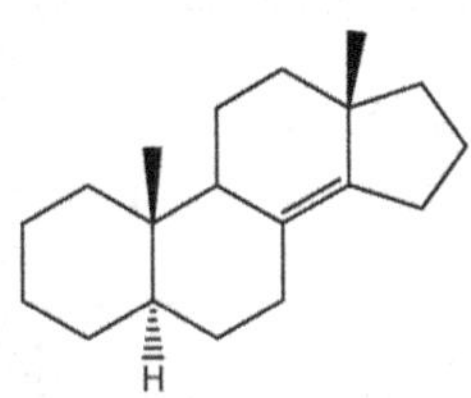

The correct name of this molecule is

(a) Sa-Androst-8-ene
(b) Sa-Progest-8-ene
c) Sa-Androst-8 (14)-ene
(d) SB-Androst-8 (14)-ene

606. Piperidine-2,6-dione is called as

(a) Hydantoin
(b) Barbituric acid
(c) GABA
(d) Glutethimide

607. Except which of the following adrenocorticoid the remaining are well-absorbed, undergo little 1st pass metabolism in the liver, & demonstrate oral bioavailability of 70%-80%.

(a) Prednisone
(b) Cortisol
(c) Triamcinolone
(d) Betamethasone

608. Prednisolone is an adrenocorticoid which is a derivative of

(a) Androstane   (b) Progestane
(c) Estrane   (d) Cholestane

609. 11, 17a, 21-trihydroxy pregnane-4-ene-3,20-dione is

(a) Cortisone
(b) Prednisone
(c) Hydrocortisone
(d) Triamcinolone

610. In methylprednisolone, the methyl group is present at ..... position

(a) i ^{h} (b) 11th
(c) 15th (d) 6th

611. The difference between cortisone & prednisone is

(a) Number of double bonds
(b) Number of keto groups
(c) Number of hydroxyl groups
(d) Number of carbon atoms

612. In triamcinolone or in fludrocortisone the fluorine atom is present at .... position

(a) 1st (b) 9th
(c) 12th (d) 16th

613. In the structure of 11-epicortisol, the stereochemistry (configuration) of hydroxyl group is

(a) a
(b) B
(c) In plane
(d) Configuration is not know

614. In the structure of adrenocorticoids, the stereochemistry (configuration) of hydroxyl group at 1i ^{h} position is

(a) a
(b) B
(c) In plane
(d) Configuration is not known

615. An introduction of double bond between 1,2-positions in the structure of cortisol
    (a) Increases anti-inflammatory activity
    (b) Decreases anti-inflammatory activity
    (c) Cannot predict
    (d) No change in activity

616. Which of the following in the structure of hydrocortisone is of major importance im binding to the receptors?
    (a) 11a-OH   (b) 11B-OH
    (c) 3-Keto   (d) 21-OH

617. Isopropylidinedioxy group is called as
    (a) Carbamate   (b) Lactam
    (c) Choline   (d) Acetonide

618. Which of the following adrenocorticoid is an antagonist of aldosterone
    (a) Mifepristone
    (b) Trilostane
    (c) Spironolactone
    (d) Aminoglutethimide

619. All of the following are adrenocorticoid antagonists, among the following which one is an antifungal agent
    (a) Glycyrrhetic acid
    (b) Spironolactone
    (c) Ketoconazole
    (d) Metyrapone

620. Which of the following is the only progestin with antimineralocoticoid activity?
    (a) Levonorgestrel

    (b) Drospirenone
    (c) Ethisterone
    (d) Dimethisterone

621. Which of the following adrenocorticoid antagonist is a derivative of 19-nor testosterone?
    (a) Mifepristone
    (b) Trilostane
    (c) Spironolactone
    (d) Aminoglutethimide

622. Which of the following hormone increases the reabsorption of Na^+ ions?
    (a) Thyroid stimulating hormone
    (b) Aldosterone
    (c) ACTH
    (d) Testosterone

623. Which of the following statement is correct regarding the SAR of Spironolactone?
    (a) The 3-keto-4-ene a ring is essential for its aldosterone antagonistic activity
    (b) Opening of the lactone ring dramatically decreases the activity
    (c) 7a-substituent increases both intrinsic activity & oral activity
    (d) All the above

624. An adrenocorticoid antagonist which inhibits 3B-hydroxysteroid dehydrogenase & which is used in the treatment of Cushing's syndrome with an epoxy linkage is
    (a) Mifepristone
    (b) Trilostane
    (c) Spironolactone
    (d) Aminoglutethimide

625. Which of the following that is an active component of 'licorice' acts as an adrenocorticoid antagonist by inhibiting 3P-hydroxysteroid dehydrogenase
    (a) Glycyrrhetic acid
    (b) Spironolactone
    (c) Ketoconazole
    (d) Metyrapone

626. Which of the following inhibits 3P-hydroxysteroid dehydrogenase & such enzyme inhibitors may be useful in the treatment of metabolic syndrome to reduce elevated glucose concentrations & as possible antidiabetic agents
    (a) Chenodeoxycholic acid
    (b) Lithocholic acid
    (c) Nonsteroidal arylsulfoamido-thiazoles
    (d) All the above

627. 17p-hydroxy androst-4-ene-3-one is
    (a) Testosterone   (b) Estrogen
    (c) Progesterone   (d) Cholesterol

628. In Oxymesterone which is an androgen the hydroxyl group ls present at .... position
    (a) 1st (b) 6th
    (c) 4th (d) 11th

629. In Fluoxymesterone, a fluorine group is present at .... position
    (a) 1st (b) 6th
    (c) 4th (d) 9th

630. The androgen with a C=C between 1,2-positions is
    (a) 17a-Methyltestosterone
    (b) Oxymesterone
    (c) Methandrostenolone
    (d) Fluoxymesterone

631. Which of the following statement/s is or are correct regarding 5a-androstane?
    (P) It is a 19 carbon containing steroid
    (Q) This basic nucleus is itself has androgenic activity
    (R) It is an 18 carbon containing steroid
    (S) This basic nucleus is itself doesn't have an androgenic activity
    (a) p & Q   (b) R & S
    (c) P & S   (d) Q & R

632. Which of the following statement/s is or are correct regarding SAR of 5a-androstane?
    (a) Changing the configuration at 5th position to p eliminates androgenic & anabolic activities
    (b) Both ring expansion or ring contraction decreases activity
    (c) Introduction of a 3-ketone function or 3a-OH group increases androgenic activity
    (d) All the above

633. Which of the following statement/s is or are correct regarding SAR of 5a-androstane?
    (a) Compounds with 17a-OH group are inactive
    (b) The 17P-oxygen atom is important for attachment to the steroid receptor site
    (c) Compounds with 17P-OH group are active
    (d) All the above

634.

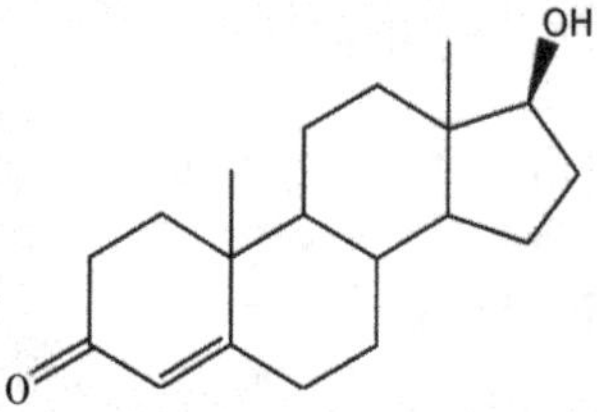

Introduction of which of the following group into the above molecule prevents the metabolic changes that takes place at 17B-OH position
(a)   9a-fluoro
(b)   17a-alkyl (methyl)
(c)   17a-OH
(d)   6a-alkyl (methyl)

635.

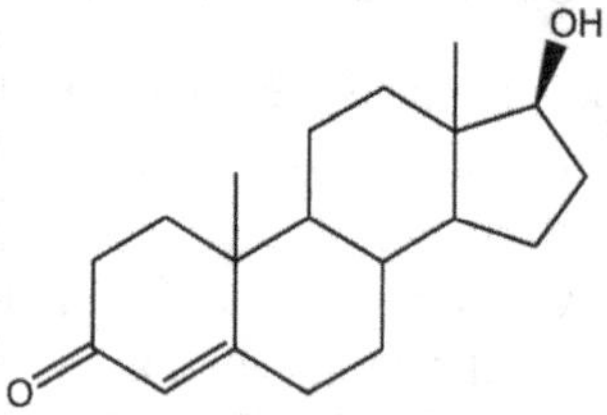

Introduction of which of the following group at 17th position in the above molecule produces a compound (ethisterone) with useful progestational activity (progestin)
(a)   /C $\equiv$ CH
(b) 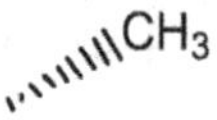   ,,,,,,||CH_3
(c) 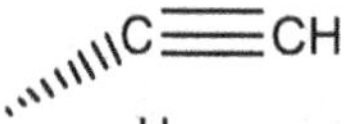   ,,,,,||C $\equiv$ CH
(d) 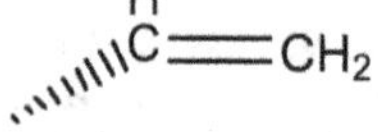   ,,,,,||C(H) $=$ CH_2

636.   The heterocyclic ring that is present in Danazole a potent antigonadotropic drug produced from ethisterone by the indroduction of that heterocyclic ring
(a)   Oxazole   (b)   Isoxazole
(c)   Pyrazole   (d)   Imidazole

637.   2-Hydroxymethylethisterone   is   an inactive   compound   which   is   a metabolite of ....
(a)   Ethisterone   (b)   Stanzolol
(c)   Testosterone   (d)   Danzol

638.

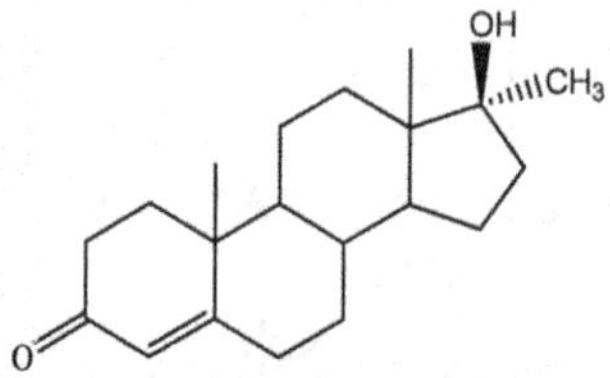

Introduction of oxygen atom with in the ring into the above molecule at which position produces potent anabolic agents (oxasteroids)
(a) 2nd (b)   1st
(c) 11th (d) 6th

639.   Oxidation of which of the following by 'selenium dioxide' produces methandrostenolone   an   anabolic steroidal agent
(a)   Stanozolol
(b)   Oxandrolone
(c)   17a-methyl testosterone
(d)   Oxymetholone

640.   The heterocyclic ring that is present in stanozolol, an anabolic steroidal agent
(a)   Imidazole   (b)   Pyrrole
(c)   Pyrazole   (d)   Oxazole

641. A lactone ring containing anabolic steroidal agent is
    (a) Stanozolol
    (b) Oxandrolone
    (c) I?a-methyl testosterone
    (d) Oxymetholone

642. A 'hydroxymethylidene' group at 2nd position containing anabolic steroidal agent is
    (a) Stanozolol
    (b) Oxandrolone
    (c) I?a-methyl testosterone
    (d) Oxymetholone

643. Which of the following anabolic steroidal agent is a 18-0xasteroid (D-homo oxandrostandiene dione analogue)
    (a) Testolactone
    (b) Methenolone
    (c) Nandrolone
    (d) Oxandrolone

644. The lactone ring that is present in testolactone which is an anabolic steroidal agent is
    (a) a-lactone   (b) B-lactone
    (c) y-lactone   (d) o-lactone

645. An anabolic agent chlortestosterone acetate contains chlorine at .... position
    (a) 1st (b) 2nd
    (c) 3rd (d) 4th

646. The removal of which of the following group of androgen results in reduction of its androgenic properties but retention of its anabolic, tissue-building properties
    (a) 18th -CH_3 group
    (b) 17th -OH group
    (c) 19th -CH_3 group
    (d) 3-Keto group

647. Ethylestrenol an anabolic steroidal agent contains an ethyl group at ..... position in its structure
    (a) 3rd (b) 7th
    (c) 10th (d) 17th

648. Which of the following anabolic steroidal agent lacks 19th -CH_3 group
    (a) Testolactone
    (b) Norethandrolone
    (c) Oxandrolone
    (d) Stanozolol

649. An anabolic agent which contains estrane as a basic steroidal nucleus
    (a) Nandrolone
    (b) Norethandrolone
    (c) Ethylestrenol
    (d) Testolactone

650. In which of the following compounds 'A' ring is completely unsaturated (presence of three double bonds)
    (a) Androgens
    (b) Progestational agents
    (c) Cholesterol
    (d) Estrogens

651. Which of the following 'endogenous estrogen' is the more potent one?
    (a) Estrone
    (b) Estradiol
    (c) Estriol
    (d) Ethinyl estradiol

652.

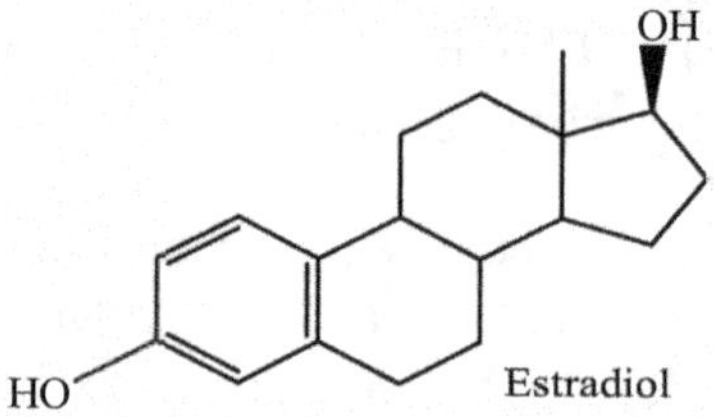

Estradiol

Introduction of 'ethynyl' group at which position in the above molecule prevents metabolic oxidation at C-17 position to form estrone

(a) 17th (b) 16th
(c) 14th (d) 18th

653. In the structure of 'Ethinyl estradiol' an estrogen the 'ethynyl' group is located at

(a) 17th (b) 16th
(c) 14th (d) 18th

654. Which of the following estrogen undergoes 'enterohepatic recycling' by GI bacteria?

(a) Estrone
(b) Estradiol
(c) Estriol
(d) Ethinyl estradiol

655. Which of the following drugs have an adverse effect on oral contraceptive efficacy of ethinyl estradiol by decreasing its 'enterohepatic recycling'?

(a) Antidiarrheal
(b) Antiulcer
(c) Antibacterial (antibiotics)
(d) Antipyretic

656. An 'ether' group containing estrogen is
(a) Ethynyl estradiol
(b) Mestronol

(c) Equilin
(d) Equilenin

657.

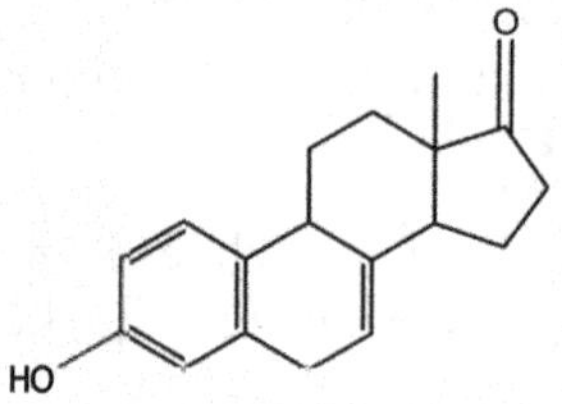

This is ....
(a) Ethinyl estradiol
(b) Mestronol
(c) Equilin
(d) Equilenin

658. Heterocyclic ring that is present in 'Estropitate' a conjugated estrogen is
(a) Pyrazine   (b) Pyrimidine
(c) Pyridazine   (d) Piperazine

659.

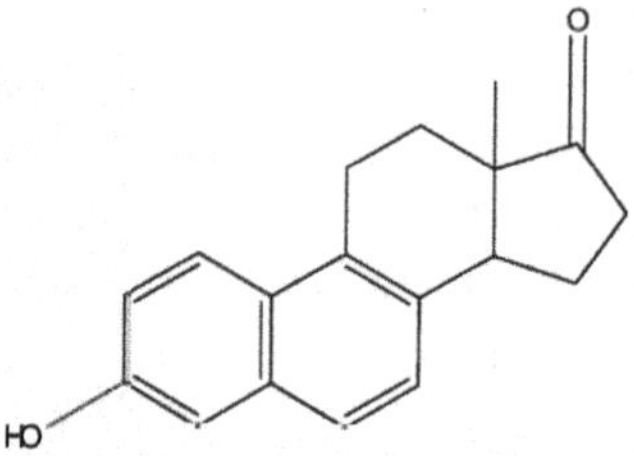

This is .....
(a) Ethinyl estradiol
(b) Mestronol
(c) Equilin
(d) Equilenin

660. Progesterone contains
(a) 21 Carbons   (b) 19 Carbons
(c) 18 Carbons   (d) 27 Carbons

661. Pregnane-4-ene-3,20-dione is
(a) Estrone   (b) Testosterone

(c) Progesterone (d) Cholesterol

662. Ethisterone is the 1st androgen found to be effective as a progestin contains
   (a) 17 -Ethynyl (b) 17a-Ethynyl
   (c) 17a-Ethyl (d) 17 -Ethyl

663. Norethisterone a synthetic progestin lacks
   (a) 18th methyl group
   (b) 17th - OH group
   (c) 17a-Ethynyl
   (d) 19th methyl group

664. In 'levonorgesrtel' a synthetic progestin, the configuration of 18th carbon atom is
   (a) a (b)
   (c) Unknown (d) Inplane

665.

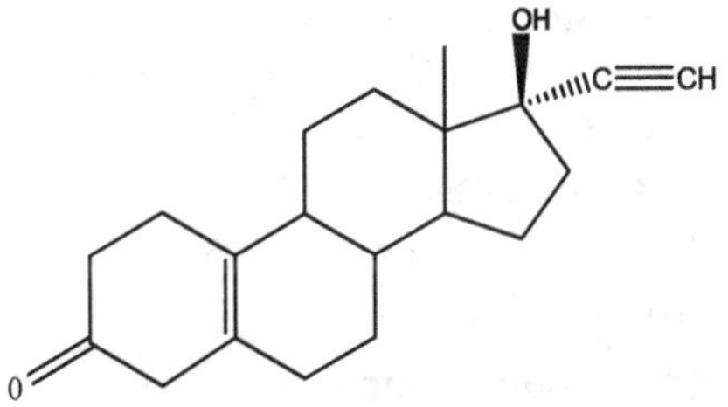

It is a synthestic progestin, what is it
   (a) Norethynodrel
   (b) Norethisterone
   (c) Norgestrel
   (d) Levonorgesrtel

666. An imine containing synthetic progestin is
   (a) Norgestimate
   (b) Desogestrel
   (c) Gestodene
   (d) Levonorgesrtel

667. A synthetic progestin without a 3-keto group ls
   (a) Norethisterone
   (b) Desogestrel
   (c) Gestodene
   (d) Levonorgesrtel

668. A nitrile or cyanide group containing synthetic progestin is
   (a) Norethisterone
   (b) Desogestrel
   (c) Gestodene
   (d) Dienogest

669. A synthetic progestin which contains a double bond between C15-C16
   (a) Norethisterone
   (b) Desogestrel
   (c) Gestodene
   (d) Dienogest

670. In Desogestrel & Etonogestrel which are synthetic progestins a 'methylidene' group ====CH2 is present at .... position
   (a) 6th (b) 12th
   (c) 15th (d) 11th

671. Progesterone is obtained from diosgenin through the following sequence of chemical reactions:
   (P) Acetylation, CrO_3 (oxidation), Acetolysis, H_2/Pd, Hydrolysis and Oppenauer oxidation
   (Q) Oppenauer oxidation, Acetylation, CrO_3 (oxidation), Acetolysis, H_2/Pd, and Hydrolysis

(R) CrO_3 (oxidation), Acetolysis, Acetylation, Oppenauer oxidation, Hydrolysis and H_2/Pd

(S) Acetylation, H_2/Pd, Hydrolysis, CrO_3 (oxidation), Oppenauer oxidation and Acetolysis

Choose the correct sequence of reactions
  (a) P
  (b) Q
  (c) R
  (d) S

672. Luteinizing hormone (LH) is responsible for ovulation. When combination oral contraceptive pills are taken which of the following component of them suppresses the release of LH & therefore blocks ovulation
  (a) Estrogen component
  (b) Progestin component
  (c) Both (a) & (b)
  (d) None

673. When combination oral contraceptive pills are taken which of the following component of them suppresses the release of FSH from hypothalamus
  (a) Estrogen component
  (b) Progestin component
  (c) Both (a) & (b)
  (d) None

674. Which of the following are enzyme inducers, when they given in combination with oral contraceptive pills decreases the efficacy of pills by decreasing the circulating levels of hormone
  (a) Primidone, carbamazepine
  (b) Topiramate, rifampin
  (c) Ritonavir, St.John's wort
  (d) All the above

675. Which of the following statement/s is/are correct regarding antibiotics?
  (a) Antibiotics alter the entero-hepatic recycling of progestins
  (b) Antibiotics alter the entero-hepatic recycling of estrogens
  (c) Antibiotics alter the entero-hepatic recycling of both progestins & estrogens
  (d) Antibiotics do not alter the enterohepatic recycling of both progestins & estrogens

676. Which of the following drugs bind to 'heat shock proteins' which are present in the cytosol of a cell
  (a) Anticancer drugs
  (b) Penicillins
  (c) **NSAIDS**
  (d) Steroidal drugs

677. Prontosil rubrum ----------X------->Sulfanilamide. X=?
  (a) Oxidative metabolism
  (b) Reductive metabolism
  (c) Conjugation
  (d) Acylation

678. Pyrimidine-2-yl containing sulphonamide is
  (a) Sulphamethoxazole
  (b) Sulphisoxazole
  (c) Sulphadiazine
  (d) Sulphacetamide

679. Which of the following is an azo compound?
  (a) Promazine
  (b) Probucol
  (c) Probenicid
  (d) Prontosil

680. Identify the metabolite of prontosil responsible for its antibacterial activity
    (a) Sulphacetamide
    (b) Sulphanilamide
    (c) p-Amino benzoic acid
    (d) Probenecid

681. Find the process by which the conversion of sulphasalazine to sulphapyridine and 5-amino salicylic acid takes place in the colon?
    (a) Hydrolysis
    (b) Deamination
    (c) Acetylation
    (d) Azoreduction

682. Multivitamin tablet containing PABA + Sulphonamide. When this combination is given to a patient, the activity of sulphonamide?
    (a) Increases
    (b) Decreases
    (c) No change
    (d) Difficult to predict

683. Stevens-Johnson syndrome characterized by fatal erythema multiforme & ulceration of mucous membranes of the eye, mouth & urethra is associated with
    (a) Sertaline
    (b) Selegiline
    (c) Sulphadiazine
    (d) Sulphonylureas

684. Sulphasalazine ------ Azoreduction -------> sulphapyridine and X. X is a/an?
    (a) Anti-inflammatory agent

    (b) Antifungal agent
    (c) Anticancer agent
    (d) Antihelminthitic agent

685. Histamine is chemically
    (a) 2-(4-amino ethyl)-imidazole
    (b) 3-(2-amino ethyl)-imidazole
    (c) 2-(2-amino ethyl)-imidazole
    (d) 4-(2-amino ethyl)-imidazole

686. Histaminic receptor found in blood vessels and blocked by mepyramine is
    (a) H1 receptor
    (b) H2 receptor
    (c) H3 receptor
    (d) All of the above

687. Histaminic receptor involved in the immuno regulatory system is
    (a) H1 receptor
    (b) H2 receptor
    (c) H3 receptor
    (d) Both a & b

688. Pheniramine belongs to the chemical class of
    (a) Ethylenediamines
    (b) Aminoethyl compounds
    (c) Cyclizines
    (d) Aminopropyl compounds

689. In Diphenhydramine series, antihistaminic property is retained in
    (a) Ortho substituted compounds
    (b) Para substituted compounds
    (c) Meta substituted compounds
    (d) All of the above

690. In propylamine derivatives like chlorpheniramine, the isomer that exhibits greater potency is
(a) Levo rotatory
(b) Dextro rotatory
(c) Racemic mixture
d) Both a & b

691. Isomer of Triprolidine which is about 1000 times more potent than its corresponding isomer is
(a) Z-isomer   (b) E-isomer
(c) Both   (d) None

692. Cimetidine is

(a) N'-cyano-N-methyl-N"-2-(5-methylimidiazol-4-yl)methyl-thioethyl guanidine

(b) N'-cyano-N-ethyl-N"-2-(5-methylimidiazol-4-yl)ethylthio-ethyl guanidine

(c) N'-cyano-N-ethyl-N"-2-(5-methylimidiazol-4-yl)methylthio-ethyl guanidine

(d) N'-nitrile-N-methyl-N"-2-(5-methylimidiazol-4-y l)methylthio-ethyl guanidine

693.

$$Ar\text{-}NH_2 + A \xrightarrow[\text{-HCI}]{NaNH_2} B \xrightarrow{C} Ar\text{-}NH_3\text{-}CH_2CH_2N(CH_3h$$
$$CH_2Ar$$

A= ClCH2CH2N(CH3)

(a)
B = ArNHCH2CH2N(CH3)
C = ArCH2Cl / NaNH2

(b)
A= ArNHCH2CH2N(CH3)
B = ArCH2Cl/NaNH2
C = ClCH2CH2N(CH3)

(c)
A= ClCH2CH2N(CH3)
B = ArCH2Cl / NaNH2
C = ArNHCH2CH2N(CH3)

(d)
A = ArNHCH2CH2N(CH3)
B = ArNHCH2CH2N(CH3)
C = ClCH2CH2N(CH3)

694. Tarry feces due to oxidized iron from hemoglobin is also called
(a) Hematemesis
(b) Haemolysis
(c) Melena
(d) None

695. Example of prostaglandin analogue
(a) Propanthelin
(b) Misopostol
(c) Pirenzepine
(d) Oxyphenonium

696. Example of Ulcer protectives
(a) Sucralfate
(b) Colloidal Bismuth Citrate(CBS)
(c) Both
(d) None

697.

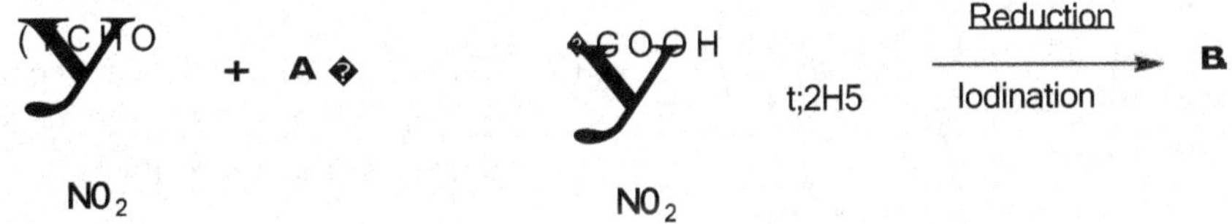

is

(a) Lamitidine
(b) Loxtidine
(c) Tiotidine
(d) Oxmetidine

698. Gynaecomastia is occurs with ---------
----type of H_2 antagonist in patients
treated for a month or more
(a) Famotidine
(b) Cimetidine
(c) Ranitidine
(d) Etintidine

701.

(a) A. Butyricacid B. Iopanoicacid
(b) A. Butyricacid B. Iodipamide
(c) A. Butyricanhydride B. Iodipamide
(d) A. Butyricanhydride B.Iopanoicacid

702. One of the following dye is used for
liver functioning test
(a) Fluroscein sodium
(b) Phenol sulphonphthlein
(c) Sulphobromophthalein sodium
(d) Congo red

703. The dye is a bright red to dark red
crystalline powder, used for test of
renal function by estimating the rate
of excretion in the urine

699. Radiopaque agents are drugs used to
diagnose certain medical problems,
they are called as
(a) X-ray contrast media
(b) Oral Cholecytographic agents
(c) Both
(d) None

700. Sodium diatriazoate is chemically
(a) 2,3,4-triacetamido-5,6-diiodo-
benzoicacid
(b) 2,3-diacetamido-4,5,6-triiodo-
benzoicacid
(c) 3,4,5-triacetamido-2,4-diiodo-
benzoicacid
(d) 3,5-diacetamido-2,4,5-triiodo-
benzoicacid

(a) Fluroscein sodium
(b) Phenol sulphonphthlein
(c) Sulphobromophthalein sodium
(d) Congo red

704. Evan blue is used for the
determination of blood volume, it is
also called as
(a) Indigo carmine
(b) Cango red
(c) Azovan blue
(d) Congo blue

705. Wood sugar is
    (a) Mannitol
    (b) Xylose
    (c) D- Glucose
    (d) Lactose

706. An aliphatic unsaturated acid used as a preservative
    (a) Sorbicacid
    (b) Phenoxy ethanol
    (c) Bronopol
    (d) None

707. Amaranth is a synthetic azodye, it is chemically
    (a) 3-hydroxy-4-(3-sulphonato-naphthylazo)naphthalene-2,7-disulphonate
    (b) 4-hydroxy-4-(4-sulphonato-naphthylazo)naphthalene-2,7-disulphonate
    (c) 3-hydroxy-4-(4-sulphonato-naphthylazo)naphthalene-2,7-disulphonate
    (d) 3-hydroxy-4-(3-sulphonato-naphthylazo)naphthalene-2,7-disulphonate

708. One of the below aromatic aldehyde gives bitter almond oil odour
    (a) Cinnamaldehyde
    (b) P-Amino benzaldehyde
    (c) Benzaldehyde
    (d) Anisaldehyde

709. One of the below compound is used as a preservative in shampoos,which is a derivative of propane-1,3-diol
    (a) Phenyl mercuriaacid
    (b) Chlrobutanol
    (c) Bronopol

(d) Phenoxy ethanol

710. A sweetening agent used as plasticizer in the manufacturing of gelatin capsules
    (a) Sucose   (b) Sorbitol
    (c) Saccharin   Fructose

711. An agent is used as a detergent and a wetting agent in shampoos
    (a) Sodium dodecyl sulphate
    (b) Sodium lauryl sulphate
    (c) Cetostearyl alcohol
    (d) Glyceryl monostearate

712. One of the Stabilizing agent is a polyuronicacid composed of residu:s of D-mannuronic and L-Guluromc acid
    (a) Pectin   (b) Celluose
    (c) Acacia   (d) Alginicacid

713. Name two of the below agents which are used as suspending agent in pharmaceutical prepations.
    (a) Carbomer and Povidone
    (b) Carbomer and Cellulose
    (c) Povidone and Cellulose
    (d) None

714. The mixtures of semisolid hydrocarbons obtained from petroleum called as
    (a) Paraffin
    (b) Camauba Wax
    (c) Bees Wax
    (d) Petroleum Wax

715. An ointment base is obtained from the honey comb of the common honey bee i.e. Apis species
    (a) Camuba Wax

   (b) Bees Wax
   (c) Microcrystalline Wax
   (d) Paraffin Wax

716. Which bases used for water soluble ointments, lotions, creams are a special class of glycol ethers of high molecular weights called
   (a) Macrogols
   (b) Polymers
   (c) Glycerides
   (d) None

71 7. An antifoaming agent is employed for the prevention of bed sores and napkin rashes
   (a) Lanolin
   (b) Dimethicone
   (c) Methicone
   (d) None

718. An agent is acts as solvent for surface coatings, Plastics, and toilet preparations
   (a) Isopropyl alcohol
   (b) Ethyl alcohol
   (c) Diethyl ether
   (d) Methylated spirit

719. Which solvent used as a emollient, water retaining agent and as a vehicle for some ear drops.
   (a) Acetone
   (b) Diethyl ether
   (c) Glycerine
   (d) Chloroform

720. Wheat is obtained from the source of
   (a) Zea mays
   (b) Oryza sativa
   (c) Triticum aestivum
   (d) Solanum tuberosum

721. Which agent is used as a lubricant in tablet making
   (a) Stearic acid
   (b) Zinc stearate
   (c) Magnesium stearate
   (d) All

722. Meglumine is an aminosugar, it is chemically
   (a) l-deoxy-1-methylamino-D-Glucitol
   (b) 1-deoxy-1-methylamino-D-Glucose
   (c) l-ethoxy-1-methylamino-D-Glucitol
   (d) l-ethoxy-1-methylamino-D-Glucose

723. Which anticoagulant agent is used for haematological investigations? Therapeutically, it is administered by slow intravenous inJection in emergency treatment of hypercalcemia and to reduce serum calcium concentration.
   (a) Di sodium Acetate
   (b) Di sodium Edetate
   (c) Di sodium Phosphate
   (d) Di sodium Tartarate

724. The metal cylinders containing the compressed liquid form of the halogenated hydrocarbons should be stored at a temperature of
   (a) 8° C-15° c   (b) 0° c -10° c
   (c) 10° C -15° C   (d) 6° C -14° C

725. One of the sweetening agent is a peptide, is about 180-200 times as sweet as surose.
 (a) Alanine dipeptide
 (b) Muramyl dipeptide
 (c) Aspartame
 (d) None

726. Prostaglandins and its related compounds are also called as
 (a) Prostacyclines
 (b) Thromboxanes
 (c) Leucotrienes
 (d) Eicosanoids

727. A compound ls synthesized from prostate gland, that stimulates the uterine contractions and reduces the blood pressure
 (a) Prostaglandins
 (b) Prostacyclins
 (c) Eicosanoids
 (d) All

728. Suicidal enzyme is
 (a) Phospholipase A2
 (b) PGI2
 (c) Cycloxygenase
 (d) Thromboxane synthase

729. The maJor site of Prostaglandin Degradation
 (a) Lungs   (b) Liver
 (c) Both   (d) None

730. Prostaglandins serve as agent in the treatment of
 (a) Hypotension
 (b) Hypertension
 (c) Both
 (d) None

731. The below agent acts as vasoconstrictor
 (a) PG!i   (b) PGA2
 (c) TXA2   (d) None

732. Immunosuppressive drugs disrupt the synthesis of DNA and RNA as well as the process of cell division
 (a) Cyclosporins
 (b) Azothioprine
 (c) Corticosteroids
 (d) None

733. ____ drugs suppress the inflammation associated with transplant rejection
 (a) Cyclosporins
 (b) Antibodies
 (c) Corticoids
 (d) None

734. The drugs used in combination with such other drugs as cyclosporine and corticosteroids in kidney transplants
 (a) Basiliximib
 (b) Muromonab
 (c) Tacrolimus
 (d) Orthodone OKT_3

735. The drug which ls used in the treatment of relapsing-remitting multiple sclerosis
 (a) Mycopehnolate
 (b) Imuran
 (c) Glatiramer Acetate
 (d) Neroral

736. Identify the immunophilin-binding drugs
    (a) Leflunomide   (b) Tacrolimus
    (c) Sirolimus   (d) None

737. Many NSAIDs can lead to gastrointestinal disturbances and they are considered to be a main factor in the etiology of peptic ulcers. What is the main cause of most peptic ulcers?
    (a) Helicobacter pylori
    (b) NSAIDs
    (c) Alcohol
    (d) Nicotine

738. Which drug-drug combination would probably best help to prevent peptic ulceration?
    (a) Aspirin/famotidine
    (b) Aspirin/omeprazole
    (c) Aspirin/aluminium hydroxide
    (d) Aspirin/misoprotosol

739. Which NSAIDs should not be used for long-term treatment of inflammatory conditions?
    (a) Diclofenac
    (b) Aspirin
    (c) Indomethacin
    (d) Mefenamic acid

740. The main action of capsaicin is
    (a) As a rubefacient
    (b) As an analgesic
    (c) As an anti-inflammatory
    (d) Through substance P

741. Which of the following local anaesthetics has the shortest duration of action
    (a) Bupivacaine
    (b) Procaine
    (c) Lidocaine
    (d) Cinchocaine

742. What would be the usual drugs used in neuroleptoanalgesia?
    (a) Midazolam, morphine and haloperidol
    (b) Midazolam, pethidine and droperidol
    (c) Fentanyl, midazolam and droperidol
    (d) Midazolam, pethidine and morphine

743. Local anaesthetics are often given together with adrenaline. Why?
    (a) To constrict blood vessels
    (b) To dilate blood vessels
    (c) To lessen the pain of injection
    (d) To act as a potentiator

744. What is the equivalent dose of fentanyl when compared with 10 mg of morphine?
    (a) 200-250 mcg of fentanyl
    (b) 150-200 mcg offentanyl
    (c) 100-150 mcg of fentanyl
    (d) 50-100 mcg of fentanyl

745. For clients receiving naltrexone, the ... should be monitored before starting treatment and monthly for the first three months.
    (a) Clotting function
    (b) Visual acuity
    (c) Renal function
    (d) Liver function

746. Which of the following opioid drugs is a useful analgesic in labour because it does not suppress uterine contractions?
    (a) Pethidine
    (b) Dextropropoxyphene
    (c) Pentazocine
    (d) Tramadol

747. For better control of acute pain
    (a) An analgesic should be always administered first time in the momïng
    (b) An analgesic should be always administered just before bedtime
    (c) Regular administration of an analgesic is required
    (d) p.r.n. (as required) administration should be followed

748. Which of the following is the most appropriate first line medication for most people with osteoarthritis?
    (a) Cox
    (b) Non-specific NSAID
    (c) Paracetamol + codeine
    (d) Regular paracetamol

749. Which NSAID has been linked with possibly negating the protective effect of aspirin?
    (a) Diclofenac
    (b) Ibuprofen
    (c) Indomethcin
    (d) Naproxen

750. What effect do NSAIDs usually have on blood pressure?
    (a) Increase by 5mmHg
    (b) Decreases by 5 mmHg
    (c) Increases with increased doses
    (d) None

751. Which of the following is the most appropriate strategy for decreasing risk of **NSAID** related GI adverse events in at-risk people?
    (a) Co-prescribe Omeprazole
    (b) Co-prescribe Ranitidine
    (c) Use Enteric-coated formulation
    (d) None

752. Which NSAID appears to have the lowest risk of causing GI bleeding?
    (a) Diclofenac
    (b) Indomethacin
    (c) Ibuprofen
    (d) Naproxen

753. Elderly people are at increased risk of which of the following adverse effects of NSAID use?
    (a) Cardiac
    (b) Gastrointestinal
    (c) Renal
    (d) All of these

754. The maJor role in chronic management of arthritis:
    (a) Glucocorticoids
    (b) Mineralocorticoids
    (c) NSAIDs
    (d) None

755. Mechanism of action: aspirin-platelet effects
    (a) Promotes platelet aggregation
    (b) Activates thromboxane synthesis
    (c) Both
    (d) Neither

756. Mediator most likely to promote pain
   (a) Serotonin
   (b) Histamine
   (c) Bradykinins
   (d) Leukotrienes

757. At low doses required to inhibition of thymidylate synthase, an enhanced adenosine release
   (a) Chloroquine
   (b) Methotrexate
   (c) Cyclophosphamide
   (d) Ketorolac

758. Mediator promoting greatest increase in vascular permeability, associated with acute inflammation
   (a) Serotonin
   (b) Prostaglandins
   (c) Bradykinins
   (d) Leukotrienes

759. Isozyme primarily responsible for prostaglandin production by cells involve an inflammation
   (a) Leukotrienes   (b) COX-I
   (c) COX-II   (d) None

760. Effective in managing acute gouty arthritis and ankh losing spondylitis also accelerates closure of patent duct us arteriosus in premature infants
   (a) Ketorolac
   (b) Phenylbut azone
   (c) Methotrexate
   (d) Indomethacine

761. In rheumatoid arthritis: primary effect of this mediator is on prostaglandin production

   (a) PDGF (platelet-derived growth factor)
   (b) GM-CSF
   (c) TNF a
   (d) None

762. Analgesic effects of aspirin
   (a) Peripheral action (inflammation)
   (b) Subcortical site of action
   (c) Both
   (d) None

763. NSAID primarily promoted as an analgesic, not as an anti-inflammatory agent
   (a) Piroxicam
   (b) Ibuprofen
   (c) Naproxen
   (d) Ketorolac

764. Drug associated with the hepatic/renal toxic metabolite: N-acetyl-p-benzoquinone
   (a) Acetaminophen
   (b) Diclofenac
   (c) Meclofenamate
   (d) Indomethacin

765. Thyroid gland 'ls controlled and maintained by
   (a) Pitutary gland
   (b) Hypothalamus
   (c) Both
   (d) None

766. The ratio of thyroxine and triiodo thyronine released into blood circulation is
   (a) 20:1   (b) 1:20
   (c) 10:8   (d) 8:20

767. Thyronine is treating with million's reagent------- colour produces
    (a) Red   (b) Yellow
    (c) Green   (d) Brown

768. Due to presence of aminoacid, thyronine on treating with ------- gives blue colour
    (a) Millon's   (b) Ninhydrin
    (c) Starch   (d) None

769. Hypothyroidism in infants/during foetal stage due to the presence of ectopic thyroid/Iodine deficiency are called
    (a) Cretinism
    (b) Myxoedema
    (c) Hashimot's Thyroiditis
    (d) None

770. Auto-immune destruction of thyroid is called
    (a) Grave's Disease
    (b) Muxoedema
    (c) Hashimoto's Thyroiditis
    (d) None

771. Moecular formula of lith$_{yr}$onine sodium
    (a) ClsH11I4NNa04
    (b) ClsH11I3NNa04
    (c) ClsH11I4NNa04
    (d) C14H11I3NNa04

772. Thiourea is -------- derivative of anti thyroid drug
    (a) Anion inhibitor
    (b) Iodinated contrast
    (c) Thioamide
    (d) None

773. Thiocyanates are------
    (a) Thioamide derivatives
    (b) Anion inhibitor
    (c) Iodinated contrast
    (d) Poly hydric phenol

774. The serious adverse effect of carbimazole is
    (a) Hypertension
    (b) Agranulocytosis
    (c) Tremors
    (d) Migrain headache

775. Structure of methimazole is
    (a)   (b)

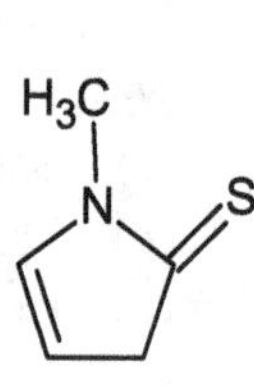

    (c)   (d)

776. Hyperth$_{yr}$oidism occurs due to the viral infection
    (a) Grave's Disease
    (b) Goiter
    (c) Myxoedema
    (d) Subcute Thyroditis

777. If thyroid gland is non-tender it is called
    (a) Thyrotoxicosis
    (b) Thyroiditis
    (c) Silent Thyroiditis
    (d) None

778. Mechanism of Iodinated contrast media
     (a) Inhibit 3'-deiodinase enzyme, thus prevents conversion of T_4 and T_3 in liver, Kidney and Brain
     (b) Inhibit 5'-deiodinase enzyme, thus prevents conversion of T_4 and T_3 in liver, Kidney and Brain
     (c) Inhibit 3'-deiodinase enzyme, thus prevents conversion of T_4 in liver
     (d) Inhibit 5'-deiodinase enzyme, thus prevents conversion of T_4 in liver

779. Preproinsuln is composed of
     (a) 86 Aminoacid
     (b) 110 Aminoacid
     (c) 51 Aminoacid
     (d) None

780. Proinsulin is composed of
     (a) 86 Aminoacid
     (b) 110 Aminoacid
     (c) 51 Aminoacid
     (d) None

781. In proinsulin connecting peptide consist of
     (a) 21 Amino acid
     (b) 30 Amino acid
     (c) 86 Amino acid
     (d) None

782. In Bovine insulin Aminoacid in Chain A at 8th and 10th position
     (a) Alanine and Valin
     (b) Valine and Alanine
     (c) Threonine and Isoleucine
     (d) Threonine and Valine

783. In Chain B, the first six(phe to leu), last three (Pro, Lys, Thr) amino acid, residues are removed that shows ----- activity
     (a) Increases
     (b) Decreases
     (c) Without significant loss
     (d) None

784. Glucagon is a ------- ammo acid containing single chain polypeptide
     (a) 51 Amino acid
     (b) 21 Amino acid
     (c) 29 Amino acid
     (d) 30 Amino acid

785. Insulin analogue obtained by replacing asparagmes at A_2, with glycine and by adding two arginine residue at the carboxy terminus of chainB
     (a) Lentin insulin
     (b) Human insulin
     (c) Insulin glargine
     (d) Isophane Insulin

786. Duration of action ____ subarachnoid injection of ester type local anesthetics
     (a) Short
     (b) Extremely long
     (c) Extremely short
     (d) None

787. Consequences of vasodilatory local anesthetic property
     (a) Reduced systemic absorption
     (b) Shorter duration of action
     (c) Both
     (d) None

788. Highest local anesthetic blood levels associated with this type of regional anesthesia
    (a) Epidural
    (b) Brachia! plexus
    (b) Sciatic
    (d) Intercostal

789. Consequencas of fetal acidosis (sometimes associated with prolonged labor) on local anesthetic accumulation in the fetus
    (a) Enhanced
    (b) Reduced
    (c) Slowly decreases
    (d) None

790. Plasma concentration of local anesthetics determined by
    (a) Rate of tissue distribution
    (b) Rate of drug clearance
    (c) Both
    (d) Neither

791. Ester type local anesthetic-most rapid hydrolysis
    (a) Tetracine
    (b) Procaine
    (c) Chloroprocaine
    (d) None

792. Enhancement of spinal anesthesia by the presence of epinephrine in local anesthesics-Reasons
    (a) Increased substance P release
    (b) Increaased dorsal horn neuronal activity
    (c) Decreased local neuronal uptake
    (d) None of the above

793. Consequence of clonidine(catapres) addition to local anesthetic solutions-----
    (a) Increases local anesthetic effect
    (b) Reduces local anesthetic effect
    (c) Gradually increases the local anesthetic effect
    (d) Gradually decreases the local anesthetic effect

794. Clearance mechanism for local anesthetics
    (a) Amides-mainly renal
    (b) Ester-rapid clearance,hydrolysis
    (c) Both
    (d) None

795. Ester-type local anesthetic
    (a) Lidocaine
    (b) Tetracaine
    (c) Ropivacaine
    (d) Bupivacaine

796. Amide-type oflocal anesthetic
    (a) Cocaine   (b) Prilocaine
    (c) Tetracaine   (d) Lidocaine

797. Local anesthetic used in greater than 50% of rhinolaryngologic cases
    (a) Prilocaine   (b) Cocaine
    (c) Mepivacaine   (d) Bupivacaine

798. Mechanism of local anesthetic action in epidural anesthesia
    (a) Direct local anesthetic action on nerve roots and spinal cord following local anesthetic diffusion across the dura
    (b) Diffusion of local anesthetic into para vertebral regions through the intravertebral for amina

(c) Both
(d) None

799. Primary side effect/toxicities associated with local anesthetic use
(a) Allergic reactions
(b) Systemic toxicity
(c) Both
(d) None

800. Typically a zone of differential sympathetic nevous system blocked
(a) Epidural   (b) Spinal
(c) Both   (d) None

801. Neurotoxicity associate with local anesthesia: sensory anesthesia, bowell & bladder spincter dysfunction, paraplegia------ may because by non homogeneous local anesthetic distribution
(a) Anterior spinal artery syndrome
(b) Cauda equine syndrome
(c) Transient radical irritation
(d) None

802. Neurotoxicity------moderate/severe lower back, buttocks, posterior side pain
(a) Anterior spinal artery syndrome
(b) Cauda equine syndrome
(c) Transient radical irritation
(d) None

803. Common eutectic mixture of local anesthetics(EMLA)
(a) Tetracaine and epinephrine
(b) Lidocaine and tetracaine
(c) Prilocine and bupivacaine
(d) Lidocaine and Prilocaine

804. Most frequent local anesthetic clinical use
(a) Treatment of grand mal seizure
(b) Analgesia
(c) Management of cardiac arrhythmias
(d) Regional anesthesia

805. Lidocaine effect on ventilation response to hypoxia
(a) Enhanced response
(b) Depressed response
(c) First depressed then slowly enhances
(d) None

806. Least likely to exhibit cross-sensitivity with amide or ester local anesthetics
(a) Lidocaine   (b) Tetracaine
(c) Mepivacaine   (d) Dyclonine

807. Local Anesthetic which produces localized vasoconstriction and anesthesia
(a) Tetracaine
(b) Lidocaine
(c) Cocaine
(d) Chlorococaine

808. Which agents not recommended for Bier block
(a) Chloroprocaine
(b) Mepivacaine
(c) Bupivacaine
(d) All the above

809. Local anesthetic most likely to cause cyanosis secondary to reduced oxygen transport
(a) Lidocaine   (b) Bupivacaine

(c) Prilocaine   (d) Procaine

810. This amide-type local anesthetic is used to assess the possible presence of atypical cholinesterase
(a) Ropivacaine
(b) Procaine
(c) Dibucaine
(d) Chloroprocaine

811. Toxicities associated with systemic epinephrine absorption following local anesthetic solution
(a) Hypertension   (b) Arrhythmias
(c) Both   (d) None

812. Neurotoxicity following local anesthesia: lower extremity paresis-----predisposing conditions may include advanced age peripheral vascular disease
(a) Anterior spinal artery syndrome
(b) Cauda equine syndrome
(c) Transient radical irritation
(d) None

813. Local anesthetic not recommended for peripheral nerve blocked
(a) Lidocaine   (b) Bupivacaine
(c) Ropivacaine   (d) Tetracaine

814. Frequently used amide-type local anesthetic for Bier block
(a) Chloroprocaine
(b) Prilocaine
(c) Bupivacaine
(d) Ropivacaine

815. Cutaneous necrosis was reduced protein C activity occurs during the first weeks of therapy with

(a) Streptokinase
(b) Abciximab
(c) Warfarin
(d) Aspirin

816. Thrombus type most likely to be formed in low pressure veins
(a) White thrombus
(b) Red thrombus
(c) Both
(d) None

817. Synonym for factor VII
(a) Proaccelerin
(b) Prothrombin
(c) Proconvertin
(d) Christmas factor

818. Immediate haemostatic responds to the damage vessel
(a) Platelet Aggregation
(b) Platelet viscous metamorphosis
(c) White thrombus formation
(d) Vasospasm

819. Mouse/human chimeric monoclonal antibody------block IIb/IIIb platelet receptor
(a) Ticlopidine
(b) Timolol
(c) Abciximab
(d) eicosapentaenoic acid

820. The cessation of blood loss from a damaged vessel
(a) Hemostasis
(b) Hematemesis
(c) Haemolysis
(d) None

821. One of the below synthetic neurotransmitter of adrenergic system
     (a) Norepinephrine (b) Epinephrine
     (c) Dopamine   (d) Isoprenaline

822. Catecholamine is
     (a) Benzene ring with two adjacent hydroxyl group and an amide side chain
     (b) Phenol ring with one adjacent hydroxyl group and an amide side chain
     (c) Catechol moiety and an amide side chain
     (d) All

823. The enzymes play a vital role in the metabolism of Norepinephrine and epinephrine
     (a) MAO and DOPA decarboxylase
     (b) COMT and DOPA decarboxylase
     (c) MAO and COMT
     (d) None

824. The iris of eye contains-------- type of adrenergic receptors
     (a) al & a2   (b) al & Pl
     (c) P1&P2   (d) a1&P2

825. An example of indirectly acting sympathomimetic drug
     (a) Epinephrine
     (b) Amphetamine
     (c) Clonidine
     (d) Salbutamol

826. One of the directly acting sympathomimetic drug , is consists of only one hydroxx group which is used to postpone premature labour
     (a) Phenylephrine

     (b) Isoproterenol
     (c) Ritodrine
     (d) None

827. A selective p_2 adrenergic agonist
     (a) Salbutamol
     (b) Dobutamine
     (c) Phenylephrine
     (d) Methyldopa

828. Which of the below is used as a base in aerosol inhalers
     (a) Salbutamol
     (b) Dobutamine
     (c) Phenylephrine
     (d) Methyldopa

829. Dobutamine act by stimulates p_1 adrenergic receptors results in
     (a) Positive ionotropic effect
     (b) Positive chronotropic effect
     (c) Negative ionotropic effect
     (d) None

830. Directly acting Non-selective sympathomimetic agent ,that dilates the renal vessels results in the treatment of renal and liver failure
     (a) Isoprenaline
     (b) Ephedrine
     (c) Dopamine
     (d) None

831. Directly and indirectly acting sympathomimetic, widely used as nasal decongestant
     (a) Ephedrine
     (b) Amphetamine
     (c) Pseudoephedrine
     (d) None

832. Benzedrine is
   (a) Amphetamine
   (b) Epinephrine
   (c) Nor epinephrine
   (d) None

833. The compounds that effect the synthesis, storage and release of neurotransmitter/ catecholamines and this reduce the amount of neurotransmitter reaching the adrenergic receptor are called as
   (a) Adrenergic neuron blocking agents
   (b) Adrenergic receptor blockers
   (c) Adrenergic blockers
   (d) None

834. a_2 - selective adrenergic antagonists is
   (a) Prazosine   (b) Terazosine
   (c) Yohimbine   (d) None

835. One of the example of B-haloalkoylamines of non-selective a-adrenergic receptor blockers
   (a) Tolazoline
   (b) Prazosine
   (c) Yohimbine
   (d) Phenoxy benzamine

836. Which type of adrenergic blocking agents blocks to prevent the endothelial vasoconstriction of arterioles and venous thus decreasing vascular resistant and increasing venous capairtance
   (a) Non selective a_2 blockers
   (b) Non selective a_1 blockers
   (c) Selective a_2 blockers
   (d) Selective a_1 blockers

837. Which type of non-selective adrenergic blockers is used to treat pulmonary h_{yp} ertension occurring in neonates
   (a) Tolazoline
   (b) Phentolamine
   (c) Phenoxy benzamine
   (d) Dibenzamine

838. Except one quinazoline derivative of a_1 - selective antagonists contains 4-amino-6,7 -di methoxy quinazoline ring attached to piperazine ring as the basic structure
   (a) Prazosine   (b) Trazosine
   (c) Alphuzosine   (d) Doxazosine

839. Identify the below examples of indole alkaloid which acts as a arselective blockers
   (a) Reserpine
   (b) Yohimbine
   (c) Terazosin
   (d) Prazosine

840. Structures of isoproterenol and pronethalol

(a)

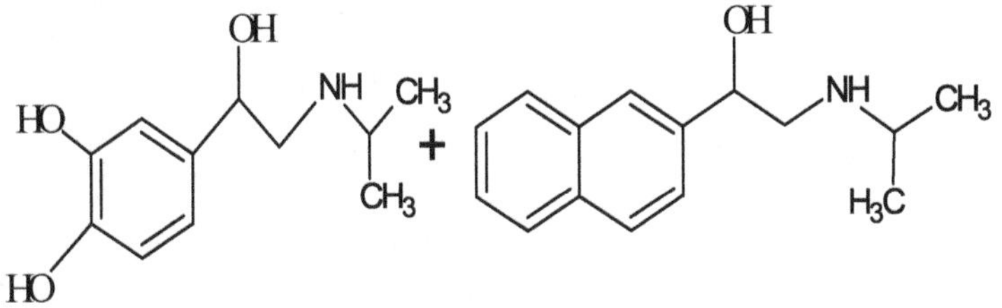

(b)

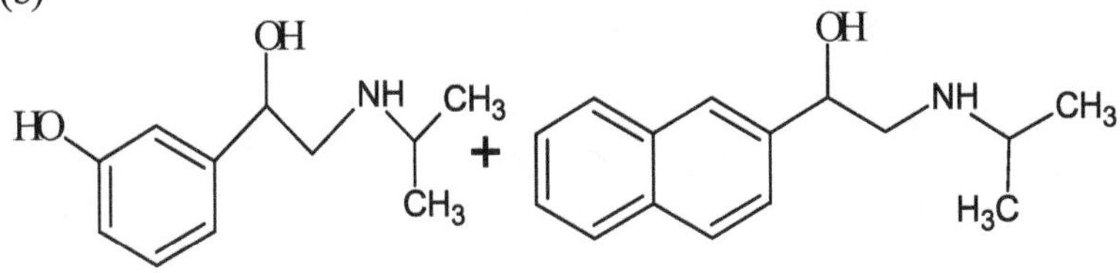

(c)

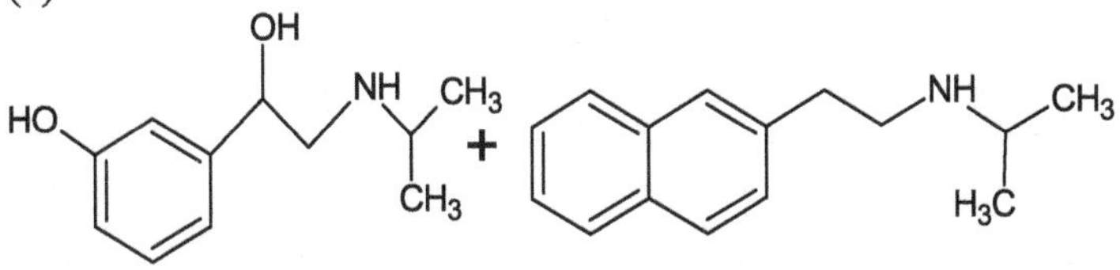

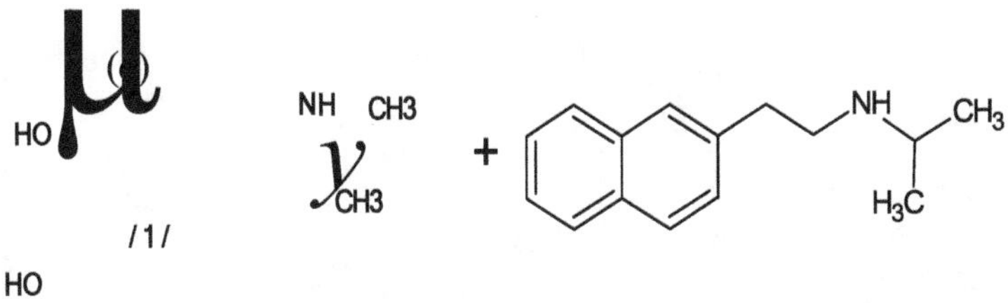

(d)

/1/

841. Propanolol is a competitive antagonists at B-receptors which inhibits cAMP levels then shows
    (a) Negative chronotropic effect
    (b) Negative inotropic effect
    (c) Both
    (d) None

842.

$$\text{C6} + \begin{array}{c} Cl \\ H_2C\text{---}\triangle\text{O} \end{array} \xrightarrow[-HCl]{aq.Alkali} A \xrightarrow[isopropylamine]{HCl} B.$$

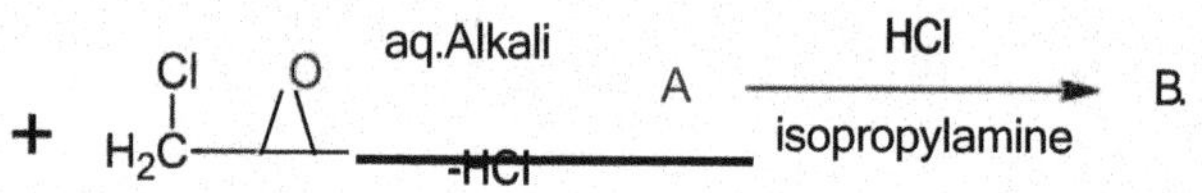

A andB?

(a)

H₃C

OH   NH   (CH₃)₂   HCl

+

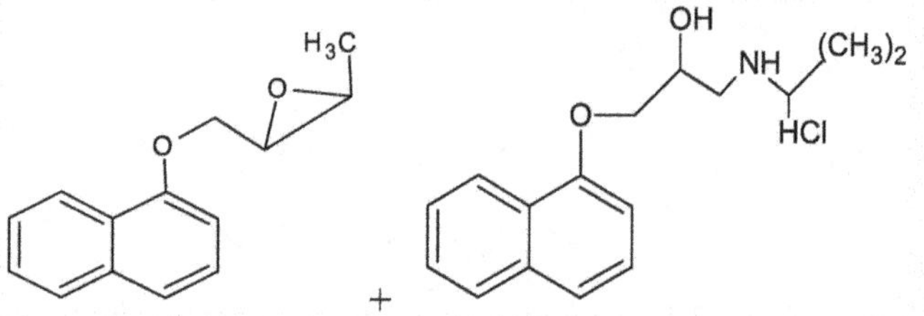

(b)

OH

♦CH3)2   HCl

HOC()O♦

I

c60

+

(c)

OH   NH   (CH₃)₂   HCl

+

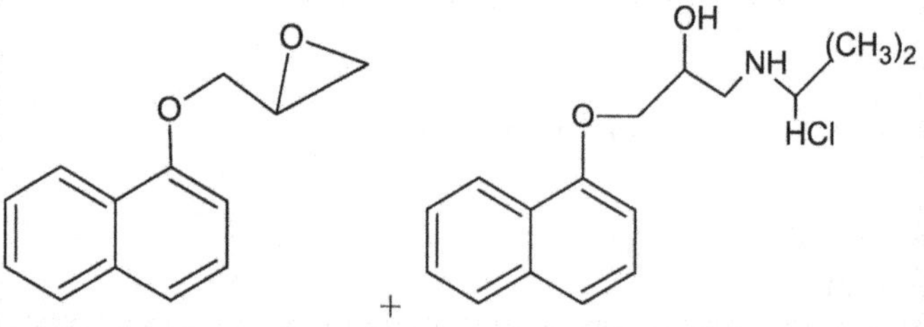

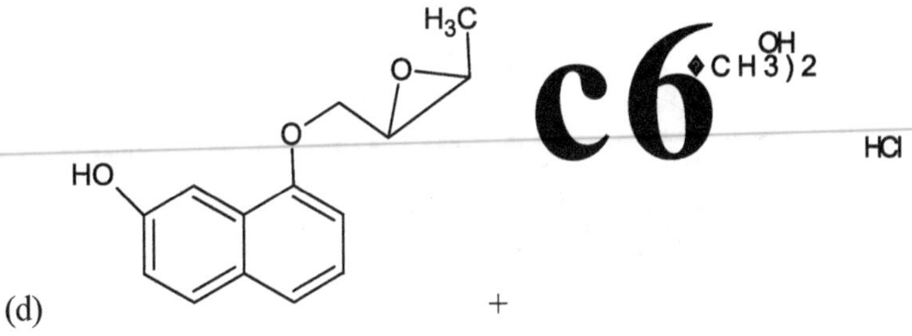

(d)   +

843. Carvediol possess antioxidant and antiproliferative effects on
   (a) Skeletal muscle
   (b) Smooth muscle
   (c) Both
   (d) None

844. Scalp tingling is a disorder occur with ___ therapy
   (a) Athenol   (b) Trazosin
   (c) Labetalol   (d) Carvediol

845. The natural neurotransmitter of parasympathetic nervous system
   (a) Adrenaline   (b) Atropine
   (c) Acetycholine (d) Atenol

846. In cholinergic system, the replacement of terminal methyl molecule of acyl oxy group with___ amine gives
   (a) Calbomic esters
   (b) Carboxylic acid
   (c) Carboxyl compound
   (d) None

847. In cholinergic system, the addition methyl group at -position to the quaternary ammonium group of acetyl choline shows
   (a) Increased muscamic activity, decreases nicotinic activity
   (b) Increases muscarnic activity, increases nicotinic activity
   (c) Decreases muscarnic activity, increases nicotinic activity
   (d) Decreases muscarnic activity, decreases nicotinic activity

848. In cholinergic system, the addition methyl group at a-position to the quaternary ammonium group of acetyl choline shows
   (a) Increased muscamic activity, decreases nicotinic activity
   (b) Increases muscarnic activity, increases nicotinic activity
   (c) Decreases muscarnic activity, increases nicotinic activity
   (d) Decreases muscarnic activity, decreases nicotinic activity

849.

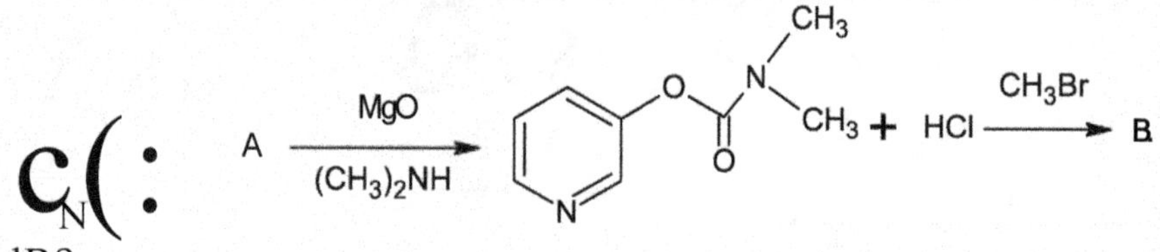

A and B ?

(a)

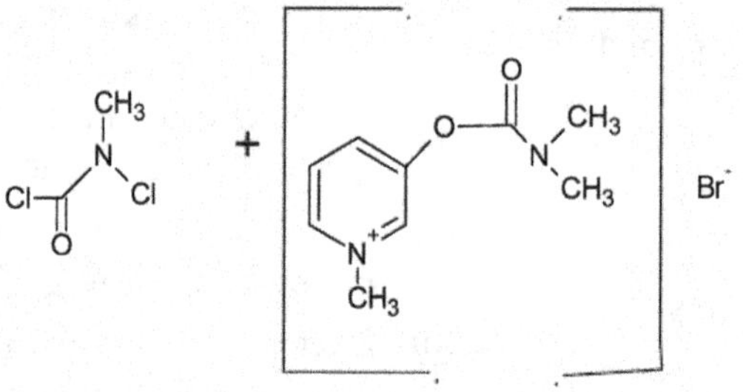

(b)

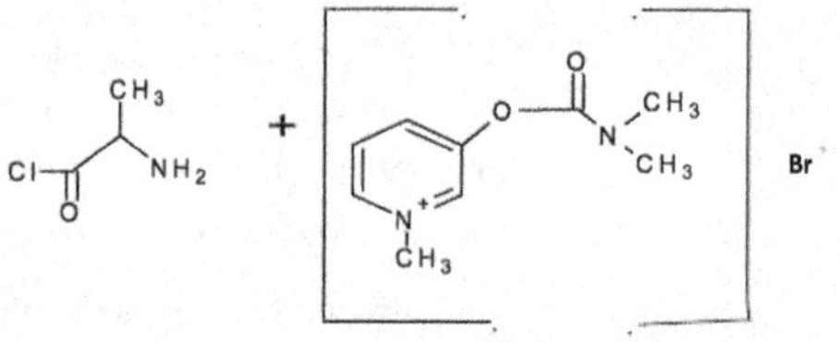

(c)

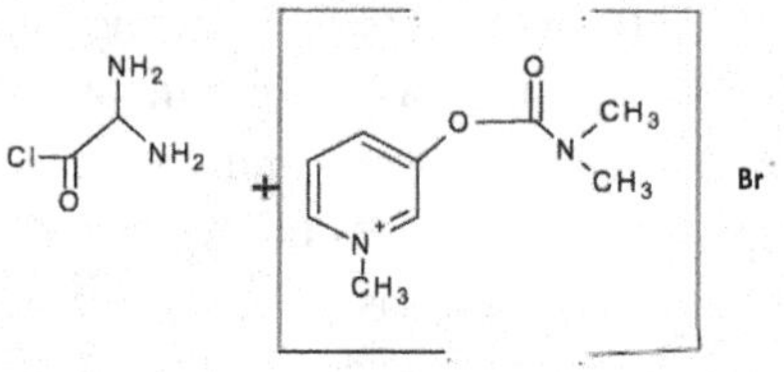

(d)

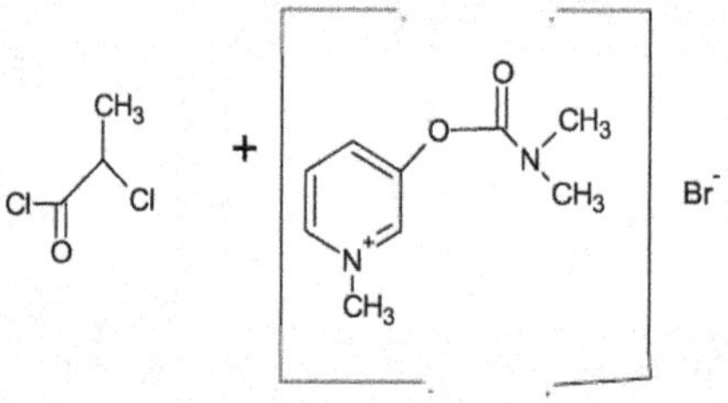

850. One of the below is used along with atropine in the treatment of poisoning associated with organophosphorus copounds
   (a) Neostigmine
   (b) Pyridostigmine
   (c) Pralidoxime
   (d) Propantheline

851. NMJ receptor are blocked by
   (a) Hexamethonium
   (b) Tubocurarine
   (c) Pralidoxime
   (d) None

852. Ganglionic receptors are blocked by
   (a) Hexamethonium

   (b) Tubocurarine
   (c) Pralidoxime
   (d) None

853. One of the below depolarizing NMJ blocking agents
   (a) Vecuronium
   (b) Pancuronium
   (c) Mivacurium
   (d) Succinyl choline

854. Source of pilocarpine is
   (a) Leaves of plant jobamdi
   (b) Seeds of plant jobamdi

   (c) Roots of plant jobamdi
   (d) Stems of plant jobamdi

855. The compounds which block the action of acetylcholine at parasympathetic system are called
   (a) Adrenergic agents
   (b) Cholinergic agents
   (c) Antiadrenergic agents
   (d) Anticholineregic agents

856. Parasympatholytic drugs antagonize the __ of Acetylcholine.
   (a) Muscarinic action
   (b) Nicotinic action
   (c) Both muscarinic and nicotinic
   (d) Cholinergic action.

857. One of the below is not effect produced by anticholinergic
   (a) Mydratic   (b) Miosis
   (c) Cycloplegic   (d) None.

858. An alkaloid used as antispasmodic and antiuler agent
   (a) Morphine   (b) Atropine
   (c) Ergotamin   (d) Vincristine.

859. A Compound is used as gastrointestinal antispasmodic agent in irritable bowel syndrome.
   (a) Dicyclomine
   (b) Tropicamide
   (c) Metaclopramide
   (d) Mebeverine.

860. Metaclopramide is chemically
   (a) 4-Amino,4-chloro,N-(2-Diethy-lamino ethyl) -2-methoxy benzamide.
   (b) 5-Amino,4-chloro,N-(2-Diethy-lamino ethyl)-2-ethoxy benzamide.

(c) 4-Amino,5-chloro,N-(2-Diethy-lamino ethyl)- 2- methoxy benzamide.

(d) 5-Amino,5-chloro,N-(2-Diethyl-amino ethyl)-2-ethoxy benzamide.

861. The drug of the choice in reflux oesophagitis and for Zollinger-Ellison Syndrone
(a) Omeprazole
(b) Lansoprazole
(c) Pantoprazole
(d) Rabeprazol.

862. An agent is a quaternary ammonium compound formed by the introduction of an isopropyl group to the nitrogen of atropine.
(a) Homatropine hydrobromide
(b) Hyoscine hydrobromide
(c) Ipratropium bromide
(d) Ipratropum hydrobromide

863. Name the heterocyclic ring system present in cimetidine.
(a) Furan   (b) Thiazole
(c) Pyrrolidine   (d) Imidazole

864. Antimalarials: dihydro   folate reductase inhibitors
(a) Chloroquine
(b) Chloroguanide
(c) Pyrimethamine
(d) Trrimethoprim

865. Factors which determine antimalarial agent efficacy
(a) Species
(b) Life-cycle stage-dependencies
(c) Both
(d) None

866. Which of the plasmodium species causative for human malaria, the one producing most serious complications
(a) Plasmodium vivax
(b) Plasmodium malariae
(c) Plasmodium ovale
(d) Plasmodium falciparum

867. Chloroquine (Aralen) is
(a) Effective against gametocytes of *P. falciparum*
(b) Used to treat *P. vivax, P. ovale, P.malariae* attacks
(c) Both
(d) None

868. Chloroquine   (Aralen)   is contraindications
(a) Patients with retinal/visual field abnormalities
(b) In patients predisposed to porphyria
(c) Both
(d) None

869.

H₂N
OCH₃
N
H₂N— —CH₂- OCH₃
N
OCH₃

Is
(a) Pyrimethamine
(b) Pamaquine
(c) Trimethoprim
(d) None

870. Clinical use of primaquine
(a) Treatment of Pneumocystis carinii pneumomia
(b) Radical cure of acute malaria
(c) Both

(d) None

871. Clinical use of chloroguanide
   (a) Malarial chemoprophylaxis
   (b) Toxoplasmosis
   (c) Both
   (d) None

872. The disease that is non-communicable
   is....
   (a) Malaria   (b) Marasmus
   (c) AIDS   (d) Jaundice

873. Malaria is caused by a
   (a) Protozoan   (b) Fungi
   (c) Virus   (d) Bacteria

874. In antimalarial drugs, The substitution
   of a hydroxyl group on one of the
   ethyl groups on the 3° amine shows----
   ------- toxicity
   (a) Reduces
   (b) Increases
   (c) Slowly decreases
   (d) None

875. Sulphonamides   blocks   the
   incorporation of PABA to form
   (a) Di hydro folicacid
   (b) Di hydro ptero acid
   (c) Tetra hydro folicacid
   (d) None

876. Plaquenil is
   (a) Amodiquine
   (b) Chlroquine
   (c) Primaquine
   (d) Hydroxy chloroquine

877. Malaria is caused by several species
   of the protozoan
   (a) Anopheles   (b) Plasmodium

(c) Ovale   (d) Microzoan

878. Two protozoal organisms: Entamoeba
   histolytica and Giardian lamblia,
   frequently cause
   (a) Thrush
   (b) Dysentery
   (c) Dermatophyte infections
   (d) Malaria

879. The   most   commonly   reported
   intestinal protozoal infection in the
   united states is
   (a) Colitis   (b) Dysentery
   (c) Amebiasis   (d) Giardiasis

880. Characteristics of quinine(Quinamm)
   antimalarial activity
   (a) Slow onset
   (b) Poorly effective blood
        schizonticide against
        Plasmodium vivax
   (c) Gametocidal for *Plasmodium
        ovale*
   (d) None

881. Diloxanide Furoate is chemically
   (a) 4-(2,2-dichloro-N-methyl
        acetamido) phenyl thiophene-2-
        carboxylate
   (b) 4-(2,2-dichloro-N-methyl
        acetamido) phenyl furan-2-
        carboxylate
   (c) 4-(2,3-dichloro-N-methyl
        acetamido) phenyl thiophene-2-
        carboxylate
   (d) 4-(2,3-dichloro-N-methyl
        acetamido) phenyl furan-2-
        carboxylate

882. Metronidazole is consist of _______
   heterocyclic ring

(a) Oxazole   (b) Thiazole
(c) Imidazole   (d) None

883. ______ is used in the treatment of intestianal and hepatic amoebisis
(a) Metronidazole (b) Tinidazole
(c) Both   (d) None

884.

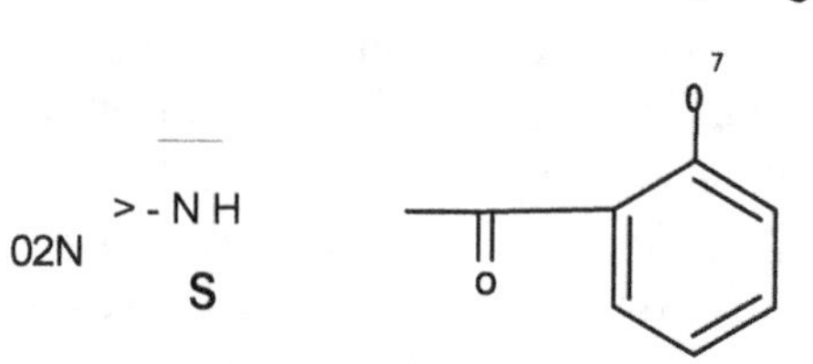

(a) Nitazoxamide
(b) Metronidazole
(c) Tinidazole
(d) Nimorazole

885. Albendazole is ______ derivative
(a) Imidazole   (b) Purine
(c) Benzimidazole (d) None

886. Vermox is
(a) Mebendazole
(b) Flubendazole
(c) Albendazole
(d) None

887. Thiabendazole is chemically
(a) 3-(Thiazo1-4-y l)-1 H-
     benzimidazole
(b) 2-(Thiazol-4-yl)-lH-
     benzimidazole
(c) 3-(Oxazol-4-yl)-lH-
     benzimidazole
(d) 2-(Oxazol-4-yl)-lH-
     benzimidazole

888. Biltricide is

(a) Albendazole
(b) Flubendazole
(c) Praziquantel
(d) None

889. Schistosoma mansom is highly susceptible to
(a) Vermizine   (b) Vellocome
(c) Oxamniquine   (d) None

890. ---------stimulate ganglion in the worms, cause tonic paralysis which results in the expulsion of live worms
(a) Niridazole   (b) Levanmisol
(c) Mectizan   (d) None

891. Gametes are
(a) Egg cells   (b) Liver cells
(c) Germ cells   (d) Sperm cells

892. "Trichomonas Vaginalis" causes "Trichomoniasis" which is common in the U.S and is transmitted
(a) By spores

(b) By Contact with infected skin of another person
(c) Sexually
(d) By insects

893. Amphotericin-B is obtained from____________
(a) Streptomyces nodosus
(b) Streptomyces noursei
(c) Streptomyces meditarani
(d) None

894. Mechanism of griseofulvin
(a) It shows fungicidal properties there by leading to cell death

(b)   It causes disruption of the mitotic spindle by interacting with polymerized microtubules

(c)   It inactivates the microsomal enzymes by leading to cell death

(d)   None

895. _ _ _ is a heterocyclic ring is present in the miconazole
(a)   Oxazole
(b)   Pyridine
(c)   Imidazole
(d)   Thiazole

896. Ketaconazole is active against-------- species
(a)   Candida spp
(b)   Cryptococcus neoformans
(c)   Both
(d)   None

897. Terconazole is ... derivative
(a)   Imidazole
(b)   Pyrole
(c)   Oxazole
(d)   Triazole

898. An _ _ _ agent is extensively used for the control of vulvovaginal moniliasis caused by candida albicans
(a)   Ketaconazole
(b)   Clotrimazole
(c)   Terconazole
(d)   Econazole

899. Ketaconzole is _ _ _ _ compound
(a)   Highly lipophilic
(b)   Highly hydrophilic
(c)   Highly hygroscopic
(d)   None

900.

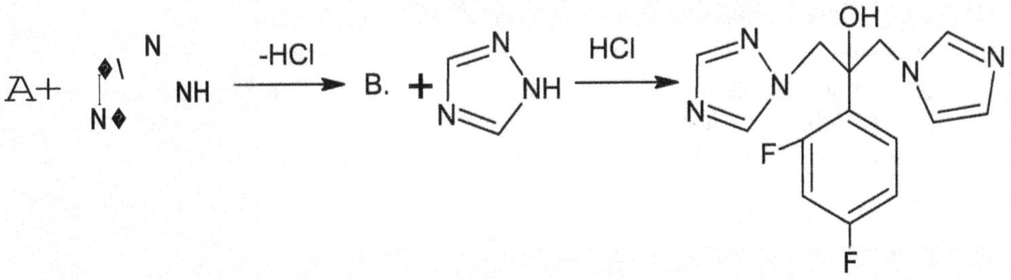

A and B ?

(a)

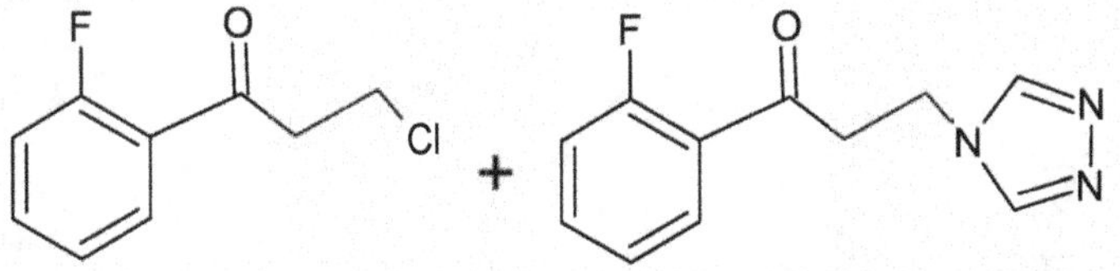

(b)

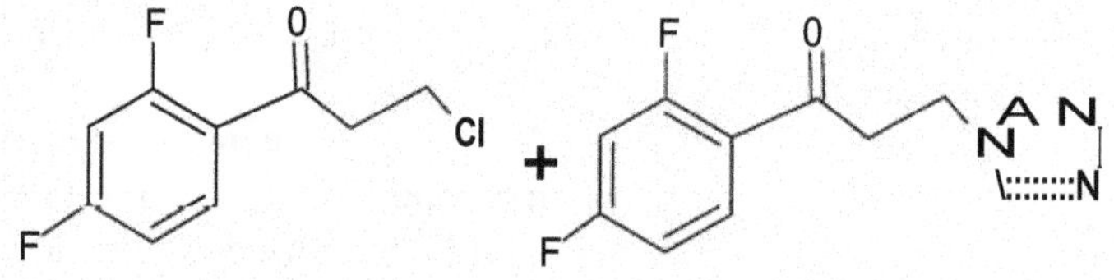

(c)

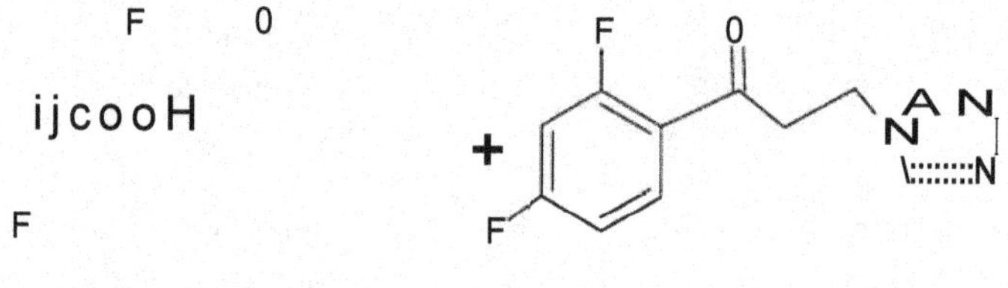

ijcooH

(d)

(YCOOH

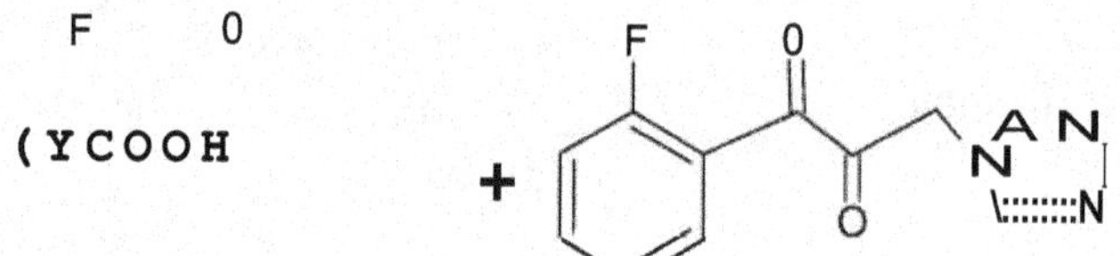

901. Fluconazole has useful activity against
   (a) Coccidioides immitis
   (b) Candida species
   (c) Cryptococcus species
   (d) All

902. Zinococonazole is consists of two heterocyclic rings
   (a) Thiazole and Pyrole
   (b) Thiophene and Pyrole
   (c) Thiophene and Imidazole
   (d) Thiazole and Imidazole

903.

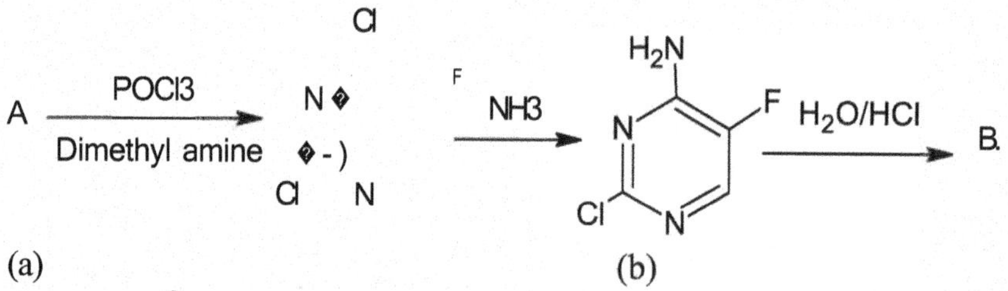

(a)

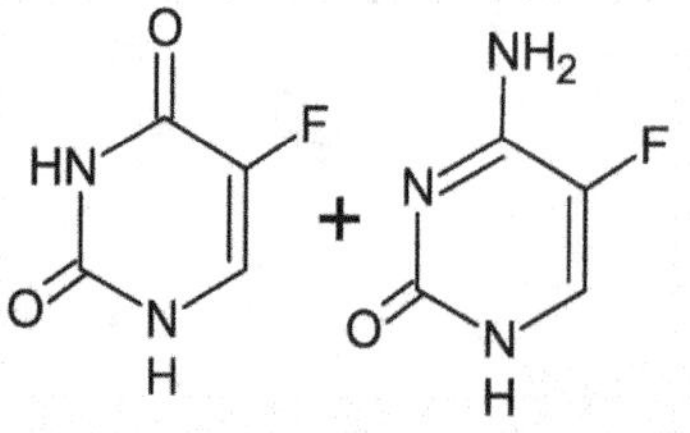

(b)

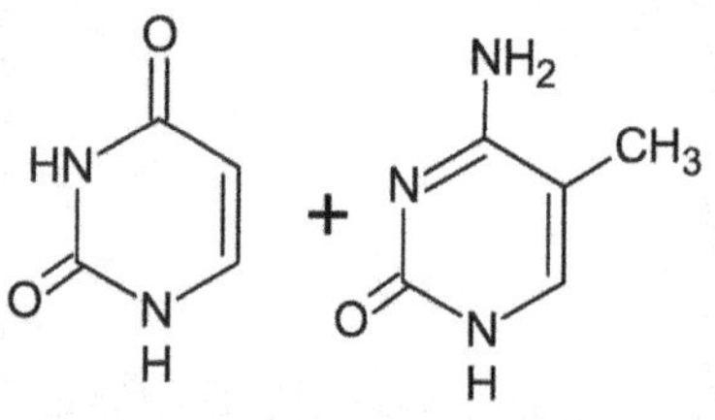

(c)   (d)

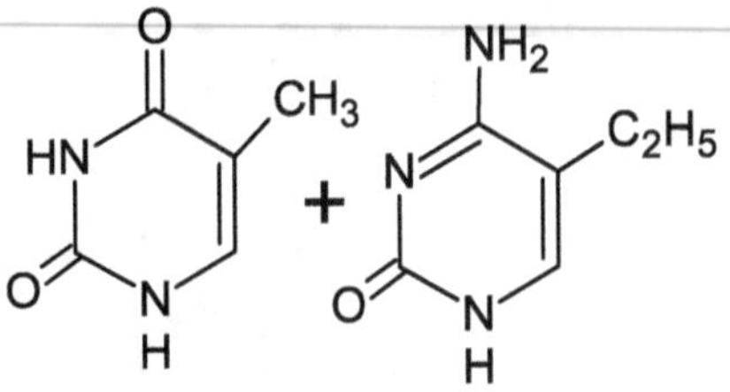

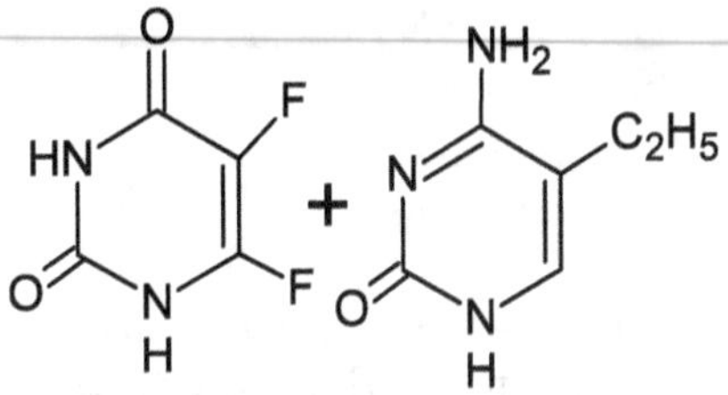

904. Nikomycin act by inhibit
  (a) Thymidylate synthase
  (b) Chitin Synthase
  (c) Glucosamine-6-phosphate
  (d) None

905. Naftifine is antifungal drug has fungicidal activity against
  (a) Tinea cruris
  (b) Streptomyces tendae
  (c) Coccidioides immitis
  (d) None

906. A common Candidiasis infection of the mouth is known as
  (a) Thrush
  (b) Gossypol
  (c) Aspergillosis
  (d) Thrombophlebitis

907. An organism that lives on or in another, drawing its nourishment from its host, is known as a
  (a) Fungi
  (b) Bacterium
  (c) Virus
  (d) Parasite

908. The most serious adverse effect of Amphotericin-B is
  (a) Renal damage
  (b) Loss of hearing
  (c) Thrombophlebitis
  (d) Fever

909. Fungal super infections usually occur in the anal, genital and
  (a) Eye areas   (b) Oral areas
  (c) Ear areas   (d) Skin areas

910. A fungal is termed a
  (a) Phagocytosis
  (b) Filamentos
  (c) Mycosis
  (d) Local infection

911. Conjuctivites caused by
  (a) Arena Virus
  (b) Adenovirus
  (c) Herpes virus
  (d) Reo virus

912. Acyclovir is a _______
  (a) Purine nucleoside analogue
  (b) Pyrimidine nucleoside analogue
  (c) Benzimidazole derivative
  (d) None

913. Idoxuridine is a ---------
  (a) Purine nucleoside analogue
  (b) Pyrimidine nucleoside analogue
  (c) Benzimidazole derivative
  (d) None

914. ------- antiviral agent is used as dopamine receptor agonist
    (a) Gancyclovir
    (b) Idoxuridine
    (c) Amantidine
    (d) Acyclovir

915. Which antiviral agent is used in the treatment of Parkinson's disease
    (a) Gancyclovir   (b) Amantidine
    (c) Acyclovir   (d) Idoxuridine

916. Ribavirin structure consisting ------- heterocyclic ring
    (a) Imidazole   (b) Thiazole
    (c) Oxazole   (d) Triazole

917. Virazole is
    (a) Amantidine   (b) Rimantidin
    (c) Ribavirin   (d) Nevirapine

918. Structure of Didanosine
    (a)

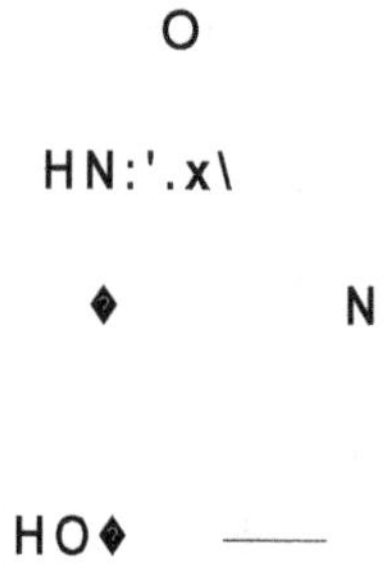

    (b)

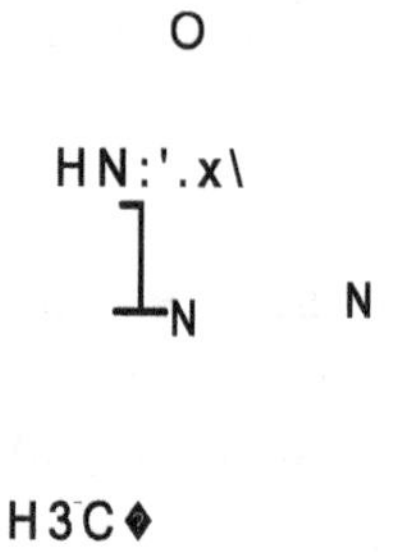

(c)

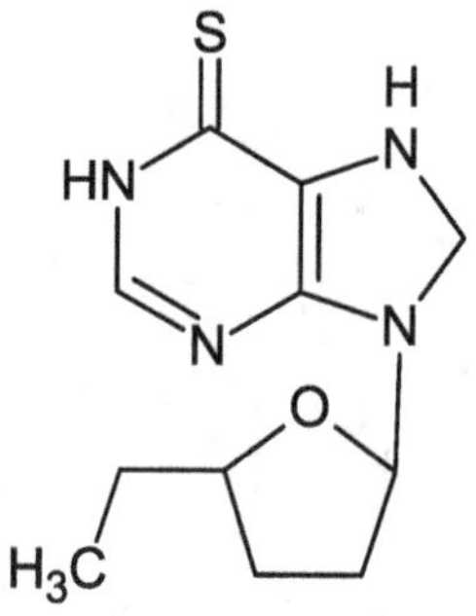

(d)

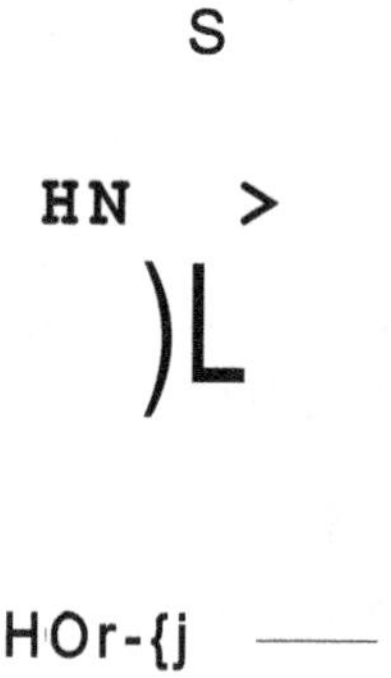

919. Lamivudine is chemically
    (a) 4-Amino-1-((2S, 5R)-2-(hydroxymethyl-1,3-oxathiolan-4-y l)purine-2(1H)-one
    (b) 4-Amino-1-((2S, 5R)-2-(hydroxymethyl-1,3-oxathiolan-5-yl)pyramidine-2(1H)-one
    (c) 4-Amino-1-((2S, 5R)-2-(hydroxymethyl-1,3-oxathiolan-4-yl)pyramidine-2(1H)-one
    (d) 4-Amino-1-((2S, 5R)-2-(hydroxymethyl-1,3-oxathiolan-5-y l)purine-2(1H)-one

920. Ritonavir is a derivative of
    (a) HIV protease inhibitor
    (b) RT inhibitor
    (c) Nucleoside analogue
    (d) Non- Nucleoside analogue

921.

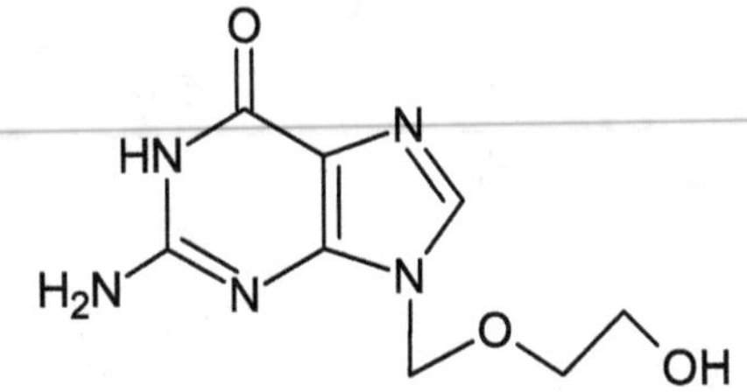

(a) Abacavir   (b) Lamivudine
(c) Acuclovir   (d) None

KEY

1.	(d)	2.	(b)	3.	(c)	4.	(a)	5.	(d)
6.	(c)	7.	(a)	8.	(c)	9.	(c)	10.	(c)
11.	(c)	12.	(a)	13.	(a)	14.	(a)	15.	(d)
16.	(b)	17.	(d)	18.	(a)	19.	(d)	20.	(c)
21.	(d)	22.	(b)	23.	(b)	24.	(c)	25.	(d)
26.	(a)	27.	(a)	28.	(a)	29.	(d)	30.	(b)
31.	(d)	32.	(b)	33.	(d)	34.	(c)	35.	(d)
36.	(b)	37.	(c)	38.	(c)	39.	(a)	40.	(d)
41.	(a)	42.	(c)	43	(a)	44.	(d)	45.	(b)
46.	(d)	47.	(a)	48.	(c)	49.	(d)	50.	(b)
51.	(b)	52	(d)	53.	(c)	54.	(a)	55.	(d)
56.	(b)	57.	(c)	58.	(c)	59.	(c)	60.	(c)
61.	(a)	62.	(d)	63.	(b)	64.	(d)	65	(c)
66.	(a)	67.	(c)	68.	(d)	69.	(a)	70.	(c)
71.	(b)	72.	(b)	73.	(d)	74.	(a)	75.	(b)
76.	(c)	77.	(d)	78.	(b)	79.	(c)	80.	(d)
81.	(a)	82.	(b)	83.	(c)	84.	(c)	85.	(d)
86.	(d)	87	(d)	88.	(a)	89.	(d)	90.	(d)
91.	(c)	92.	(b)	93.	(b)	94.	(d)	95.	(c)
96.	(c)	97.	(d)	98.	(d)	99.	(a)	100.	(c)
101.	(a)	102.	(a)	103	(b)	104.	(b)	105.	(a)
106.	(a)	107.	(a)	108.	(d)	109.	(c)	110.	(d)
111.	(b)	112.	(c)	113.	(b)	114.	(a)	115.	(c)
116.	(a)	117.	(b)	118.	(b)	119.	(d)	120.	(d)
121.	(b)	122.	(a)	123	(d)	124.	(d)	125.	(b)
126.	(c)	127.	(a)	128.	(d)	129	(d)	130.	(a)
131.	(b)	132.	(a)	133.	(b)	134.	(a)	135.	(c)
136.	(d)	137.	(a)	138.	(b)	139.	(c)	140.	(a)
141.	(a)	142.	(a)	143.	(c)	144.	(b)	145.	(c)
146.	(b)	147.	(d)	148.	(b)	149.	(d)	150.	(c)

151. (d)	**152.** (d)	**153.** (a)	**154.** (d)	**155.** (c)
156. (c)	**157.** (a)	**158.** (a)	**159.** (b)	**160.** (b)
161. (b)	**162.** (a)	**163.** (d)	**164.** (d)	**165.** (c)
166. (c)	**167.** (a)	**168.** (d)	**169** (b)	**170.** (d)
171. (a)	**172.** (d)	**173.** (a)	**174.** (c)	**175.** (d)
176. (d)	**177.** (b)	**178.** (d)	**179.** (a)	**180.** (d)
181. (b)	**182.** (c)	**183.** (c)	**184.** (b)	**185.** (c)
186. (c)	**187.** (a)	**188.** (b)	**189.** (d)	**190.** (c)
191. (c)	**192.** (b)	**193.** (d)	**194.** (a)	**195.** (d)
196. (b)	**197.** (b)	**198.** (d)	**199.** (c)	**200.** (b)
201. (a)	**202.** (d)	**203.** (b)	**204.** (d)	**205.** (a)
206. (c)	**207.** (c)	**208.** (b)	**209.** (b)	**210.** (d)
211. (b)	**212.** (d)	**213.** (c)	**214.** (c)	**215.** (a)
216. (a)	**217.** (d)	**218.** (d)	**219.** (d)	**218.** (a)
221. (a)	**222.** (c)	**223.** (b)	**224.** (b)	**225.** (c)
226. (c)	**227.** (a)	**228.** (a)	**229.** (c)	**230.** (a)
231. (b)	**232.** (c)	**233.** (a)	**234.** (b)	**235.** (d)
236. (d)	**237.** (c)	**238.** (b)	**249.** (a)	**240.** (c)
241. (a)	**242.** (a)	**243.** (a)	**244.** (a)	**245.** (b)
246. (b)	**247.** (c)	**248.** (a)	**249.** (b)	**250.** (d)
251. (c)	**252.** (d)	**253.** (b)	**254.** (d)	**255.** (a)
256. (d)	**257.** (c)	**258.** (b)	**259.** (d)	**260.** (c)
261. (b)	**262.** (d)	**263.** (a)	**264.** (c)	**265.** (c)
266. (d)	**267.** (c)	**268.** (b)	**269.** (d)	**270.** (b)
271. (a)	**272.** (d)	**273.** (c)	**274.** (b)	**275.** (a)
276. (a)	**277.** (d)	**278.** (c)	**279.** (b)	**280.** (a)
281. (d)	**282.** (a)	**283.** (d)	**284.** (a)	**285.** (c)
286. (b)	**287.** (d)	**288.** (d)	**289.** (c)	**290.** (a)
291. (b)	**292.** (c)	**293.** (c)	**294.** (c)	**295.** (a)
296. (d)	**297.** (d)	**298.** (a)	**299.** (b)	**300.** (d)
301. (d)	**302.** (a)	**303.** (d)	**304.** (c)	**305.** (c)
306. (d)	**307.** (d)	**308.** (c)	**309.** (b)	**310.** (a)

311.	(a)	**312.**	(b)	**313.**	(c)	**314.**	(d)	**315.**	(b)
316.	(a)	**317.**	(a)	**318.**	(c)	**319.**	(b)	**320.**	(d)
321.	(a)	**322.**	(b)	**323.**	(c)	**324.**	(b)	**325.**	(b)
326.	(d)	**327.**	(a)	**328.**	(c)	**329.**	(a)	**330.**	(d)
331.	(b)	**332.**	(c)	**333.**	(c)	**334.**	(b)	**335.**	(a)
336.	(d)	**337.**	(d)	**338.**	(a)	**339.**	(c)	**340.**	(a)
341.	(b)	**342.**	(a)	**343.**	(b)	**344.**	(c)	**345.**	(d)
346.	(c)	**347.**	(b)	**348.**	(d)	**349.**	(b)	**350.**	(d)
351.	(d)	**352.**	(a)	**353.**	(d)	**354.**	(c)	**355.**	(b)
356.	(b)	**357.**	(a)	**358.**	(a)	**359.**	(b)	**360.**	(a)
361.	(c)	**362.**	(b)	**363.**	(a)	**364.**	(d)	**365.**	(d)
366.	(a)	**367.**	(b)	**368.**	(c)	**369.**	(b)	**370.**	(c)
371.	(b)	**372.**	(c)	**373.**	(c)	**374.**	(c)	**375.**	(d)
376.	(a)	**377.**	(b)	**378.**	(b)	**379.**	(c)	**380.**	(d)
381.	(b)	**382.**	(c)	**383.**	(a)	**384.**	(c)	**385.**	(d)
386.	(c)	**387.**	(d)	**388.**	(c)	**389.**	(c)	**390.**	(c)
391.	(d)	**392.**	(d)	**393.**	(c)	**394.**	(c)	**395.**	(b)
396.	(d)	**397.**	(a)	**398.**	(c)	**399.**	(d)	**400.**	(c)
401.	(b)	**402.**	(c)	**403.**	(b)	**404.**	(a)	**405.**	(a)
406.	(c)	**407.**	(b)	**408.**	(a)	**409.**	(d)	**410.**	(d)
411.	(a)	**412.**	(d)	**413.**	(d)	**414.**	(d)	**415.**	(d)
416.	(a)	**417.**	(c)	**418.**	(b)	**419.**	(d)	**420.**	(d)
421.	(d)	**422.**	(d)	**423.**	(d)	**424.**	(c)	**425.**	(a)
426.	(a)	**427.**	(a)	**428.**	(b)	**429.**	(c)	**430.**	(d)
431.	(b)	**432.**	(b)	**433.**	(c)	**434.**	(a)	**435.**	(b)
436.	(b)	**437.**	(a)	**438.**	(c)	**439.**	(a)	**440.**	(d)
441.	(b)	**442.**	(b)	**443.**	(c)	**444.**	(d)	**445.**	(a)
446.	(c)	**447.**	(d)	**448.**	(a)	**449.**	(b)	**450.**	(c)
451.	(b)	**452.**	(d)	**453.**	(a)	**454.**	(d)	**455.**	(c)
456.	(a)	**457.**	(d)	**458.**	(c)	**459.**	(a)	**460.**	(b)
461.	(c)	**462.**	(d)	**463.**	(b)	**464.**	(c)	**465.**	(d)
466.	(c)	**467.**	(b)	**468.**	(b)	**469.**	(d)	**470.**	(c)

471. (a)	**472.** (b)	**473.** (a)	**474.** (d)	**475.** (d)
476. (d)	**477.** (c)	**478.** (a)	**479.** (b)	**480.** (a)
481. (d)	**482.** (c)	**483.** (d)	**484.** (c)	**485.** (d)
486. (b)	**487.** (c)	**488.** (d)	**489.** (b)	**490.** (c)
491. (d)	**492.** (b)	**493.** (d)	**494.** (c)	**495.** (d)
496. (a)	**497.** (b)	**498.** (c)	**499.** (d)	**500.** (c)
501. (b)	**502.** (a)	**503.** (d)	**504.** (a)	**505.** (c)
506. (d)	**507.** (b)	**508.** (c)	**509.** (d)	**510.** (d)
511. (a)	**512.** (c)	**513.** (b)	**514.** (d)	**515.** (a)
516. (d)	**517.** (a)	**518.** (d)	**519.** (d)	**520.** (a)
521. (b)	**522.** (c)	**523.** (c)	**524.** (c)	**525.** (b)
526. (c)	**527.** (a)	**528** (a)	**529.** (c)	**530.** (d)
531. (d)	**532.** (c)	**533.** (d)	**534.** (c)	**535.** (d)
536. (a)	**537.** (b)	**538.** (d)	**539.** (d)	**540.** (a)
541. (a)	**542.** (d)	**543.** (c)	**544.** (c)	**545.** (a)
546. (b)	**547.** (c)	**548.** (c)	**549.** (b)	**550.** (a)
551. (a)	**552.** (a)	**553.** (a)	**554.** (c)	**555.** (d)
556. (d)	**557.** (b)	**558.** (c)	**559.** (c)	**560.** (b)
561. (c)	**562.** (d)	**563.** (c)	**564.** (d)	**565.** (b)
566. (a)	**567.** (a)	**568.** (b)	**569.** (b)	**570.** (d)
571. (d)	**572.** (a)	**573.** (b)	**574.** (c)	**575.** (a)
576. (d)	**577.** (a)	**578.** (a)	**579.** (d)	**580.** (d)
581. (c)	**582.** (b)	**583.** (b)	**584.** (d)	**585.** (a)
586. (a)	**587.** (c)	**588.** (d)	**589.** (d)	**590.** (c)
591. (d)	**592.** (d)	**593.** (a)	**594.** (d)	**595.** (d)
596. (c)	**597.** (c)	**598.** (d)	**599.** (a)	**600.** (b)
601. (b)	**602.** (a)	**603.** (a)	**604.** (a)	**605.** (c)
606. (d)	**607.** (c)	**608.** (b)	**609.** (c)	**610.** (d)
611. (a)	**612.** (b)	**613.** (a)	**614.** (a)	**615.** (a)
616. (b)	**617.** (d)	**618.** (c)	**619.** (c)	**620.** (b)
621. (a)	**622.** (b)	**623.** (d)	**624.** (b)	**625.** (a)
626. (d)	**627.** (a)	**628.** (c)	**629.** (d)	**630.** (c)

631.	(a)	**632.**	(d)	**633.**	(d)	**634.**	(b)	**635.**	(c)
636.	(b)	**637.**	(d)	**638.**	(a)	**639.**	(c)	**640.**	(c)
641.	(b)	**642.**	(d)	**643.**	(a)	**644.**	(d)	**645.**	(d)
646.	(c)	**647.**	(d)	**648.**	(b)	**649.**	(c)	**650.**	(d)
651.	(b)	**652.**	(a)	**653.**	(a)	**654.**	(d)	**655.**	(c)
656.	(b)	**657.**	(c)	**658.**	(d)	**659.**	(d)	**660.**	(a)
661.	(c)	**662.**	(b)	**663.**	(d)	**664.**	(b)	**665.**	(a)
666.	(a)	**667.**	(b)	**668.**	(d)	**669.**	(c)	**670.**	(d)
671.	(a)	**672.**	(b)	**673.**	(a)	**674.**	(d)	**675.**	(b)
676.	(d)	**677.**	(b)	**678.**	(c)	**679.**	(d)	**680.**	(b)
681.	(d)	**682.**	(b)	**683.**	(c)	**684.**	(a)	**685.**	(d)
686.	(a)	**687.**	(b)	**688.**	(d)	**689.**	(b)	**690.**	(b)
691.	(b)	**692.**	(a)	**693.**	(a)	**694.**	(c)	**695.**	(b)
696.	(c)	**697.**	(a)	**698.**	(b)	**699.**	(c)	**700.**	(d)
701.	(d)	**702.**	(c)	**703.**	(b)	**704.**	(c)	**705.**	(b)
706.	(a)	**707.**	(c)	**708.**	(c)	**709.**	(c)	**710.**	(b)
711.	(a)	**712.**	(d)	**713.**	(a)	**714.**	(a)	**715.**	(b)
716.	(a)	**717.**	(b)	**718.**	(d)	**719.**	(c)	**720.**	(c)
721.	(d)	**722.**	(a)	**723.**	(b)	**724.**	(a)	**725.**	(c)
726.	(d)	**727.**	(d)	**728.**	(c)	**729.**	(c)	**730.**	(b)
731.	(c)	**732.**	(b)	**733.**	(c)	**734.**	(a)	**735.**	(c)
736.	(b)	**737.**	(a)	**738.**	(b)	**739.**	(d)	**740.**	(d)
741.	(b)	**742.**	(c)	**743.**	(a)	**744.**	(b)	**745.**	(d)
746.	(a)	**747.**	(c)	**748.**	(d)	**749.**	(b)	**750.**	(d)
751.	(a)	**752.**	(c)	**753.**	(d)	**754.**	(c)	**755.**	(d)
756.	(c)	**757.**	(b)	**758.**	(d)	**759.**	(c)	**760.**	(d)
761.	(c)	**762.**	(c)	**763.**	(d)	**764.**	(a)	**765.**	(c)
766.	(a)	**767.**	(a)	**768.**	(b)	**769.**	(a)	**770.**	(c)
771.	(b)	**772.**	(c)	**773.**	(b)	**774.**	(b)	**775.**	(c)
776.	(d)	**777.**	(c)	**778.**	(b)	**779.**	(b)	**780.**	(a)
781.	(d)	**782.**	(a)	**783.**	(c)	**784.**	(c)	**785.**	(c)
786.	(b)	**787.**	(b)	**788.**	(d)	**789.**	(a)	**790.**	(c)

791.	(c)	**792.**	(d)	**793.**	(d)	**794.**	(b)	**795.**	(b)
796.	(d)	**797.**	(b)	**798.**	(c)	**799.**	(c)	**800.**	(b)
801.	(b)	**802.**	(c)	**803.**	(d)	**804.**	(d)	**805.**	(b)
806.	(d)	**807.**	(c)	**808.**	(d)	**809.**	(c)	**810.**	(c)
811.	(c)	**812.**	(a)	**813.**	(d)	**814.**	(b)	**815.**	(c)
816.	(b)	**817.**	(c)	**818.**	(d)	**819.**	(a)	**820.**	(a)
821.	(d)	**822.**	(d)	**823.**	(c)	**824.**	(b)	**825.**	(b)
826.	(c)	**827.**	(a)	**828.**	(a)	**829.**	(a)	**830.**	(c)
831.	(c)	**832.**	(a)	**833.**	(a)	**834.**	(c)	**835.**	(d)
836.	(b)	**837.**	(a)	**838.**	(c)	**839.**	(b)	**840.**	(a)
841.	(c)	**842.**	(c)	**843.**	(b)	**844.**	(c)	**845.**	(c)
846.	(a)	**847.**	(a)	**848.**	(c)	**849.**	(a)	**850.**	(c)
851.	(b)	**852.**	(a)	**853.**	(d)	**854.**	(a)	**855.**	(d)
856.	(a)	**857.**	(b)	**858.**	(b)	**859.**	(d)	**860.**	(c)
861.	(a)	**862.**	(c)	**863.**	(d)	**864.**	(c)	**865.**	(c)
866.	(d)	**867.**	(b)	**868.**	(c)	**869.**	(c)	**870.**	(c)
871.	(c)	**872.**	(b)	**873.**	(a)	**874.**	(a)	**875.**	(b)
876.	(d)	**877.**	(b)	**878.**	(b)	**879.**	(d)	**880.**	(c)
881.	(b)	**882.**	(c)	**883.**	(c)	**884.**	(a)	**885.**	(c)
886.	(a)	**887.**	(b)	**888.**	(c)	**889.**	(c)	**890.**	(b)
891.	(c)	**892.**	(c)	**893.**	(a)	**894.**	(b)	**895.**	(c)
896.	(c)	**897.**	(d)	**898.**	(c)	**899.**	(a)	**900.**	(b)
901.	(d)	**902.**	(c)	**903.**	(a)	**904.**	(b)	**905.**	(a)
906.	(a)	**907.**	(d)	**908.**	(a)	**909.**	(b)	**910.**	(c)
911.	(b)	**912.**	(a)	**913.**	(b)	**914.**	(c)	**915.**	(b)
916.	(d)	**917.**	(c)	**918.**	(a)	**919.**	(b)	**920.**	(a)
921.	(c)								

III   PHARMACOLOGY

1. Old, comlmon, easy route of administration of drugs?
   - (a) Parenteral
   - (b) Sublingual
   - (c) Oral
   - (d) Rectal

2. Disadvantage is with oral route....
   - (a) Slower action-not suitable in emergency
   - (b) Cause nausea, vomiting & degradation of drugs in GIT
   - (c) Unpalatable drugs difficult to administer
   - (d) All the above

3. Which drugs are administered by sublingual route....
   - (a) Water soluble
   - (b) Lipid soluble
   - (c) Non-irritating
   - (d) Both b & c

4. Advantage of sublingual route
   - (a) Rapid absorption
   - (b) Action produced within minutes
   - (c) No first pass metabolism directly absorbed into systemic circulation
   - (d) All the above

5. Dosage form with faster onset of action...
   - (a) Tablets **(b)** Capsules
   - (c) Syrups (d) Parenterals

6. Dosage forms given by rectal route
   - (a) Tablets **(b)** Capsules
   - (c) Suppositories (d) Syrups

7. Nitro-glycerin (Glyceryl-trinitrate) is administered through which of the following route?
   - (a) Oral route
   - (b) Sublingual route
   - (c) Parenteral route
   - (d) Rectal route

8. Drug is delivered at constant & predictable rate irrespective of site of application by
   - (a) Rectal route
   - (b) Parenteral route
   - (c) Sublingual route
   - (d) Transdermal route

9. Drug absorption takes place by the surface of alveoli of lungs is by
   - (a) Oral route
   - (b) Inhalation
   - (c) Sublingual route
   - (d) Cutaneous route

10. Drug administered through sublingual route is/are...
    - (a) Nitro-glycerin
    - (b) Isoprenaline
    - (c) Clonidine
    - (d) All the above

11. Example for transdermal patches...
    - (a) Fentanyl
    - (b) Estradiol

(c) Testosterone

(d) All the above

12. Desmopressin and GnRH agonists are administered by
    (a) Oral route
    (b) Rectal route
    (c) Parentral route
    (d) Nasal spray

13. Route with faster action and no first pass metabolism...
    (a) Oral route
    (b) Rectal route
    (c) Cutaneous route
    (d) Parentral route

14. Disadvantage with parental route
    (a) Preparation is sterilised & costlier
    (b) Painful
    (c) Local tissue injury
    (d) All the above

15. BCG vaccine administered by
    (a) Subcutaneous route
    (b) Intradermal route
    (c) Intravenous route
    (d) Intra-muscular route

16. Intramuscular injection is given to ....
    (a) Deltoid
    (b) Gluteus maximus
    (c) Rectus femoris
    (d) All the above

17. Deep penetration is needed for ....
    (a) IM   (b) IV
    (c) SC   (d) IP

18. Thrombophlebitis is caused by
    (a) IM   (b) IV
    (c) SC   (d) IP

19. Dorzolamide & timolol are given by
    (a) Oral route
    (b) IV
    (c) Inhalation route
    (d) Eye drops

20. Injection to subarachnoid space via lumber puncture needle is called ....
    (a) IV
    (b) IM
    (c) IP
    (d) Intrathecal route

21. Following physical action is responsible for drug mechanism of action ....
    (a) Adsorptive property of charcoal & Kaolin
    (b) Radioactivity of I_{131} & other isotopes
    (c) Mass of the bulk laxatives (Bran)
    (d) All the above

22. Example for mechanism of action of drug by chemical action
    (a) Antacids neutralise gastric HCl
    (b) Acidifying and alkalinising agents alters the urine p^H
    (c) Chelating agents sequester toxic metals
    (d) All the above

23. IP3 & cAMP are the second messengers in
    (a) Ligand gated ion channels
    (b) G-Protein couple receptors

(c) Kinase linked receptors

(d) Nuclear receptors

24. One drug affecting the absorption, metabolism & excretion of the other drug is called as
    (a) Chemical antagonism
    (b) Competitive antagonism
    (c) Pharmacokinetic antagonism
    (d) Physiological antagonism

25. Both drugs binding at the same receptor is known as
    (a) Chemical antagonism
    (b) Competitive antagonism
    (c) Pharmacokinetic antagonism
    (d) Physiological antagonism

26. Two drugs producing produce opposing physiological effects is known as
    (a) Physiological antagonism
    (b) Chemical antagonism
    (c) Both a & b
    (d) None

27. Efficacy is zero for
    (a) Agonists   (b) Antagonists
    (c) Both a & b   (d) None

28. Intermediate efficacy has shown by ......
    (a) Agonist
    (b) Partial agonist
    (c) Antagonist
    (d) All the above

29. Agents show selectivity for resting state of the receptor are called as
    (a) Agonists

(b) Inverse agonists

(c) Antagonists

(d) Partial agonists

30. Example of chemical antagonism
    (a) Dimercaprol & heavy metals
    (b) Warfarin & phenobarbital
    (c) Histamine & omeprazole
    (d) None

31. Histamine stimulation of a gastric acid is inhibited by omeprazole is example for...
    (a) Chemical antagonism
    (b) Physiological antagonism
    (c) Pharmacokinetic antagonism
    (d) None

32. The action of one drug is increased by the other drug is called
    (a) Antagonism
    (b) Synergism
    (c) Agonism
    (d) Competitive antagonism

33. Nicotinic acetylcholine receptors are example for?
    (a) G-Protein couple receptors
    (b) Ligand gated ion channels
    (c) Kinase linked receptors
    (d) Nuclear receptors

34. Acetylcholinesterase enzyme is target for the following drug?
    (a) Acetylcholine
    (b) Neostigmine
    (c) Carbachol
    (d) None

35. Muscarinic acetylcholine receptors are example for. ..?
    (a) Ligand gated ion channels

(b)   GPCRs
(c)   Kinase linked receptors
(d)   Nuclear receptors

36.   Insulin receptors are example for?
(a)   Ligand gated ion channels
(b)   GPCRs
(c)   Kinase linked receptors
(d)   Nuclear receptors

37.   Fast synaptic transmission is carried out by?
(a)   Ligand gated ion channels
(b)   GPCRs
(c)   Kinase linked receptors
(d)   All the above

38.   Rhodopsin family belongs to
(a)   Ligand gated ion channels
(b)   GPCRs
(c)   Kinase linked receptors
(d)   Nuclear receptors

39.   In GPCRs which subunit possess GTPase activity
(a)   a   (b)
(c)   y   (d)   None

40.   Targets for G-protein
(a)   Adenyl cyclase enzyme
(b)   Phospholipase C enzyme
(c)   Ion Channels
(d)   All the above

41.   Jak/Stat pathway belongs to
(a)   Ligand gated ion channels
(b)   GPCRs
(c)   Kinase linked receptors
(d)   Nuclear receptors

42.   Aspirin inhibits the following enzyme
(a)   Cyclooxygenase
(b)   AChE
(c)   Xanthine oxidase
(d)   ACE

43. Na^+/K^+ ATP ase pump is inhibited by
(a)   Cardiac glycosides
(b)   Anti-ulcer drugs
(c)   Proton pump inhibitors
(d)   Reserpine

44.   Use ofbioassay
(a)   To measure the pharmacological activity of new substance
(b)   To investigate the function of endogenous mediator
(c)   To measure the drug toxicity & unwanted effects
(d)   All the above

45.   Bio-assay normally involves
(a)   Comparison of unknown preparation with a standard
(b)   Comparison of unknown preparation with control
(c)   Both a & b
(d)   None

46.   Acid drugs bind to
(a)   Albumin
(b)   Globulin
(c)   a-Acid glycoprotein
(d)   All the above

47.   Pharmacologically active
(a)   Free drug
(b)   Protein binding drug

(c) Both a & b

(d) None

48. Addition of adrenaline to local anaesthetics leads to

(a) Reduction in absorption

(b) Increase in absorption

(c) Reduction of distribution

(d) Reduction of plasma protein binding

49. Minute vesicles produced by sonication of aqueous suspension of phospholipids are called as

(a) Prodrugs

(b) Liposome's

(c) Coated device

(d) Microspheres

50. Inactive precursors on metabolism converted to active precursors are called as...

(a) Liposome's

(b) Pro-drugs

(c) Microspheres

(d) All the above

51. Phase-I reactions

(a) Oxidation

(b) Reduction

(c) Hydrolysis

(d) All the above

52. Following drugs undergo first pass metabolism except

(a) Aspirin

(b) Glyceryl trinitrate

(c) Lidocaine

(d) Pantoprazole

53. Active metabolite of paracetamol

(a) Mercaptopurine

(b) N-acetyl-p-benzoquinone

(c) Acetyl-p-benzoquinone imine

(d) N-acetyl-p-benzamide

54. Acrolein is the toxic metabolite of

(a) Diazepam

(b) Cyclophosphamide

(c) Cisplatin

(d) Chlorambucil

55. Halothane toxic metabolite

(a) Acetic acid

(b) Difluoroacetic acid

(c) Trifluoroacetic acid

(d) All the above

56. Drug undergoes first pass metabolism belongs to the class of B-adrenoceptor antagonist

(a) Propranolol

(b) Aspirin

(c) Glyceryl trinitrate

(d) Levodopa

57. Calcium channel blocker undergo first pass metabolism

(a) Nifedipine

(b) Amlodipine

(c) verapamil

(d) Diltiazem

58. Type of drugs cross blood brain barrier

(a) Lipid soluble drugs

(b) Water soluble drugs

(c) Ionisable drugs

(d) All the above

59. The drugs reabsorbed by tubular reabsorption
    (a) Water soluble drugs
    (b) Lipid soluble drugs
    (c) Both a & b
    (d) None

60. Weak acids more rapidly excreted in
    (a) Alkaline urine
    (b) Acidic urine
    (c) Neutral urine
    (d) All the above

61. Pharmacological effect of isoniazid in slow acetylators is
    (a) High   (b) Less
    (c) Intermediate   (d) None

62. Harmful, sometimes fatal reactions that occur in some individuals are called as
    (a) Idiosyncratic reactions
    (b) Harmful reactions
    (c) Allergic reactions
    (d) Pharmacokinetic reactions

63. Factors responsible for idiosyncratic reactions
    (a) Genetic Factors
    (b) Immunological factors
    (c) Both a & b
    (d) None

64. Which of the following drug is enzyme inhibitor?
    (a) Ciprofloxacin
    (b) Chloramphenicol
    (c) Cimetidine
    (d) All the above

65. Probenecid inhibits the following drug excretion?
    (a) Penicillin
    (b) Cephalosporin
    (c) Aminoglycosides
    (d) Ciprofloxacin

66. Enzyme inducer has anti-epileptic activity?
    (a) Rifampicin   (b) Phenytoin
    (c) Ethosuximide   (d) Tiagabine

67. High therapeutic index drug is
    (a) Safe   (b) Toxic
    (c) Both a & b   (d) None

68. Dummy medicine containing no active ingredient is called as ...
    (a) Test drug
    (b) Standard drug
    (c) Placebo
    (d) None

69. Calcium release is regulated by?
    (a) IP3
    (b) Ryanodine receptors
    (c) Both a & b
    (d) None

70. All of the following are drug absorption mechanisms except
    (a) Passive diffusion
    (b) Facilitated diffusion
    (c) Active transport
    (d) Osmosis

71. Neurotransmitter in somatic nervous system
    (a) Adrenaline
    (b) Acetylcholine
    (c) Nor-adrenaline
    (d) All the above

72. Neurotransmitter in parasympathetic nervous system?
    (a) Adrenaline
    (b) Acetylcholine
    (c) Nor-adrenaline
    (d) All the above

73. Neurotransmitter in sympathetic nervous system ganglia
    (a) Nor-adrenaline
    (b) ACh
    (c) Adrenaline
    (d) All the above

74. Neurotransmitter in sympathetic nervous system at target organs
    (a) Nor-adrenaline
    (b) ACh
    (c) Adrenaline
    (d) All the above

75. Resting membrane potential is
    (a) $-40\,mV$ (b) $-30\,mV$
    (c) $-70\,mV$ (d) $-50\,mV$

76. Depolarisation means
    (a) Na^+ enters in & K^+ move out
    (b) Na^+ enters out & K^+ move in
    (c) K^+ efflux & C r influx
    (d) All the above

77. Hyperpolarisation means
    (a) K^+ efflux & er influx
    (b) Na^+ efflux & K^+ influx
    (c) Na^+ influx & K^+ efflux
    (d) All the above

78. Excitatory post synaptic potential (EPSP) leads to
    (a) Permeability of all cations Na^+, Ca^+ influx
    (b) Na^+, Ca^+ efflux
    (c) K^+ efflux & er influx
    (d) Both b & c

79. Inhibitory post synaptic potential (IPSP) leads to
    (a) Permeability of all cations
    (b) Na^+, Ca^+ efflux
    (c) K^+ efflux & er influx
    (d) All the above

80. Co-transmitters
    (a) ACh & ATP
    (b) Nor-adrenaline
    (c) Both a & b
    (d) ACh & nor-adrenaline

81. Co-transmitters
    (a) ACh & NA
    (b) Purine & ATP
    (c) 5-HT & ACh
    (d) Neuropeptide Y & NA

82. M1 selective antagonist used in the treatment of peptic ulcer
    (a) Acetylcholine
    (b) Propanthelin
    (c) Oxyptenonium
    (d) Pirenzepine

83. Select the alkaloid, muscarinic agonist used in the treatment of glaucoma
    (a) Muscarinic
    (b) Arecoline
    (c) Oxotremorine
    (d) Pilocarpine

84. Drugs used to dilate the pupil and to block muscarinic receptors?
    (a) Pilocarpine
    (b) Tropicamide

(c) Cyclopent
(d) Both b & c

85. Semisynthetic derivative, muscarinic antagonist used to treat asthama and COPD
(a) Homatropine
(b) Tiotropium
(c) Ipratropium
(d) Both b & c

86. Sympathetic action of Heart (decreasing heart rate) is due to the mediation of following adrenergic receptor
(a) a1
(b) a2
(c) P1
(d) p2

87. Cholinergic receptor involved in the heart rate regulation
(a) **M1**
(b) M2
(c) M3
(d) M4

88. Adrenergic & cholinergic receptors involved in pupil dilation & constriction respectively
(a) a1 & M3
(b) a1 & M1
(c) a1 & M2
(d) None

89. Branchal smooth muscle is dilated & constricted by following adrenergic & cholinergic receptors respectively
(a) P1 & M2
(b) P2 & M3
(c) p3 & M1
(d) None

90. Functions of ANS
(a) Smooth muscle contraction and relaxations
(b) Exocrine and endocrine secretions
(c) Control of the heart beat
(d) All the above

91. Membrane bound enzyme responsible for the degradation of ACh
(a) AChE
(b) Butyrylcholinesterase
(c) Both a & b
(d) None

92. Type of muscarinic receptors present in glandular & smooth muscle?
(a) M1
(b) M2
(c) M3
(d) M4

93. Edrophonium binding site
(a) Anionic site of AChE
(b) Cationic site of AChE
(c) Both a & b
(d) None

94. Anticholinesterase drug used in diagnosis of myasthenia gravis
(a) Ecothiopate
(b) Edrophonium
(c) Parathion
(d) Dyflos

95. Anticholinesterase Drug used as eye drops
(a) Edrophonium
(b) Ecothiopate
(c) Neostigmine
(d) Dyflos

96. Binding site of parathion
(a) Anionic site of AChE
(b) Cationic site of AChE
(c) Esteratic site of AChE
(d) All the above

97. Irreversible anticholinesterases
form with AChE
    (a) Acetylated Enzyme
    (b) Carbonylated enzyme
    (c) Phosphorylated Enzyme
    (d) None

98. Antidote in organophosphate
p01sonimg
    (a) Physostigmine
    (b) Pyridostigmine
    (c) Pralidoxime
    (d) Neostigmine

99. The action of pralidoxime is due to
the presence of
    (a) Oxide group
    (b) Oxime group
    (c) Both a & b
    (d) Acetyl group

100. Anticholinesterase drug used in the
treatment of alzheimer's disease?
    (a) Neostigmine
    (b) Pyridostigmine
    (c) Donepezil
    (d) Ecothiopate

101. DMPP is
    (a) Ganglionic stimulant
    (b) Ganglionic blocker
    (c) Both a & b
    (d) None

102. Ganglionic stimulant isolated from
the frog skin
    (a) Nicotine   (b) Lobeline
    (c) Epibatadine   (d) DMPP

103. Drugs acts as both ganglionic
stimulant & blocker?
    (a) Nicotine
    (b) Lobeline
    (c) DMPP
    (d) All the above

104. Effect of Ganglionic blockers
    (a) Loss of cardiovascular reflexes
    (b) Gastrointestinal paralysis
    (c) Postural hypotension
    (d) All the above

105. Only one drug in the ganglionic
blocker used clinically as
intravenous infusion to produce
hypotension
    (a) Nicotine
    (b) Trimethaphan
    (c) DMPP
    (d) Neostigmine

106. Drug belongs to the depolarising
neuromuscular blocking agents?
    (a) Tubocurarine
    (b) Suxamethonium
    (c) Pancuronium
    (d) Vecuronium

107. Fasciculations are produced by
    (a) Tubocurarine
    (b) Pancuronium
    (c) Suxamethonium
    (d) Mivacurium

108. Tetanic fade is the result of
    (a) Tubocurarine
    (b) Suxamethonium
    (c) Both a & b
    (d) None

109. Following non-depolarising neuro-muscular blocking agent is hydro-lysed by plasma cholinesterase?
    (a) Pancuronium
    (b) Mivacurium
    (c) Tubocurarine
    (d) Vecuronium

110. Drug having fast onset of action
    (a) Tubocurarine
    (b) Mivacurium
    (c) Vecuronium
    (d) Gallamine

111. Adverse effect of non-depolarising agents
    (a) Bronchoconstriction
    (b) Hypotension
    (c) Double vision
    (d) All the above

112. Drug cause tachycardia due to blockade of muscarinic receptor belongs to non-depolarising neuromuscular blocker?
    (a) Pancuronium
    (b) Vecuronium
    (c) Atracurium
    (d) Tubocurarine

113. Following drug cause extensor spasm in chick?
    (a) Suxamethonium
    (b) Pancuronium
    (c) Vecuronium
    (d) Atracurium

114. Bradycardia induced by neuro-muscular blocking agents is treated with?

    (a) Atropine
    (b) Tubocurarine
    (c) Pirenzepine
    (d) Oxyphenonium

115. Potassium (cation) ion permeability at end plate regions is increased by
    (a) Ganglionic blockers
    (b) Neuromuscular blocking agents
    (c) Muscarinic blockers
    (d) Adrenergic blockers

116. Malignant hyperthermia is the adverse effect of
    (a) Neuromuscular blocking agents
    (b) Ganglionic blockers
    (c) Muscarinic blockers
    (d) Adrenergic blockers

117. Drugs prevent the release of Ca^{2+} release from sarcoplasmic reticulum used in the treatment of malignant hyperthermia?
    (a) Tubocurarine
    (b) Pancuronium
    (c) Dopamine
    (d) Dantroline

118. Malignant hyperthermia is caused by
    (a) Mutations in K^+ release channel
    (b) Mutations in Ca^{2+} release channels
    (c) Mutations in Na^+ release channels
    (d) All the above

119. nor-adrenaline co-transmitted with
    (a) ATP
    (b) Neuropeptide Y
    (c) Both a & b
    (d) None

120. Following receptor agonists are used in the treatment of asthama
    (a) Pl   (b) a2
    (c) al   (d) p2

121. Inhibition of insulin release by following adrenoceptor mechanism?
    (a) Pl   (b) al
    (c) a2   (d) p2

122. Which type of receptors is present in heart?
    (a) Pl   (b) al
    (c) a2   (d) p2

123. Skeletal muscle consist of
    (a) p1 receptors
    (b) p2 receptors
    (c) a l receptors
    (d) a2 receptors

124. p3 receptors are present in
    (a) Skeletal muscle
    (b) Smooth muscle
    (c) Blood vessels
    (d) Adipose tissue

125. Location of al receptors
    (a) Blood vessels (b) Bronchi
    (c) GI tract   (d) All the above

126. Actions of al receptors
    (a) GI constriction
    (b) GI relaxation

(c) Vasodilation
(d) Glucogenesis

127. Location of a2 receptors
    (a) GI tract
    (b) Pancreatic islets
    (c) Platelets
    (d) All the above

128. Autoinhibitory receptors
    (a) a l   (b) a2
    (c) Pl   (d) p2

129. Histamine release is inhibited by following receptors
    (a) a l   (b) a2
    (c) Pl   (d) p2

130. al-selective adrenoceptor agonist
    (a) Nor-adrenaline
    (b) Phenylephrine
    (c) Methoxamine
    (d) Both b & c

131. p2 selective adrenoceptor agonist
    (a) Salbutamol
    (b) Terbutaline
    (c) Both a & b
    (d) None

132. a2 selective agonists
    (a) Clonidine
    (b) Terbutaline
    (c) Methoxamine
    (d) Dobutamine

133. Adrenoceptor inhibits the neuro-transmitter release?
    (a) a l   (b) a2
    (c) Pl   (d) p2

134. Following receptor agonists are used in the treatment of premature labour
   (a) a1
   (b) a2
   (c) P1
   (d) p2

135. Action of adrenoceptor agonist
   (a) Metabolism of fats & glycogen
   (b) Insulin secretion is inhibited
   (c) Stimulation of lipolysis
   (d) All the above

136. p2 agonist used in the treatment of asthama
   (a) Salbutamol
   (b) Methoxamine
   (c) Terbutaline
   (d) Both a & c

137. Drug of choice in anaphylactic shock
   (a) Atropine
   (b) Acetylcholine
   (c) Adrenaline
   (d) Propranolol

138. Drug of choice in nasal decongestion
   (a) Adrenaline
   (b) Dobutamine
   (c) Ephedrine
   (d) Isoprenaline

139. a2 agonist used to treat hypertension
   (a) Clonidine
   (b) Adrenaline
   (c) Isoprenaline
   (d) Salbutamol

140. p2 agonist used in the treatment of premature labour
   (a) Salbutamol
   (b) Adrenaline
   (c) Propranolol
   (d) Methoxamine

141. a2 selective antagonist
   (a) Prazosin
   (b) Terazosin
   (c) Yohimbine
   (d) Phentolamine

142. a+ P antagonist
   (a) Labetalol
   (b) Carvedilol
   (c) Both a & b
   (d) Prazosin

143. Non-selective a-adrenoceptor antagonist
   (a) Phenoxybenzamine
   (b) Prazosin
   (c) Yohimbine
   (d) Ergotamine

144. Drug of choice for benign prostate hypertrophy
   (a) Tamsulosin
   (b) Prazosin
   (c) Doxazosin
   (d) Terazosin

145. Drug used in the treatment of pheochromocytoma
   (a) Phenoxybenzamine
   (b) Prazosin
   (c) Terazosin
   (d) Carvedilol

146. Excitatory neurotransmitter in the **CNS**
   (a) Glutamate
   (b) **GABA**
   (c) Glycine
   (d) ACh

147. Inhibitory neurotransmitter in the CNS
     (a) GABA
     (b) Glycine
     (c) Both a & b
     (d) Glutamate

148. GABA-A is a
     (a) Ligand gated ion channel
     (b) G-Protein couple receptor
     (c) Nuclear receptor
     (d) All the above

149. Prolactin release is inhibited & growth hormone release is stimulated by
     (a) Ach
     (b) Noradrenaline
     (c) Dopamine
     (d) GABA

150. 5HT-1A receptor agonist used in the treatment of anxiety
     (a) Buspirone
     (b) Ondansetron
     (c) Fluoxetine
     (d) Sumatriptan

151. Hypnotic drugs
     (a) Reduce anxiety & exert calming effect
     (b) Induce absence of sensation
     (c) Produce drowsiness, encourage the onset and maintenance of sleep
     (d) Increase anxiety

152. Which of the following agents used in the treatment of insomnia
     (a) Benzodiazepines
     (b) Imidazopyridines
     (c) Barbiturates
     (d) All the above

153. Select a hypnotic drug, which is imidazopyridine derivative
     (a) Pentobarbital
     (b) Temazepam
     (c) Zolpidem
     (d) Chloral hydrate

154. Which of the following hypnotic is absorbed slowly?
     (a) Phenobarbital
     (b) Temazepam
     (c) Zolpidem
     (d) Chloral hydrate

155. Which of the following hypnotic drugs increase the activity of hepatic drug metabolising enzyme systems?
     (a) Phenobarbital   (b) Zolpidem
     (c) Flurazepam   (d) Zaleplon

156. Hepatic microsomal drug-metabolising enzyme induction leads to
     (a) Barbiturate tolerance
     (b) Cumulative effects
     (c) Development of physical dependence
     (d) Hangover effects

157. Which of the following hypnotic is preferred for elderly patients?
     (a) Phenobarbital
     (b) Flurazepam
     (c) Temazepam
     (d) Secobarbital

158. Which of the following hypnotic used in patients with limited hepatic function?
    (a) Zolpidem
    (b) Amobarbital
    (c) Flurazepam
    (d) Pentobarbital

159. Indicate the mechanism of barbiturates?
    (a) Increase the duration of the GABA gated chloride channel openings
    (b) Directly activating chloride ion channels
    (c) Increasing the frequency of chloride channel opening events
    (d) All the above

160. Imidazopyridines are
    (a) Partial agonists at brain 5-HT1A receptors
    (b) Selective agonist of the Bz1 subtype of Bz receptors
    (c) Competitive antagonist of Bz receptors
    (d) Nonselective agonists of both Bz1 & Bz2 receptor

161. Which of the following hypnotic agent is competitive antagonist of Bz receptors
    (a) Flumazenil
    (b) Picrotoxin
    (c) Zolpidem
    (d) Temazepam

162. Barbiturates are being replaced by benzodiazepines because of
    (a) Low therapeutic index
    (b) Suppression of REM sleep
    (c) High potential of Physical dependence & abuse
    (d) All the above

163. Indicate the usual cause of death due to overdose of hypnotics?
    (a) Depression of the medullar respiratory centre
    (b) Hypothermia
    (c) Cerebral edema
    (d) All the above

164. MOA of antidepressants
    (a) Stabilisation of dopamine & -adrenergic receptors
    (b) Inhibition of the storage of serotonin & epinephrine in the vesicles of presynaptic nerve endings
    (c) Blocking Serotonin & adrenaline reuptake pumps
    (d) All the above

165. Which of the following antidepressant is an unselective MAO blocker & produces extremely long lasting inhibition of the enzyme
    (a) Moclobemide
    (b) Tranylocypramine
    (c) Selegiline
    (d) Fluxeotine

166. Indicate irreversible MAO inhibitor, which is a hydrazide derivative
    (a) Moclobemide
    (b) Selegiline
    (c) Tranylcypramine
    (d) Phenelzine

167. Which of the following MAO
     Inhibitor has amphetamine like
     activity & related to nor-hydrazine
     derivatives?
     (a) Phenelzine
     (b) Moclobemide
     (c) Tranylcypramine
     (d) All the above

168. Which synapses are involved in
     depression?
     (a) Dopaminergic synapses
     (b) Serotonergic synapses
     (c) Cholinergic synapses
     (d) All the above

169. Most dangerous pharmacodynamic
     interaction is between MAO
     inhibitors?
     (a) **SSRI**
     (b) Trycyclics
     (c) Sympathomimetics
     (d) All the above

170. Which of the following ANS effect
     is common for trycyclic
     antidepressants?
     (a) Antimuscarinic action
     (b) Antistomachic action
     (c) a-adrenoceptorreceptor
          blocking action
     (d) All the above

171. Indicate an effective antidepressant
     minimal autonomic toxicity
     (a) Amitriptyline
     (b) Fluoxetine
     (c) Imipramine
     (d) Doxepin

172. Which of the following tricyclic &
     heterocyclic antidepressants has
     greatest sedation?
     (a) Doxepin
     (b) Amitriptyline
     (c) Trazodone
     (d) All the above

173. Which of the following
     antidepressants has significant a-2
     adrenoceptor antagonism?
     (a) Amitriptyline
     (b) Nefazodone
     (c) Mirtazepine
     (d) Doxepin

174. Which of the following drug is least
     likely to be prescribed to patients
     with prostatic hypertrophy,
     glaucoma, coronary &
     cerebrovascular disease?
     (a) Amitriptyline
     (b) Paroxetine
     (c) Bupropion
     (d) Fluoxetine

175. Which of the following
     antidepressants are used for
     treatment of eating disorders
     especially buliemia?
     (a) Amitriptyline
     (b) Fluoxetine
     (c) Imipramine
     (d) Tranylcypramine

176. Most common mediated
     complication of alcohol abuse is
     (a) Liver failure including liver
          cirrhosis
     (b) Tolerance & Physical
          dependence

(c) Generalized symmetric peripheral nerve injury ataxia & dementia

(d) All the above

177. Effect of moderate consumption of alcohol on plasma lipoproteins is

(a) Raising serum levels of high density lipoproteins

(b) Increasing serum concentration of low density lipoproteins

(c) Decreasing the serum levels of high density lipoproteins

(d) All the above

178. Which of the following agents is an inhibitor of aldehyde dehydrogenase?

(a) Fomepizole

(b) Ethanol

(c) Disulfiram

(d) Naltrexone

179. Alcohol causes an acute increase in the local concentrations of

(a) Dopamine

(b) Opioid

(c) Serotonin

(d) All the above

180. The symptoms resulting from the combination of disulfiram & alcohol are

(a) Hypertensive crisis leading to cerebral ischemia & oedema

(b) Nausea & vomiting

(c) Respiratory depression & seizures

(d) Acute Psychotic reactions

181. The combination of disulfiram & ethanol leads to accumulation of

(a) Formaldehyde

(b) Acetate

(c) Formic acid

(d) Acetaldehyde

182. Indicate the specific modality of treatment for severe methanol poisoning?

(a) Dialysis to enhance removal of methanol

(b) Alkalinisation to counteract metabolic acidosis

(c) Suppression of metabolism by alcohol dehydrogenase to toxic products

(d) All the above

183. Which of the following agents may be used as an antidote for ethylene glycol & methanol poisoning?

(a) Disulfiram

(b) Fomepizol

(c) Naltrexone

(d) Amphetamine

184. The principal mechanism of fomepizole is associated with inhibition of

(a) Aldehyde dehydrogenase

(b) Acetylcholinesterase

(c) Alcohol dehydrogenase

(d) **MAO**

185. Which of the following CNS stimulants are the agents of selective effect?

(a) Analeptics

(b) General tonics

(c) Psychostimulants

(d) Actoprotectors

186. Which of the following agents belongs to psychostimulants?
    (a) Meridil
    (b) Camphor
    (c) Piracetam
    (d) Pantocrin

187. Indicate the nootropic agent
    (a) Sydnocarb
    (b) Eleuterococcus extracts
    (c) Fluoxetine
    (d) Piracetam

188. Actoprotectors are
    (a) Stimulators, improving physical efficiency
    (b) Cognition enhancers
    (c) Stimulants, raising non-specific resistance towards stresses
    (d) Agents, stimulating the vasomotor centres

189. Indicate the CNS stimulants which mitigate conditions of weakness or lack of tone within the entire organism or in particular organs?
    (a) Psychostimulants
    (b) Analeptics
    (c) General tonics
    (d) Antidepressants

190. General tone increasing drug, which is an animal origin?
    (a) Pantocrin
    (b) Amphetamine
    (c) Sydnocarb
    (d) Camphor

191. CNS stimulant, which is a piperidine derivative
    (a) Meridil
    (b) Amphetamine
    (c) Caffeine
    (d) Sydnophen

192. Which of the following psychostimulants acts centrally mainly by blocking adenosine receptors?
    (a) psychostimulants
    (b) Caffeine
    (c) Amphetamine
    (d) Sydnophen

193. Caffeine can produce all of the following effect except?
    (a) Coronary vasodilation
    (b) Relaxation of bronchial & biliary tract smooth muscles
    (c) Vasodilation of cerebral vessels
    (d) Reinforcement of the contractions & increase of the striated muscle work

194. Therapeutic uses of caffeine include all of the following except
    (a) Cardiovascular collapse & respiratory insufficiency
    (b) Migraine
    (c) Somnolence
    (d) Gastric ulceration

195. Principal properties of cordiamine include all of the following except
    (a) Cardiac analeptic
    (b) Respiratory analeptic
    (c) Coronary dilator
    (d) Significant abuse potential

196. Cordiamine is useful in the treatment of
    (a) Hypotension
    (b) Coronary insufficiency
    (c) Respiratory insufficiency
    (d) All the above

197. Bemegride
    (a) Stimulates the medullar respiratory centre
    (b) Stimulates chemoreceptor of the carotid sinus zone
    (c) Is a mixed agent
    (d) Is a spinal analeptic

198. Which of the following CNS stimulants belongs to nootropics?
    (a) Camphor   (b) Pantocrin
    (c) Sydnocarb   (d) Piracetam

199. Piracetam can produce all of the following effects except
    (a) Antipsychotic
    (b) Anticonvulsant
    (c) Psychometabolic
    (d) Antihypoxic

200. Piracetam widely used for the treatment of
    (a) Senile dementia
    (b) Asthenia
    (c) Chronic alcoholism
    (d) All the above

201. Indicate the CNS stimulant which is used in pediatric medicine, as it im_proves the communication with the child, increases the ability to study and communication with peers, improves school performance?

    (a) Meridil
    (b) Piracetam
    (c) Bemegride
    (d) Amphetamine

202. Which of the following CNS stimulants is used for the cerebral stroke treatment?
    (a) Pantocrin
    (b) Sydnocarb
    (c) Piracetam
    (d) Caffeine

203. Psychologic dependence is
    (a) Decrease response to a drug following repeated exposure
    (b) A combination of certain drugs-specific sy_{mp}toms that occur on sudden discontinuation of drug
    (c) Co_{mp}ulsive drug seeking behaviour
    (d) None

204. Substances causing narco & glue sniffings are all of the following except
    (a) Stimulants
    (b) Antipsychotic drugs
    (c) Psychedelics
    (d) Sedative drugs

205. Which of the following abused drugs do not belong to sedative agents?
    (a) Barbiturates
    (b) Tranquilisers
    (c) Cannabinoids
    (d) Opioids

206. In contrast to morphine heroin is
 (a) Used clinically
 (b) More addictive & fast acting
 (c) More effective orally
 (d) Less potent & long acting

207. Sedative hypnotic agent, which has the highest abuse potential
 (a) Buspirone   (b) Diazepam
 (c) Phenobarbitol   (d) Zolpidem

208. Which one of the following tranquilizers belongs to strong euphorizing agents?
 (a) Mebicarum
 (b) Buspirone
 (c) Diazepam
 (d) Chlordiazepoxide

209. Which of the following abused drug is related to stimulants?
 (a) Cocaine
 (b) Amphetamine
 (c) Caffeine
 (d) All the above

210. Cocaine exerts its central actions by
 (a) Inhibiting Phosphodiesterase
 (b) Increasing the release of catecholamine neurotransmitters, including dopamine
 (c) Inhibiting dopamine & norepinephrine reuptake
 (d) Altering serotonin turnover

211. Crack is derivative of
 (a) Opium   (b) LSD
 (c) Cocaine   (d) Cannabis

212. Overdoses of cocaine are usually rapidly fatal form
 (a) Respiratory depression
 (b) Arrhythmias
 (c) Seizures
 (d) All the above

213. LSD decreases in brain
 (a) 5-HT2 receptor densities
 (b) GABA-A benzodiazepine receptor densities
 (c) Adrenergic receptor densities
 (d) D2-Receptor densities

214. The early stage of cannabis intoxication is characterised by
 (a) Euphoria, uncontrolled laugher
 (b) Alteration of the time sense, depersonalisation
 (c) Sharpened vision
 (d) All the above

215. Which of the following physiological signs is a characteristic of cannabis intoxication?
 (a) Bradycardia
 (b) Reddening of the convective
 (c) Miosis
 (d) Nausea & vomiting

216. MOA of anti-seizure drug is
 (a) Enhancement of GABAergic transmission
 (b) Inhibition of Glutaminergic transmission
 (c) Modification of ionic conductance
 (d) All the above

217. Which of the following anti-seizure drugs produces enhancement of GABA-mediated inhibition?
    (a) Ethosuximide
    (b) Carbamazepine
    (c) Phenobarbitol
    (d) Lamotrigine

218. Indicate an anti-seizure drug, which has an impotent effect on the T-type of calcium channels in thalamic neurons
    (a) Carbamazepine
    (b) Lamotrigine
    (c) Ethosuximide
    (d) Phenytoin

219. Anti-epileptic drug inhibiting central effects of excitatory amino acids
    (a) Ethosuximide
    (b) Lamotrigine
    (c) Diazepam
    (d) Tiagabine

220. The drug for partial & generalized tonic-clonic seizures is
    (a) Carbamazepine
    (b) Valproate
    (c) Phenytoin
    (d) All the above

221. Indicate an anti-absence drug
    (a) Valproate
    (b) Phenobarbital
    (c) Carbamazepine
    (d) Phenytoin

222. The drug against Myoclonic seizure is
    (a) Primidone

    (b) Carbamazepine
    (c) Clonazepam
    (d) Phenytoin

223. Most effective drug for stopping generalized tonic-clonic status epilepticus in adults is
    (a) Lamotrigine
    (b) Ethosuximide
    (c) Diazepam
    (d) Zonisamide

224. Phenytoin is used in the treatment of
    (a) Petitmal epilepsy
    (b) Grandmal epilepsy
    (c) Myoclonic seizures
    (d) All the above

225. Anti-epileptic drug which induces hepatic microsomal enzymes
    (a) Lamotrigine   (b) Phenytoin
    (c) Valproate   (d) None

226. Which of the following anti-epileptic drug is also effective in treating trigeminal neuralgia?
    (a) Primidone
    (b) Topiramate
    (c) Carbamazepine
    (d) Lamotrigine

227. Drug of choice for status epilepticus in infants
    (a) Phenobarbital sodium
    (b) Clonazepam
    (c) Ethosuximide
    (d) Phenytoin

228. Which of the following anti-seizure drug binds to allosteric regulatory site on GABA-Bz receptor increases the duration of chloride channel opening?
    (a) Diazepam
    (b) Valproate
    (c) Phenobarbital
    (d) Topiramate

229. Which of the following anti-seizure drug is a pro-drug metabolised to phenobarbital
    (a) Phenytoin
    (b) Primidone
    (c) Felbamate
    (d) Vigabatrine

230. The anti-seizure drug which is a phenyl triazine derivative
    (a) Phenobarbital
    (b) Clonazepam
    (c) Lamotrigine
    (d) Carbamazepine

231. Irreversible inhibitor of GABA aminotransferase (GABA-T)
    (a) Diazepam
    (b) Phenobarbital
    (c) Vigabatrin
    (d) Felbamate

232. Mechanism of action both topiramate & felbamate is
    (a) Reduction of excitatory glutaminergic neurotransmission
    (b) Inhibition of voltage sensitive Na^+ channels
    (c) Potentiation of GABAergic neuronal transmission
    (d) All the above

233. Drug of choice for petitmal epilepsy (Absence seizures)
    (a) Phenytoin
    (b) Ethosuximide
    (c) Phenobarbital
    (d) Carbamazepine

234. Drug of choice for the treatment of myoclonic seizure is
    (a) Valproate
    (b) Phenobarbital
    (c) Phenytoin
    (d) Felbamate

235. Reason for preferring ethosuximide to valproate for uncomplicated absence seizure is
    (a) More effective
    (b) Valproate's idiosyncratic
    (c) Greater CNS depressant activity
    (d) All the above

236. Anti-epileptic drug which is a sulfonamide derivative blocking Na^+ channels & having additional ability to inhibit T-type Ca^{2+} channels
    (a) Tiagabine
    (b) Zonisamide
    (c) Ethosuximide
    (d) Primidone

237. Long acting drug against both absence & myoclonic seizure is
    (a) Primidone
    (b) Carbamazepine
    (c) Clonazepam
    (d) Phenytoin

238. Which of the following anti-epileptic drug may produce teratogenicity?
(a) Phenytoin
(b) Valproate
(c) Topiramate
(d) All the above

239. Most dangerous effect of anti-seizure drug after large overdose is
(a) Respiratory Depression
(b) GI irritation
(c) Alopecia
(d) Sedation

240. Hormone released by anterior pituitary which is inhibited by dopamine release
(a) Growth Hormone
(b) Prolactin
(c) ACTH
(d) TSH

241. Hormone secreted by posterior pituitary has action on uterus
(a) Vasopressin   (b) Oxytocin
(c) Both a & b   (d) None

242. Hormone released by pancreas which decreases blood glucose level
(a) Somatostatin   (b) Glucagon
(c) Insulin   (d) b & c

243. Hormone released by pancreas and co secreted with insulin
(a) Glucagon
(b) Somatostatin
(c) Somatotropin
(d) Amylin

244. Pancreatic hormone which inhibit the release of insulin & glucagon?
(a) Somatotropin
(b) Amylin
(c) Both a & b
(d) Somatostatin

245. Actions of Insulin
(a) Increase glucose uptake
(b) Increase protein synthesis
(c) Increase fat synthesis
(d) All the above

246. Due to the deficiency of insulin resulting from auto-immune destruction of -cells cause
(a) Type I diabetes
(b) Type-II diabetes
(c) Juvenile onset diabetes
(d) Both a & c

247. Glucose enters into the   cells via the transport
(a) Glut-2
(b) Na^+-k^+ ATPase
(c) ion channels
(d) None

248. Second generation sulphonyl ureas?
(a) Glipizides
(b) Biguanides
(c) Glitazones
(d) All the above

249. Lactic acidosis is the adverse effect of following drugs?
(a) Sulphonyl ureas
(b) Biguanides
(c) Glitazones
(d) All the above

250. Hepatotoxicity is the adverse effect of following drugs
    (a) Sulphonyl ureas
    (b) Biguanides
    (c) Glitazones
    (d) All the above

251. Mechanism of sulphonyl ureas & meglitinide analogues?
    (a) Increase the uptake of glucose by muscles
    (b) Inhibition of a-glucosidase
    (c) Block K-ATP channels
    (d) Binds to PPARy leads to insulin signalling

252. Rosiglitazone act by
    (a) Block K-ATP channels
    (b) Increase the uptake of glucose by muscles
    (c) Inhibition of a-glucosidase
    (d) Binds to PPARy leads to insulin signal and release

253. Calcium homeostasis regulated by following substance
    (a) Parathyroid hormone
    (b) VitaminD
    (c) Calcitonin
    (d) All the above

254. Etidronate belongs
    (a) Biguanides
    (b) Sulphonyl ureas
    (c) Bisphosphonates
    (d) All the above

255. Example for nitrogen containing bisphosphonate?
    (a) Alendronate
    (b) Residronate

    (c) Zoledronate
    (d) All the above

256. Food absorption is impaired by following calcium homeostatic drug?
    (a) Parathyroid hormone
    (b) Calcitonin
    (c) Calcitriol
    (d) Residronate

257. Peptic ulcer is the adverse effect of below calcium homeostatic drug?
    (a) Calcitriol
    (b) Salcatonin
    (c) Etidronate
    (d) None

258. Hormone released from th$_y$$_r$oid gland action on calcium homeostasis?
    (a) Thyroxine
    (b) Trilodothyronin
    (c) Calcitonin
    (d) All the above

259. Modified version of growth hormone prepared by recombinant DNA technology acts as antagonist?
    (a) Somatotropin
    (b) Pegvisomant
    (c) Bromocriptine
    (d) None

260. Posterior lobe of pituitary gland connected to hypothalamus by
    (a) Pars tuberralis
    (b) Pars intemedia
    (c) Infundibulaer stalk
    (d) Adenohypophysis

261. The stimulating factors for pituitary hormones are released from
    (a) Thalamus
    (b) Hypothalamus
    (c) Cerebellum
    (d) Cerebrum

262. Insulin like growth factors is stimulated by following anterior pituitary hormone?
    (a) Somatotropin
    (b) Somatostatin
    (c) Adrenocorticotropic hormone
    (d) Prolactin

263. Pituitary hormone stimulates the release of glucocorticoids & mineralocorticoids?
    (a) Adrenocorticotropic hormone
    (b) TSH
    (c) Prolactin
    (d) Oxytocin

264. Thyroid stimulating hormone stimulates the release of
    (a) Growth hormone
    (b) calcitonin
    (c) Aldosterone
    (d) Cortisone

265. Skin darkening is depends on the following stimulating hormone of anterior pitutary
    (a) Thyroid stimulating hormone
    (b) Melanocyte stimulating hormone
    (c) ACTH
    (d) Prolactin

266. Gonadal stimulating hormones released by anterior pituitary is/are
    (a) FSH
    (b) LH
    (c) Both a & b
    (d) None

267. ADH is released from
    (a) Anterior pituitary
    (b) Posterior pitutary
    (c) Both a & b
    (d) None

268. Control of water content in the body action is showed by
    (a) ADH
    (b) Oxytocin
    (c) LH
    (d) FSH

269. Hyperprolactinemia is treated by
    (a) Somatropin
    (b) Bromocriptine
    (c) Pegvisomant
    (d) Desmopressin

270. ADH deficiency leads to
    (a) Diabetes mellitus
    (b) Diabetes insipidus
    (c) Diabetic coma
    (d) Diabetic ketoacidosis

271. ADH release is stimulated by following conditions except?
    (a) Increase in plasma osmolarity
    (b) Decrease in plasma osmolarity
    (c) Decrease in blood volume
    (d) Angiotensin release

272. ADH receptors are
    (a) GPCRs
    (b) Ligand gated
    (c) Kinase linked
    (d) Nuclear receptors

273. ADH has more affinity to the following receptor subtype
    (a) V1
    (b) V2
    (c) V3
    (d) None

274. V2 selective agonist
    (a) Vasopressin
    (b) Desmopressin
    (c) Telipressin
    (d) Felypressin

275. ADH receptor agonist short acting vasoconstrictor injected with local anaesthetic prilocaine to prolong the action
    (a) Vasopressin
    (b) Felypressin
    (c) Desmopressin
    (d) Telipressin

276. Hormones released from adrenal gland are clinically used as anti-inflammatory & Immunosuppressant?
    (a) Mineralocorticoids
    (b) Glucocorticoids
    (c) Androgens
    (d) Aldosterone

277. Adrenal gland hormone action on water & electrolyte balance
    (a) Cortisone
    (b) Hydrocortisone
    (c) Aldosterone
    (d) Testosterone

278. Actions of aldosterone except
    (a) Increase sodium reabsorption
    (b) Decrease sodium reabsorption
    (c) Increase Potassium excretion
    (d) Increase water reabsorption

279. Competitive antagonist of aldosterone?
    (a) Hydrocortisone
    (b) Spiranolactone
    (c) Acetazolamide
    (d) None

280. Antiandrogen used to treat prostatic cancer
    (a) Flutamide
    (b) Cyproterone
    (c) Finasteride
    (d) All the above

281. Iodide is transported to thyroid follicle by the transporter?
    (a) Na^+-K^+ ATP ase
    (b) Na^+/r symporter
    (C) r/Cl- transporter
    (d) Both b & c

282. Mechanism of thioureylenes?
    (a) Inhibition of Iodination of tyrosyl residues
    (b) Inhibition of thyroperoxidase
    (c) Deiodination of T_4 to T_3
    (d) All the above

283. Granulocytopenia is the adverse effect of following antithyroid drug?
    (a) Iodide
    (b) Carbimazole
    (c) Prednisone
    (d) Guanethidine

284. Synthetic estrogen
    (a) Diethylstilbestrol
    (b) Mestranol
    (c) Ethinyl estradiol
    (d) All the above

285. Adverse effect of diethylstilbestrol
    (a) Nausea
    (b) Headache
    (c) Ovarian cancer
    (d) Oedema

286. Important adverse effect of oestrogens?
    (a) Thromboembolism
    (b) Nausea
    (c) Vomiting
    (d) Oedema

287. Partial agonist of progesterone receptors
    (a) Miafepristone
    (b) Clomiphene
    (c) Tamoxifen
    (d) Raloxifene

288. Antifungal agent inhibits steroidogenesis?
    (a) Ketoconazole
    (b) Amphotericin
    (c) Nystatin
    (d) Griseofulvin

289. Moon face Fish mouth is caused by
    (a) Mineralocorticoids
    (b) Androgens
    (c) Glucocorticoids
    (d) All the above

290. Actions of glucocorticoid except
    (a) Promote lipolysis
    (b) Promote glycogen deposition in liver
    (c) Inhibit the absorption of calcium
    (d) Decrease heart rate

291. Gluco-corticoids are used in the treatment of
    (a) Rheumatoid arthritis
    (b) Asthama
    (c) Leukaemia
    (d) All the above

292. Short acting insulin preparation
    (a) Isophane insulin
    (b) Regular Insulin
    (c) Protamine zinc insulin
    (d) Extended insulin zn preparation

293. Long action insulin preparation?
    (a) Isophane insulin
    (b) Regular insulin
    (c) Protamine zinc insulin
    (d) Extended insulin zn preparation

294. Type-I diabetes is treated by
    (a) Insulin preparations
    (b) Biguanides
    (c) Sulphonyl ureas
    (d) None

295. Gastric emptying is delayed by following pancreatic hormone
    (a) Insulin   (b) Glucagon
    (C) Amylin   (d) Somatostatin

296. Precursor for the synthesis of insulin
    (a) Pre-proinsulin   (b) Proinsulin
    (c) Isophane   (d) None

297. A chain of insulin consist of
    (a) 21 amino acid residues
    (b) 30 amino acid residues

(c) 20 amino acid residues
(d) 32 amino acid residues

298. In insulin receptors following unit consist of insulin binding site
(a) a-subunit
(b) B-subunit
(c) y-subunit
(d) All the above

299. Insulin receptors are
(a) Ligand gated ion channels
(b) GPCRs
(c) Kinase linked receptors
(d) Nuclear Receptors

300. Deficiency of Insulin resulting from auto immune destruction of Beta cells called as
(a) Type-I Diabetes
(b) Type-II Diabetes
(c) Both a & b
(d) None

301. Insulin injections are used in the treatment of
(a) Type-I Diabetes
(b) Type-II Diabetes
(c) Juvenile onset diabetes
(d) Both a & c

302. a-glucosidase inhibitor
(a) Miglitol
(b) Pioglitazone
(c) Metformin
(d) Glipizide

303. Parasympathetic innervation cause
(a) Bronchoconstriction
(b) Broncho-relaxation
(c) Dilation of the bronchi
(d) None

304. Receptors involved in bronchial constriction of parasympathetic system
(a) M1
(b) M2
(c) M3
(d) M4

305. Mediators in asthama pathogenesis are
(a) Leukotriene B4
(b) Cysteinyl leukotrienes
(c) Interleukins
(d) All the above

306. First line drugs used in the treatment of asthama
(a) Cysteinyl leukotrienes
(b) Xanthine drugs
(c) B-adrenoceptor receptor agonists
(d) Muscarinic receptor antagonists

307. Symptoms of asthama
(a) Wheezing
(b) Cough
(c) Difficulty in breathing
(d) All the above

308. Mediators involved in the asthama
(a) T-lymphocytes
(b) Eosinophils
(c) IgE
(d) All the above

309. Which of the following is Spasmogens?
(a) Histamine
(b) Cysteinyl leukotrienes
(c) Prostaglandin D2
(d) All the above

310. Important mediators for asthama in both phases
    (a) Leukotrienes
    (b) Chemo toxins
    (c) Chemokines
    (d) All the above

311. Which of the following are antiasthmatic drugs except?
    (a) Salmeterol
    (b) Theophylline
    (c) Salbutamol
    (d) Propranolol

312. Short acting anti-asthmatic drug belongs to P2-adrenoceptor agonist?
    (a) Salmeterol
    (b) Formoterol
    (c) Salbutamol
    (d) Pirbuterol

313. Which of the following are inhalational antiasthmatic drugs except?
    (a) Salbutamol
    (b) Terbutaline
    (c) Salmeterol
    (d) Montelukast

314. Following P-adrenoceptor antagonist cause severe bronchoconstriction
    (a) Propranolol
    (b) Salbutamol
    (c) Salmeterol
    (d) All the above

315. Theophylline ethylene diamine is also known as
    (a) Caffeine

(b) Xanthine
(c) Aminophylline
(d) None

316. Second line drugs used to treat asthama
    (a) Cysteinyl leukotrienes
    (b) Xanthine drugs
    (c) P-antagonists
    (d) Muscarinic antagonists

317. Action of xanthine drugs on heart
    (a) Positive inotropic effect
    (b) Positive chronotropic effect
    (c) Both a & b
    (d) Negative inotropic effect

318. Action of P2 agonist
    (a) Branchodilation
    (b) Bronchoconstriction
    (c) Both a & b
    (d) None

319. Mechanism of xanthine drugs
    (a) Inhibition of phosphodiesterase
    (b) Relaxant effect of smooth muscle
    (c) Increase in cAMP
    (d) All the above

320. Adverse effect of xanthine drugs
    (a) Anorexia
    (b) Nervousness
    (c) Tremor
    (d) All the above

321. Muscarinic receptor antagonist used in the treatment of asthama?
    (a) Atropine
    (b) Hyoscine

(c) Ipratropium
(d) Scopolamine

322. Zafirlukast is
  (a)   agonist
  (b) Xanthine agonist
  (c) Cysteinyl leukotriene antagonist
  (d) Cysteinyl leukotriene agonist

323. Asprin sensitive asthama, exercise induced asthama is treated by
  (a)   2 agonist
  (b) Xanthine drugs
  (c) Muscarinic antagonists
  (d) Cysteinyl leukotriene antagonist

324. Action of cysteinyl leukotrienes
  (a) Relax airways in mild asthama
  (b) Bronchodilator activity
  (c) Reduce sputum eosinophilia
  (d) All the above

325. Adverse effect of cysteinyl leukotrienes
  (a) Headache
  (b) GI disturbances
  (c) Churg-strauss syndrome
  (d) All the above

326. Action of gluco-corticoids
  (a) Decrease formation of cytokines
  (b) Inhibit generation of vasodilators PGE2 & 12
  (c) Both a & b
  (d) None

327. All of the following drugs used in the treatment of asthama except
  (a) Beclomethasone

(b) Budesonide
(c) Fluticasone
(d) Prednisolone

328. Oropharyngeal candidiasis is the adverse effect of following antiasthmatic drugs
  (a) Loratadine
  (b) Beclomethasone
  (c) Aminophylline
  (d) Montelukast

329. Mechanism of Cromoglyclate
  (a) Mast cell stabilizer- prevent histamine release
  (b) Inhibition of PGE2 & 12
  (c) Both a & b
  (d) None

330. Unwanted effect of cromoglylate
  (a) Hypersensitivity reactions
  (b) Nausea
  (c) Vomiting
  (d) Headache

331. All of the following are respiratory diseases except
  (a) COPD   (b) CAD
  (c) Emphysema (d) Asthma

332. Destruction and damage of lung tissue is called as
  (a) COPD
  (b) Emphysema
  (c) CAD
  (d) None

333. Drug used in the treatment of both asthama & COPD
  (a) Ipratropium
  (b) Propranolol

    (c) Atropine
    (d) All the above

334. Drugs used to treat cough
    (a) Codeine
    (b) Dextromethorphan
    (c) Phalcodeine
    (d) All the above

335. Actions of codeine
    (a) Decreases secretions of bronchioles
    (b) Thicknesses the sputum and inhibit ciliary activity
    (c) Reduce the clearance of thickened sputum
    (d) All the above

336. Adverse effect of codeine
    (a) Constipation   (b) Diarrhoea
    (c) Nausea   (d) Vomiting

337. Synthetic narcotic analgesic used to treat cough
    (a) Dextromethorphan
    (b) Dexamethasone
    (c) Dacarbazine
    (d) Daunorubicin

338. Opioid analogues suppress cough by action via
    (a) u receptors
    (b) K receptors
    (c) 8 receptors
    (d) None

339. Non glycoside positive inotropic drug is
    (a) Digoxin
    (b) Strophantin K
    (c) Dobutamine
    (d) Digitoxin

340. Aglycone is essential for
    (a) Plasma protein binding
    (b) Half life
    (c) Cardiotonic action
    (d) Metabolism

341. Following drugs are used to treat initial stages of treating patients with heart failure except?
    (a) Verapamil
    (b) ACE inhibitors
    (c) Reduced salt intake
    (d) Diuretics

342. Glycone part in cardiac glycoside influence
    (a) Cardiotonic action
    (b) Pharmacokinetic properties
    (c) Toxic properties
    (d) All the above

343. Following statements are true about cardiac glycosides except?
    (a) They inhibit the Na^+/K^+ ATPase & thereby increase the intracellular Ca^{2+} in myocardial cells
    (b) They cause decrease in vagal tone
    (c) Children tolerate higher doses of digitalis than do adults
    (d) The most frequent cause of digitalis intoxication- administration of diuretics; deplete K^+

344. False statement about digoxin?
    (a) Digoxin is a mild inotrope
    (b) Digoxin increases vagal tone

(c) Has longer half life then digitoxin

(d) Acts by inhibiting Na^+/K^+ ATPase

345. Following drug is used in the treatment of digitalis intoxication
(a) Lidocaine
(b) Digibind
(c) Oral K^+ supplementation
(d) Reduce the dose of drug

346. Drug of choice for digitalis induced arrhythmias?
(a) Verapamil
(b) Amiodarone
(c) Lidocaine
(d) Propranolol

347. Selective B1 agonist
(a) Digoxin
(b) Dobutamine
(c) Amrinone
(d) Dopamine

348. Tolerance is developed with the following inotropic drug after few days?
(a) Amrinone
(b) Amiodarone
(c) Dobutamine
(d) Adenosine

349. Which of the following drug inhibit the breakdown of cAMP in vascular smooth muscle?
(a) Digoxin
(b) Dobutamine
(c) Amrinone
(d) Dopamine

350. This drug is useful for treating heart failure, because it increases the inotropic state and reduces after load?
(a) Amiodarone   (b) Amrinone
(c) Propranolol   (d) Enalapril

351. This drug act by inhibiting Type-III cyclic nucleotide phosphodiesterase
(a) Amiodarone   (b) Milrinone
(c) Propranolol   (d) Enalapril

352. All of the following drugs are used in the treatment of congestive heart failure except
(a) Verapamil
(b) Digoxin
(c) Dobutamine
(d) Dopamine

353. Drugs most commonly used in congestive heart failure except
(a) Cardiac glycosides
(b) Diuretics
(c) ACE Inhibitors
(d) All the above

354. Following effects of ACE inhibitors are useful in treating heart except
(a) They decrease after load
(b) They increase circulating catecholamines
(c) They reduce reactive myocardial hypertrophy
(d) They increase myocardial B-adreno receptor density.

355. Which of the following drug prolongs repolarization?
(a) Flecainide
(b) Sotalol

(c) Lidocaine
(d) Verapamil

356. Which of the following is class I A anti arrhythmic drug?
(a) Sotalol
(b) Propranolol
(c) Verapamil
(d) Quinidine

357. Which of the following drug is used to treat supra ventricular tachycardia
(a) Digoxin
(b) Dobutamine
(c) Amrinone
(d) Dopamine

358. Which of the following drug is associated with Torsade de pointes
(a) Flecainide
(b) Sotalol
(c) Lidocaine
(d) Verapamil

359. Which of the following drug has beta adrenergic receptor blocking activity?
(a) Flecainide
(b) Sotalol
(c) Lidocaine
(d) Verapamil

360. Drug used in terminating atrial but not ventricular tachycardia
(a) Flecainide
(b) Sotalol
(c) Lidocaine
(d) Verapamil

361. Drug of choice for treatment of ventricular tachycardia
(a) Flecainide
(b) Sotalol
(c) Lidocaine
(d) Verapamil

362. Drugs contraindicated in patients with moderate to severe heart failure
(a) Flecainide
(b) Nifedipine
(c) Verapamil
(d) Both b & c

363. Drugs with effective branchodilation action?
(a) Nifedipine
(b) Verapamil
(c) Both a & b
(d) None

364. Which of the following drug is used intravenously to treat supraventricular tachycardias?
(a) Nifedipine
(b) Verapamil
(c) Both a & b
(d) None

365. Drug no direct effect on chronotropy & dromotropy at normal doses
(a) Nifedipine
(b) Diltiazem
(c) Verapamil
(d) All the above

366. Drugs acts by inhibiting slow calcium channels in SA & AV nodes
     (a) Quinidine
     (b) Adenosine
     (c) Flecainide
     (d) Diltiazem

367. Following statements regarding the verapamil are correct except?
     (a) It Blocks L-type of calcium channels
     (b) It increases heart rate
     (c) It relaxes coronary artery smooth muscle
     (d) It depresses cardiac contractility

368. Calcium channel blockers useful in treatment of cardiac arrhythmias except
     (a) Bepridil
     (b) Diltiazem
     (c) Verapamil
     (d) Nifedipine

369. Adverse effect of calcium channel blockers except?
     (a) Skeletal muscle weakness
     (b) Dizziness
     (c) Headache
     (d) Flushing

370. Lidocaine adverse effect
     (a) Agranulocytosis, leucopenia
     (b) Extrapyramidal disorders
     (c) Hypotension, paresthesias, convulsions
     (d) Brancho spasm, dyspepsia

371. Which of the following nitrates & nitrite drugs are long acting?
     (a) Nitroglycerin, sublingual
     (b) Isosorbide dinitrate, sublingual
     (c) Amyl nitrite, inhalant
     (d) Sustac

372. Which of the following nitrates & nitrite drugs are short acting?
     (a) Nitroglycerin, sublingual
     (b) Isosorbide dinitrate, sublingual
     (c) Amyl nitrite, inhalant
     (d) Sustac

373. Duration of nitroglycerin (sublingual) is
     (a) 10-30 min   (b) 6-8 hrs
     (c) 3-5 min   (d) 1.5-2 hrs

374. Mechanism of nitrate except?
     (a) Decreased myocardial oxygen requirement
     (b) Relief of coronary artery spasm
     (c) Improved perfusion to ischaemic myocardium
     (d) Increased myocardial oxygen consumption

375. Side effect of nitrates except?
     (a) Orthostatic hypotension, tachycardia
     (b) GI disturbance
     (c) Throbbing headache
     (d) Tolerance

376. Which of the following antianginal agents is calcium channel blocker?
     (a) Nitro-glycerine
     (b) Dipyridamole
     (c) Minoxidil
     (d) Nifedipine

377. Main clinical use of calcium channel blockers
     (a) Angina pectoris
     (b) Hypertension
     (c) Supraventricular tachycardia
     (d) All the above

378. Which of the following anti-anginal agent is myotropic coronary dilator?
     (a) Dipyridamole   (b) Validol
     (c) Atenolol   (d) Alindine

379. Which of the following anti-anginal agent s are P-adrenoceptor blocking drugs?
     (a) Dipyridamole   (b) Validol
     (c) Atenolol   (d) Alindine

380. Drugs reflex coronary dilators?
     (a) Dipyridamole   (b) Validol
     (c) Atenolol   (d) Alindine

381. Which of the following anti-anginal agent is the specific bradycardia drug?
     (a) Dipyridamole   (b) Validol
     (c) Atenolol   (d) Alindine

382. Which of the following anti-anginal agent is potassium channel opener?
     (a) Dipyridamole   (b) Validol
     (c) Atenolol   (d) Minoxidil

383. Drugs reduce the blood pressure by acting on vasomotor centres in CNS
     (a) Labetolol
     (b) Clonidine
     (c) Enalapril
     (d) Nifedipine

384. Central acting anti-hypertensive drug except?
     (a) Methyl-dopa   (b) Clonidine
     (c) Moxonidine   (d) Minoxidil

385. Ganglionic blocking drug for hypertension treatment
     (a) Hydralazine
     (b) Tubocurarine
     (c) Trimethaphan
     (d) Metoprolol

386. Which of the following is sympatholythic drug?
     (a) Labetolol   (b) Prazosin
     (c) Guanethidine   (d) Clonidine

387. Drug with non-selective P-adrenoblocking activity
     (a) Atenolol
     (b) Propranolol
     (c) Metoprolol
     (d) Nebivolol

388. Selective blockers of Pl adrenoceptors?
     (a) Labetalol
     (b) Prazosin
     (c) Atenolol
     (d) Propranolol

389. a, p adrenoceptor blockers used as antih$_{y\,p}$ertensive drug?
     (a) Labetalol
     (b) Verapamil
     (c) Nifedipine
     (d) Metoprolol

390. Directly acting vasodilator?
     (a) Labetalol
     (b) Clonidine

(c) Enalapril

(d) Nifedipine

391. Diuretic agent for treatment of hypertension?

(a) Losartan

(b) Dichlothiazide

(c) Captopril

(d) Prazosin

392. Antihypertensive drug blocks a1-adrenergic receptors?

(a) Prazosin

(b) Clonidine

(c) Enalapril

(d) Nifedipine

393. Anti-hypertensive drug activates a2 adrenergic receptors?

(a) Labetolol

(b) Phentolamine

(c) Clonidine

(d) Enalapril

394. Non-peptide angiotensin II receptor antagonist?

(a) Clonidine   (b) Captopril

(c) Losartan   (d) Diazoxide

395. Potassium channel activator?

(a) Nifedipine   (b) Saralasin

(c) Diazoxide   (d) Losartan

396. Drug contraindicated in patients with bronchial asthama?

(a) Propranolol

(b) Clonidine

(c) Enlapril

(d) Nifedipine

397. Which of the following drug is converted into active metabolite after absorption?

(a) Labetalol

(b) Clonidine

(c) Enalapril

(d) Nifedipine

398. Which of the following drug produces some tachycardia?

(a) Propranolol

(b) Clonidine

(c) Enalapril

(d) Nifedipine

399. All of the following statements regarding vasodilators are true except?

(a) Hydralazine causes tachycardia

(b) Nifedipine is a dopamine receptor antagonist

(c) Nitroprusside dilates both arterioles

(d) Minoxidil can cause hypertrichosis

400. Actions of verapamil except?

(a) It blocks T-type of calcium channels

(b) It increases the heart rate

(c) It relaxes coronary artery smooth muscles

(d) It depresses cardiac contractility

401. Unwanted effect of clonidine

(a) Parkinson's syndrome

(b) Sedative & Hypnotic syndrome

(c) Agranulocytosis & aplastic anaemia

(d) Dry cough & respiratory depression

402. Reason of -blockers administration for h$_{yp}$ertension treatment is?
(a) Peripheral vasodilation
(b) Diminishing the blood volume
(c) Decreases of heart work
(d) Depression of vasomotor centre

403. Endogenous vasoconstrictor stimulates aldosterone release from glands?
(a) Angiotensinogen
(b) Angiotensin-I
(c) Angiotensin-11
(d) Angiotensin converting enzyme

404. Antihypertensive drug diminishes the metabolism of bradycardia?
(a) Ganglion blockers
(b) a-adrenoblockers
(c) Angiotensin-11
(d) ACE Inhibitors

405. Hydralazine can produce
(a) Seizures
(b) Tachycardia
(c) Hepatitis
(d) Aplastic anaemia

406. Vasodilator which releases **NO**
(a) Nifedipine
(b) Hydralazine
(c) Minoxidil
(d) Sodium nitroprusside

407. Diuretic agent aldosterone antagonist?
(a) Furosemide
(b) Spironolactone
(c) Dichlorothiazide
(d) Captopril

408. Diuretic agent having potent and rapid effect?
(a) Furosemide
(b) Spiranolactone
(c) Dichlorothiazide
(d) Indapamide

409. Hormone (Pancreatic) used in the treatment of congestive heart failure?
(a) Insulin
(b) Glucagon
(c) Somatostatin
(d) All the above

410. Increase K$^+$ ion concentration
(a) Decreases effect of cardiac glycosides
(b) Increases effect of cardiac glycosides
(c) No effect of cardiac glycosides
(d) None

411. Phosphodiesterase inhibitor used in the treatment of congestive heart failure?
(a) Amrinone
(b) Milrinone
(c) Both a & b
(d) Dobutamine

412. Digoxin excretion and tissue binding is reduced by
(a) Amiodarone
(b) Verapamil

(c) Both a & b

(d) Diltiazem

413. Angina characterized by paroxysmal pain in substemal or pericardial region of chest relieved by rest is called as
(a) Stable angina
(b) Unstable angina
(c) Variant angina
(d) None

414. Angina characterised by pain at rest
(a) Stable angina
(b) Unstable angina
(c) Variant angina
(d) None

415. Potassium channel activator
(a) Nifedipine
(b) Nicorandil
(c) Nebivolol
(d) All the above

416. Calcium channel blocker phenylalkylamines?
(a) Verapamil
(b) Nifedipine
(c) Diltiazem
(d) None

417. Following drug produce improve perfusion, reduce oxygen demand to the heart
(a) Glyceryl trinitrate
(b) Verapamil
(c) Both a & b
(d) CHF

418. P-blockers are used in the treatment of angina pectoris by the action
(a) Slow the heart rate and reduce the metabolic oxygen demand
(b) Increase heart rate and reduce oxygen demand
(c) Both a & b
(d) None

419. Antianginal action of nitrates involves
(a) Reduction of cardiac oxygen consumption by reducing preload & afterload
(b) Coronary flow towards ischaemic areas via collaterals
(c) Relief of coronary spasm
(d) All the above

420. Adverse effect of verapamil
(a) Constipation   (b) Vomiting
(c) Nausea   (d) Diarrhoea

421. Repeated administration of nitrates leads to diminished relaxation because
(a) Increase in SH groups
(b) Depletion of SH groups
(c) No change in SH groups
(d) None of the above

422. Ca^{2+} channel blocker action on both heart & smooth muscle?
(a) Verapamil
(b) Diltiazem
(c) Nifedipine
(d) Amlodipine

423. Following calcium channel blocking drug increase reflex tachycardia
    (a) Verapamil
    (b) Nifedipine
    (c) Diltiazem
    (d) All the above

424. Which of the following calcium channel blocking drug shows greater effect on smooth muscle?
    (a) Verapamil
    (b) Diltiazem
    (c) Nifedipine
    (d) All the above

425. Adverse effect of nifedipine
    (a) Headache
    (b) Flushing
    (c) Ankle swelling
    (d) All the above

426. Calcium channel blocking agent used in the treatment of hypertension?
    (a) Amlodipine
    (b) Propranolol
    (c) Glyceryl trinitrate

427. Vomiting is regulated by
    (a) Vomiting centre
    (b) Chemoreceptor trigger zone
    (c) Nucleus tractus
    (d) All the above

428. Blood brain barrier present beside
    (a) Vomiting centre
    (b) CTZ
    (c) NTS
    (d) Medulla oblongata

429. Neurotransmitters involved in the control of vomiting?
    (a) Ach & substance P
    (b) Histamine
    (c) Dopamine and 5-HT
    (d) All the above

430. Substance P is a
    (a) Muscarinic agonist
    (b) Neurokinin agonist
    (c) Neurokinin antagonist
    (d) Dopamine agonist

431. Neurokinin receptor antagonist used in the treatment of vomiting?
    (a) Cinnarizine
    (b) Aprepitant
    (c) Nabilone
    (d) Dolasetron

432. Sedation is main adverse effect of following antiemetic drug?
    (a) Cyclizine
    (b) Ondansetron
    (c) Atropine
    (d) Metoclopramide

433. Antiemetic drug used treat morning sickness in pregnancy?
    (a) Promethazine
    (b) Cyclizine
    (c) Cinnarizine
    (d) All of the above

434. Drug of choice for the treatment of motion sickness by NASA people
    (a) Ondansetron
    (b) Promethazine
    (c) Metoclopramide
    (d) Nabilone

435. Which of the following is vomiting inducing agent (emetics)
    (a) Ipecac
    (b) Apomorphine
    (c) Both a & b
    (d) None

436. Cisplatin induced vomiting is treated by
    (a) Ondansetron
    (b) Atropine
    (c) Metoclopramide
    (d) Hyoscine

437. Vomiting induced by radiation therapy in cancer treatment is treated with?
    (a) Muscarinic receptor antagonists
    (b) 5HT3 receptor antagonists
    (c) HI receptor antagonists
    (d) Dopamine receptor antagonists

438. Vomiting caused by vertigo and migraine is treated with
    (a) Muscarinic receptor antagonists
    (b) H1 receptor antagonists
    (c) Dopamine receptor antagonists
    (d) 5HT3 receptor antagonists

439. Tardive dyskinesia, dystonias are the adverse effect of following antiemetic drugs?
    (a) HI receptor antagonists
    (b) D2 receptor antagonists
    (c) 5HT3 receptor antagonists
    (d) All the above

440. Which of the following is/are prokinetic agent/agents?
    (a) Metoclopramide
    (b) Domperidone
    (c) Cisapride
    (d) All the above

441. Occulogyric crises (involuntary eye movement)are the adverse effect of?
    (a) Metoclopramide
    (b) Cisapride
    (c) Ondansetron
    (d) Nabilone

442. Prolactin release is stimulated by following antiemetic drug?
    (a) Metoclopramide
    (b) Cisapride
    (c) Ondansetron
    (d) Aprepitant

443. Galactorrhoea is the adverse effect of following antiemetic drug?
    (a) Nabilone
    (b) Granisetron
    (c) Metoclopramide
    (d) All the above

444. Hallucination is the adverse effect of following antiemetic drug?
    (a) Nabilone
    (b) Aprepitant
    (c) Cisapride
    (d) Granisetron

445. Following antiemetic drug have adverse effect of Cardiotoxicity?
    (a) Metoclopramide
    (b) Domperidone
    (c) Cisapride
    (d) Ondansetron

446. Semisynthetic disaccharide used as laxative?
    (a) Methyl cellulose
    (b) Lactulose
    (c) Sterculia
    (d) Bran

447. Salts used as laxatives (osmoti(c) except
    (a) Magnesium salts
    (b) Aluminium salts
    (c) Sodium salts
    (d) None

448. Action of bulk laxative is
    (a) Absorb water in intestine & increase water content in faeces
    (b) Promote peristalsis
    (c) Both a & b
    (d) None

449. Following osmotic laxatives are avoided in small children & patients with kidney diseases due to heart block adverse effect?
    (a) Aluminium salts
    (b) Magnesium salts
    (c) Sodium salts
    (d) All the above

450. Following laxatives shows their action by stimulating enteric nerves?
    (a) Lactulose   (b) Agar
    (c) Isapghol   (d) Bisacodyl

451. Anti-diarrhoeal drug which undergo enterohepatic circulation?
    (a) Morphine
    (b) Loperamide

    (c) Bismuth subsalicylate
    (d) Atropine

452. In addition to anti motility action the following drugs have ant secreting action?
    (a) Codeine & loperamide
    (b) Loperamide & diphenoxylate
    (c) Codeine & bismuth subsalicylate
    (d) Loperamide & bismuth subsalicylate

453. Diphenoxylate preparations contains additionally?
    (a) Codeine   (b) Atropine
    (c) Loperamide   (d) Charcoal

454. Paralytic ileus is the adverse effect of following antidiarrheal drugs?
    (a) Antimotility agents
    (b) Adsorbents
    (c) Both a & b
    (d) None

455. Blocking of faeces is the adverse effect of following anti-diarrhoeal drug?
    (a) Diphenoxylate
    (b) Codeine
    (c) Bismuth subsalicylate
    (d) Morphine

456. Action of adsorbents?
    (a) Adsorb microorganisms & toxins
    (b) Coating & protecting the intestinal mucosa
    (c) Adsorb excess fluids
    (d) All the above

457. Drugs causing gynaecomastia?
    (a) Omeprazole
    (b) Cimetidine
    (c) Metronidazole
    (d) Epoprosteno

458. Proglumide is
    (a) Gastrin agonist
    (b) Gastrin antagonist
    (c) Partial agonist
    (d) None

459. Antacids are used in combination with?
    (a) Alginates
    (b) Bismuth chelates
    (c) Simeticones
    (d) Both a & c

460. Which of the following causes belching effect?
    (a) Mg trisilicate
    (b) Aluminium hydroxide gel
    (c) NaHCO3
    (d) None

461. Which of the following is a component of a therapy of *Hpylori*?
    (a) Bismuth chelates
    (b) Aluminium hydroxide gel
    (c) NaHCO3
    (d) Mg trisilicate

462. Drug of choice for traveller's diarrhoea?
    (a) Tegaserod
    (b) Hyoscine
    (c) Loperamide
    (d) All the above

463. Which alkaloid is used in motion sickness?
    (a) Atropine
    (b) Hyoscine
    (c) Morphine
    (d) Caffeine

464. Spasmodic torticollis is unwanted effect of?
    (a) Domperidone
    (b) Metoclopramide
    (c) Haloperidol
    (d) Nabilone

465. The main approach of peptic ulcer treatment?
    (a) Neutralisation of gastric acid
    (b) Eradication of *H pylori*
    (c) Inhibition of gastric acid secretion
    (d) All the above

466. Gastric acid secretion is the under control of which of the following agents except?
    (a) Histamine   (b) Ach
    (c) Serotonin   (d) Gastrin

467. All of the following agents intensify the secretion of gastric glands except?
    (a) Pepsin   (b) Gastrin
    (c) Histamine   (d) Carbonate

468. Drug belonging Ml-receptor blocker?
    (a) Cimetidine
    (b) Ranitidine
    (c) Pirenzepine
    (d) Omeprazole

469. Drugs may cause reversible gynaecomastia?
    (a) Omeprazole
    (b) Pirenzepine
    (c) Cimetidine
    (d) Sucralfate

470. Select the drug forming a physical barrier to HCl and pepsin?
    (a) Ranitidine
    (b) Sucralfate
    (c) Pirenzepine
    (d) Omeprazole

471. Drug cause metabolic alkalosis
    (a) $NaHco_3$
    (b) Cimetidine
    (c) Carbenoxalate
    (d) Omeprazole

472. Antiulcer drug causes constipation?
    (a) $NaHco_3$
    (b) Al hydroxide
    (c) $CaCO_3$
    (d) Magnesium oxide

473. All of the following drugs stimulate appetite except?
    (a) Vitamins
    (b) Bitters
    (c) Fepranone
    (d) Insulin

474. Antiemetic drug belongs to neuroleptics?
    (a) Metoclopramide
    (b) Nabilone
    (c) Tropisetron
    (d) Prochlorperazine

475. Mechanism of stimulant purgative?
    (a) Increasing the volume of non absorbable solid residue
    (b) Increasing motility
    (c) Altering the consistency of the faeces
    (d) Increasing the water content

476. Drug irritating the gut & causing increased peristalsis
    (a) Phenolphthalein
    (b) Methyl cellulose
    (c) Proserpine
    (d) Mineral oil

477. Following histamine receptors are involved in the ulcerogenesis?
    (a) HI   (b) H2
    (c) H3   (d) None

478. Following neurotransmitter is responsible for ulcer formation?
    (a) Nor adrenaline
    (b) Adrenaline
    (c) Ach
    (d) Histamine

479. Inflammatory mediator responsible for ulcer formation?
    (a) Prostaglandin
    (b) Histamine
    (c) Leukotriene
    (d) Interleukins

480. Vitamin K reductase inhibitor?
    (a) Warfarin   (b) Heparin
    (c) Lepirudin   (d) None

481. Vitamin L deficiency leads to
    (a) Sprue
    (b) Celiac disease

(c)   Steatorrhoea
(d)   All the above

482. Fibrin converted to stabilize fibrin in the presence of?
(a) 11th factor   (b) 12th factor
(c) 5th factor   (d) 13th factor

483. Fibrinogen is converted to fibrin in the presence of
(a)   Thrombin
(b)   Prothrombin
(c) Ca^{2+} ions
(d)   Christmas factor

484. Prothrombin is converted into in the presence of?
(a)   Xa   (b)   Xia
(c)   Xlla   (d)   IXa

485. Blood coagulation is controlled by
(a)   Enzyme inhibitors
(b)   Fibrinolytics
(c)   Both
(d)   None

486. X is converted into Xa in the presence of?
(a)   IXa   (b)   Xia
(c)   Xlla   (d)   XIIIa

487. Vitamin K is essential for the formation of clotting factors?
(a)   2,7,9,10   (b)   2,8,6,10
(c)   2,5,8,9   (d)   2,7,8,10

488. Synthetic vitamin K preparation?
(a)   Tocopherol
(b)   Calciferol
(c)   Menadiol Sodium Phosphate
(d)   All the above

489. Mechanism of heparins?
(a)   Inhibits coagulation by activating antithrombin III
(b)   Inhibits coagulation by activating Prothrombin
(c)   Inhibits coagulation by inhibiting Prothrombin
(d)   All the above

490. Which of the following is /are low molecular weight heparins?
(a)   Enoxaparin
(b)   Dalteparin
(c)   Fondaparinux
(d)   All the above

491. Unwanted effect of heparin?
(a)   Haemorrhage
(b)   Thrombosis
(c)   Osteoporosis
(d)   All the above

492. Mechanism of action of warfarin?
(a)   Inhibits y-carboxylation of glutamic acid residues in clotting factor 2, 7, 8, & 10
(b)   Inhibits prothrombin
(c)   Inhibits fibrinogen
(d)   All the above

493. Anticoagulants are used in the treatment of
(a)   Deep vein thrombosis
(b)   Pulmonary embolus
(c)   Myocardial infarction
(d)   All the above

494. Soluble fibrinogen is converted insoluble fibrin strand in the presence of
(a)   Prothrombin
(b)   Thrombin

(c)   Thromboplastin

(d)   Fibrin stabilising factor

495. Vascular endothelium provide non thrombogenic surface by the presence of
(a)   Warfarin
(b)   Phenindione
(c)   Heparin
(d)   Hirudin

496. All components of the blood are present in
(a)   Extrinsic pathway
(b)   Intrinsic pathway
(c)   Both a & b
(d)   None of the above

497. Blood coagulation factor XII is
(a)   Prothrombin
(b)   Thromboplastin
(c)   Fibrin stabilising factor
(d)   Hegman factor

498. 12, 11 & 9 factors are involved in
(a)   Intrinsic pathway
(b)   Extrinsic pathway
(c)   Both a & b
(d)   None of the above

499. IX is converted to IXa in the presence of
(a)   Xia   (b)   XI
(c)   XII   (d)   XIIa

500. Vascular endothelium provide thrombogenic surface due to the presence of
(a)   Tissue factor
(b)   Von will brand factor

(c)   Plasminogen activator inhibitor
(d)   All the above

501. Vitamin involved in blood coagulation is
(a)   Tocopherol
(b)   Calciferol
(c)   Naphthoquinone
(d)   Cholicalciferol

502. Synthetic vitamin K preparation
(a)   Phenindione
(b)   Coumarin
(c)   Dicoumarol
(d)   Menadiol

503. Vitamin K is necessary for the
(a)   y-carboxylation of glutamic acid residues of factor 2, 7, 9 & 10.
(b)   y-decarboxylation of 2, 7, 9 & 10.
(c)   Inhibition of 2, 7, 9 & 10 factors
(d)   None of the above

504. In genetic disorder haemophilia which factor is deficient?
(a)   Christmas factor
(b)   Stuart factor
(c)   Antihemophilic factor
(d)   All the above

505. Injectable anticoagulant?
(a)   Warfarin
(b)   Coumarin
(c)   Heparin
(d)   Phenindione

506. Oral anticoagulant?
    (a) Heparin
    (b) Hirudin
    (c) Phenindione
    (d) Low molecular weight heparin

507. Anticoagulant present in mast cells?
    (a) Hirudin
    (b) Phenindione
    (c) Warfarin
    (d) Heparin

508. Low molecular weight heparin
    (a) Warfarin
    (b) Enoxaparin
    (c) Phenindione
    (d) Heparin sulfate

509. Fondaparinux is
    (a) Oral anticoagulant
    (b) Injectable anticoagulant
    (c) Low molecular weight heparin
    (d) Both b & c

510. Unwanted effect of heparin
    (a) Haemorrhage
    (b) Osteoporosis
    (c) Thrombosis
    (d) All the above

511. Antithrombin-III independent anticoagulant isolated from leach?
    (a) Hirudin
    (b) Argatroban
    (c) Heparin
    (d) None of the above

512. Antithrombin-III independent anticoagulant arginine based compound?
    (a) Hirudin
    (b) Hirugen
    (c) Heparin
    (d) Argatroban

513. Glycoprotein lib/Illa receptor are present on
    (a) Erythrocytes
    (b) Platelets
    (c) WBC
    (d) All the above

514. The clotting factor binds to Ilb/Illa receptors of platelets during platelet aggregation
    (a) Factor I
    (b) Factor II
    (c) Factor III
    (d) Factor IV

515. Cyclic endoperoxide involved in platelet aggregation?
    (a) LTl
    (b) LT2
    (c) TXA2
    (d) PGI2

516. Platelets on the Gp lib/Illa receptors are linked by following factor?
    (a) Fibrinogen
    (b) Prothrombin
    (c) Labile factor
    (d) Proconvertin

517. Mechanism of aspirin?
    (a) Stimulation of TXA2
    (b) Inhibition of TXA2
    (c) Both a & b
    (d) None of the above

518. Antiplatelet phosphodiesterase inhibitor?
    (a) Aspirin
    (b) Ticlopidine
    (c) Dipyridamole
    (d) Clopidogrel

519. Mechanism of ticlopidine?
  (a) Inhibition of TXA2
  (b) Inhibition of ADP dependent aggregation
  (c) Stimulation of ADP dependent aggregation
  (d) All the above

520. Antiplatelet drug congener of ticlopidine is
  (a) Aspirin
  (b) Dipyridamole
  (c) Clopidogrel
  (d) Epoprosteanol

521. Monoclonal antibody used as antiplatelet drug?
  (a) Tirofiban
  (b) Abciximab
  (c) Eptifibatide
  (d) Clopidogrel

522. Glycoprotein IIb/IIIa antagonists?
  (a) Abciximab
  (b) Tirofiban
  (c) Eptifibatide
  (d) All the above

523. Mechanism of action of clopidogrel?
  (a) Inhibit TXA2 synthesis
  (b) Inhibit ADP Dependent aggregation
  (c) Stimulate TXA2 synthesis
  (d) All the above

524. Headache is the adverse effect of following antiplatelet drug?
  (a) Dipyridamole
  (b) Ticlopidine
  (c) Clopidogrel
  (d) All the above

525. Plasminogen activator?
  (a) Kallikrien
  (b) Tissue plasminogen activator
  (c) Neutrophil elastase
  (d) All the above

526. Fibrinolytic drug?
  (a) Tranexamic acid
  (b) Aprotinin
  (c) Streptokinase
  (d) None of the above

527. Antifibrinolytic drug?
  (a) Streptokinase
  (b) Duteplase
  (c) Aprotinin
  (d) All the above

528. Fibrinolytic drug obtained from bacteria have antigenic in nature
  (a) Urokinase
  (b) Streptokinase
  (c) Alteplase
  (d) None

529. Fibrinolytic drug isolated from unne?
  (a) Alteplase
  (b) Tranexamic acid
  (c) Streptokinase
  (d) Urokinase

530. Headache is the adverse effect of following antiplatelet drug because of following action respectively?
  (a) Dipyridamole, vasodilation
  (b) Asprin, COX inhibition
  (c) Tirofiban, vasodilation
  (d) Ticlopidine, vasoconstriction

531. Which of the following synthetic steroids shows predominantly mineralocorticoid action?
    (a) Hydrocortisone
    (b) Spironolactone
    (c) Dexamethasone
    (d) Fludrocortisone

532. Major mineralocorticoids are the following except?
    (a) Aldosterone
    (b) Deoxycorticosterone
    (c) Fludrocortisone
    (d) Hydrocortisone

533. Which of the following statement is true about spiroanolactone?
    (a) Spiroanolactone reverses the many of the manifestations of spiranolactone
    (b) It is also an androgen antagonist as such is used in the treatment of hirsutism in women
    (c) It is useful as a diuretic
    (d) All the above

534. Drug inhibit the carbonic anhydrase enzyme
    (a) Acetazolamide
    (b) Furosemide
    (c) Hydrocortisone
    (d) Spiranolactone

535. Drug acts by competitively blocking NaCl co-transporters in the distal tubule?
    (a) Acetazolamide
    (b) Furosemide
    (c) Hydrochlorothiazide
    (d) Spiranolactone

536. Drug acts at proximal tubule?
    (a) Acetazolamide
    (b) Furosemide
    (c) Hydrochlorothiazide
    (d) Spiranolactone

537. Which of the following drug is potassium sparing diuretic that blocks Na^+ channels in collecting tubules?
    (a) Acetazolamide
    (b) Amiloride
    (c) Furosemide
    (d) Hydrochlorothiazide

538. Chronic use of this drug can lead to distal tubular hypertrophy, which may reduce its diuretic effect?
    (a) Acetazolamide
    (b) Amiloride
    (c) Furosemide
    (d) Hydrochlorothiazide

539. Drug has steroid like structure which is responsible for the antiandrogenic effect?
    (a) Amiloride
    (b) Furosemide
    (c) Hydrochlorothiazide
    (d) Spiranolactone

540. Sustained use of drug results in increased plasma urate concentration?
    (a) Furosemide
    (b) Acetazolamide
    (c) Both a and B
    (d) None

541. Drug used as both diuretic & to treat glaucoma?
    (a) Furosemide
    (b) Acetazolamide
    (c) Both a & b
    (d) None

542. Drug can cause ototoxicity?
    (a) Furosemide
    (b) Acetazolamide
    (c) Both a & b
    (d) None

543. Drugs acts only on the luminal side of renal tubules?
    (a) Furosemide
    (b) Acetazolamide
    (c) Both a and b
    (d) None

544. Drug promotes sodium loss in patients with low glomerular filtration rates?
    (a) Furosemide
    (b) Acetazolamide
    (c) Hydrochlorothiazide
    (d) None

545. Drug used to treat nephrogenic diabetes insipidus?
    (a) Hydrochlorothiazide
    (b) Amiloride
    (c) Furosemide
    (d) Spiranolactone

546. Drug is sometimes fixed dose combinations used to treat essential hypertension?
    (a) Hydrochlorothiazide
    (b) Amiloride
    (c) Both a and b

    (d) None

547. Drug should never be administered to patients taking potassium supplements?
    (a) Hydrochlorothiazide
    (b) Amiloride
    (c) Furosemide
    (d) None

548. Drug decreases the calcium excretion in urine
    (a) Hydrochlorothiazide
    (b) Amiloride
    (c) Furosemide
    (d) Acetazolamide

549. Drugs acts at the proximal tubule?
    (a) Loop diuretics
    (b) Thiazide diuretics
    (c) Potassium sparing diuretics
    (d) Carbonic anhydrase inhibitors

550. Drugs acts at the distal convoluted tubule?
    (a) Loop diuretics
    (b) Thiazide diuretics
    (c) Potassium sparing diuretic
    (d) Carbonic anhydrase inhibitors

551. Drug inhibits sodium and chloride transport in the cortical thick ascending limb and the early distal tubule?
    (a) Acetazolamide
    (b) Furosemide
    (c) Hydrochlorothiazide
    (d) Amiloride

552. Drug cause ototoxicity?
    (a) Acetazolamide
    (b) Furosemide

(c) Hydrochlorothiazide
(d) Amiloride

553. Drug usually given in combination
with thiazide diuretic
(a) Acetazolamide
(b) Furosemide
(c) Hydrochlorothiazide
(d) Amiloride

554. Drug least potent diuretic?
(a) Osmotic diuretics
(b) Loop diuretics
(c) Thiazide diuretics
(d) K-sparing diuretics

555. These agents given parentarally
because they are not absorbed when
given orally?
(a) Osmotic diuretics
(b) Loop diuretics
(c) Thiazide diuretics
(d) K-sparing diuretics

556. Furosemide acts at?
(a) Proximal convoluted tubule
(b) Ascending thick limb of loop
of henle
(c) Distal convoluted tubule
(d) Collecting duct

557. Metolazone acts at
(a) PCT
(b) Ascending limb of loop of
henle
(c) DCT
(d) Collecting duct

558. Drugs act by affecting tubular fluid
composition in a non-receptor
mediated fashion?

(a) Furosemide
(b) Acetazolamide
(c) Triamterene
(d) Mannitol

559. Spiraonolactone acts at this
nephron site?
(a) PCT
(b) Ascending limb of loop of
henle
(c) DCT
(d) Collecting duct

560. Amiloride acts at this nephron site?
(a) PCT
(b) Ascending limb of loop of
henle
(c) DCT
(d) Collecting duct

561. Histamine releases gastric acid by
the action on?
(a) H1 receptors
(b) H2 receptors
(c) H3 receptors
(d) None

562. Contraction of bronchi, bronchioles
caused by histamine action on
following receptors?
(a) H1 receptors
(b) H2 receptors
(c) H3 receptors
(d) None

563. Potent vasoconstrictor?
(a) Angiotensin
(b) Angiotensin II
(c) Angiotensinogen
(d) None of the above

564. PGI2 action on vascular smooth muscle?
    (a) Constriction
    (b) Relaxation
    (c) Both a & b
    (d) None of the above

565. Actions of Angiotensin-II?
    (a) Vasoconstriction
    (b) Aldosterone secretion
    (c) Tubular Na^+ absorption
    (d) All the above

566. Actions of Histamine except?
    (a) Gastric acid secretion-H2 receptor
    (b) Gastric acid secretion-H1 receptor
    (c) Contraction of smooth muscle-H1 receptor
    (d) Vasodilation-H1 receptor

567. Inflammatory mediators are derived from which of the following phospholipids?
    (a) Prostanoids
    (b) Leukotrienes
    (c) Lipoxins
    (d) All the above

568. Actions of PGD2 except?
    (a) Vasodilation
    (b) Inhibition of platelet aggregation
    (c) Relaxation of GI smooth muscle
    (d) Vasoconstriction

569. Prostaglandin analogue used in the treatment of peptic ulcer?
    (a) Prostacyclin

    (b) Misoprostal
    (c) Carboprost
    (d) All the above

570. Prostaglandin analogue used to treat glaucoma?
    (a) Latanoprost
    (b) Gemeprost
    (c) Misoprostal
    (d) Carboprost

571. Actions of PGF2alpha
    (a) Bronchoconstriction
    (b) Myometrial contraction
    (c) Both a& b
    (d) Bronchodilation

572. Platelet activating factor action?
    (a) Vasodilation
    (b) Vascular permeability
    (c) Activation of leukocytes
    (d) All the above

573. Coagulation factor involved in the synthesis of bradykinin?
    (a) Hageman factor
    (b) Stuart factor
    (c) Prothrombin
    (d) Christmas factor

574. Pharmacological actions of bradykinin except?
    (a) Vasodilation
    (b) Contraction of intestinal & uterine smooth muscle
    (c) Vasoconstriction
    (d) Stimulation of pain

575. All are cytokines except?
    (a) Interleukins
    (b) Chemokines

(c) Interferons
(d) Leukotrienes

(c) Probenecid
(d) All the above

576. Antipyretic action of NSAIDS is due to?
(a) Inhibition of prostaglandin production in hypothalamus
(b) Stimulation of prostaglandin production
(c) Both a & b
(d) None of the above

577. Analgesic action NSAIDS is due to
(a) By vasodilator action
(b) By decreasing the production of prostaglandins
(c) Both a & b
(d) By increasing the prostaglandin production

578. Unwanted effect of NSAIDS
(a) GI disturbances
(b) Skin allergy
(c) Bone marrow disturbance
(d) All the above

579. Aspirin is
(a) Antiplate drug
(b) NSAID
(c) Treat Alzheimer's disease
(d) All the above

580. Unwanted effect of aspirin?
(a) Gastric bleeding
(b) Tinnitus
(c) Reye's syndrome
(d) All the above

581. Drug interactions of aspirin with
(a) Warfarin
(b) Sulphinpyrazone

582. Action of Paracetamol
(a) Inhibition of COX-3
(b) Inhibition of Prostaglandins
(c) Both a & b
(d) None of the above

583. Salicylism is the adverse effect of following NSAID
(a) Aspirin
(b) Paracetamol
(c) Celecoxib
(d) Aceclofenac

584. Tolmetin is a
(a) NSAID
(b) Anticoagulant
(c) Antiviral drug
(d) Anti ulcer drug

585. Nabumetone is a?
(a) Anticoagulant
(b) NSAID
(c) Antimicrobial drug
(d) Antiviral drug

586. Adverse effect of mefenamic acid?
(a) Haemolytic anemia
(b) GI disturbances
(c) Diarrhoea
(d) All the above

587. Liver damage of paracetamol is due to its metabolite
(a) N-acetyl para benzoquinone imine
(b) N-acetyl muramic-p-benzoquinone
(c) Both a & b
(d) None of the above

588. Reye's syndrome is the adverse effect of following NSAID drug?
    (a) Aspirin
    (b) Paracetamol
    (c) Sulindac
    (d) Diclofenac

589. Selective COX-2 inhibitor?
    (a) Rofecoxib
    (b) Celecoxib
    (c) Both a & b
    (d) Paracetamol

590. Drug selective COX-2 inhibitor contraindicated in individuals with hypersensitivity to sulphonamides?
    (a) Celecoxib
    (b) Paracetamol
    (c) Aspirin
    (d) Rofecoxib

591. Interactions of celecoxib with
    (a) Rifampicin
    (b) Fluconazole
    (c) Leflunomide
    (d) All the above

592. Oxicam type drug which is NSAID
    (a) Piroxicam
    (b) Meloxicam
    (c) Both a & b
    (d) None of the above

593. NSAIDS are used in the treatment of?
    (a) Headache
    (b) Chronic pain
    (c) Back ache
    (d) All the above

594. Oxygen radical scavenging effect and NSAID effect is due to
    (a) Aspirin
    (b) Paracetamol
    (c) Sulindac
    (d) Diclofenac

595. NSAIDS Pharmacological action?
    (a) Anti-inflammatory effect
    (b) Antipyretic effect
    (c) Analgesic effect
    (d) All the above

596. Housekeeping role in the body is due to?
    (a) COX-1
    (b) COX-2
    (c) COX-3
    (d) All the above

597. Which of the following group of antibiotics demonstrates a bactericidal effect?
    (a) Tetracyclines
    (b) Macrolides
    (c) Penicillins
    (d) All the above

598. Which of the following group of antibiotics demonstrates a bacteriostatic effect?
    (a) Carbapenems
    (b) Macrolides
    (c) Aminoglycosides
    (d) Cephalosporins

599. Following antibiotic contain β-lactam ring in their structure?
    (a) Penicillins
    (b) Cephalosporins

   (c) Carbapenems
   (d) All the above

600. Which of the following is macrolide antibiotic?
   (a) Neomycin
   (b) Doxycycline
   (c) Erythromycin
   (d) Cefotaxime

601. Which of the following is belongs to carbapenems?
   (a) Aztreonam
   (b) Amoxicillin
   (c) Imipenem
   (d) Clarithromycin

602. All of the following antibiotics are aminoglycosides except?
   (a) Gentamicin
   (b) Streptomycin
   (c) Clindamycin
   (d) Neomycin

603. Drug belongs to nitrobenzene derivative?
   (a) Clindamycin
   (b) Streptomycin
   (c) Azithromycin
   (d) Chloramphenicol

604. Which of the following is glycopeptides antibiotic?
   (a) Vancomycin
   (b) Lincomycin
   (c) Neomycin
   (d) carbenicillin

605. Antibiotics inhibit bacterial cell wall synthesis are?
   (a) β-lactam antibiotics
   (b) Tetracyclines
   (c) Aminoglycosides
   (d) Macrolides

606. Antibiotic inhibits bacterial RNA synthesis?
   (a) Erythromycin
   (b) Rifampicin
   (c) Chloramphenicol
   (d) Imipenem

607. Antibiotics altering the permeability of cell membrane?
   (a) Glycopeptides
   (b) Polymyxins
   (c) Tetracyclines
   (d) Cephalosporins

608. All of the following antibiotics inhibit the protein synthesis except?
   (a) Macrolides
   (b) Aminoglycosides
   (c) Glycopeptides
   (d) Tetracyclines

609. Which of the following is acid resistant penicillin?
   (a) Penicillin G
   (b) Penicillin V
   (c) Carbenicillin
   (d) Procaine Penicillin

610. Drugs belong to antibiotics having polyene structure?
   (a) Nystatin
   (b) Ketoconazole
   (c) Griseofulvin
   (d) All the above

611. Polyenes
    (a) Cause nephrotoxicity
    (b) Acts against fungi
    (c) Altering the structure & functions of cell membrane
    (d) Broad spectrum antibiotic

612. Unwanted effect of amphotericin B
    (a) Psychosis
    (b) Renal impairment
    (c) Hypertension
    (d) Bone marrow toxicity

613. Mechanism of action of amphotericin B?
    (a) Inhibition of cell wall synthesis
    (b) Inhibition of DNA synthesis
    (c) Inhibition of fungal protein synthesis
    (d) Alteration of cell membrane permeability

614. All of the following antifungal drugs are antibiotics except?
    (a) Amphotericin B
    (b) Nystatin
    (c) Didanosine
    (d) Griseofulvin

615. Which of the following drug is used for the treatment of dermatomycosis?
    (a) Nystatin
    (b) Griseofulvin
    (c) Amphotericin B
    (d) Vancomycin

616. Chloramphenicol has following unwanted effect?
    (a) Nephrotoxicity
    (b) Pancytopenia
    (c) Hepatotoxicity
    (d) Ototoxicity

617. Mechanism of sulphonamides?
    (a) Inhibition of dihydropteroate reductase
    (b) Inhibition of dihydropteroate synthase
    (c) Inhibition of DNA gyrase
    (d) Inhibition of DHFR

618. Combination of sulphonamides with trimethoprim?
    (a) Decreases the unwanted effect of sulphonamides
    (b) Increases the antimicrobial activity
    (c) Decreases antimicrobial activity
    (d) Increases the elimination of sulphonamides

619. Following measures are necessary for prevention of sulphonamide precipitation and crystalluria?
    (a) Taking of drinks with acid p^H
    (b) Taking of drinks with alkaline p^H
    (c) Taking of saline drinks
    (d) Restriction of drinking

620. Mechanism of action of trimethoprim?
    (a) Inhibition of cyclooxygenase
    (b) Inhibition of dihydropteroate reductase
    (c) Inhibition of dihydropteroate synthase
    (d) Inhibition of DNA gyrase

621. Unwanted effect of sulfonamides?
   (a) Hematopoietic disturbances
   (b) Crystalluria
   (c) Nausea, vomiting & diarrhea
   (d) All the above

622. First line antimicrobial drug?
   (a) PAS
   (b) Kanamycin
   (c) Isoniazid
   (d) Pyrazinamide

623. Antimycobacterial drug belonging to antibiotics?
   (a) Isoniazid
   (b) PAS
   (c) Ethambutol
   (d) Rifampicin

624. Mechanism of action of cycloserine?
   (a) Inhibition of mycolic acid synthesis
   (b) Inhibition of RNA synthesis
   (c) Inhibition of cell wall synthesis
   (d) Inhibition of pyridoxal phosphate synthesis

625. Unwanted effect of rifampicin?
   (a) Dizziness & headache
   (b) Loss of hair
   (c) Flu like syndrome, tubular necrosis
   (d) Hepatotoxicity

626. Unwanted effect of ethambutol
   (a) Cardiotoxicity
   (b) Immunotoxicity
   (c) Retrobulbarneuritis with red-green color blindness
   (d) Hepatotoxicity

627. Following agents are first line antimycobacterial drugs except?
   (a) Rifampicin
   (b) Pyrazinamide
   (c) Isoniazide
   (d) Streptomycin

628. Fluoroquinolones are used for treatment of
   (a) Infection of urinary tract
   (b) Bacterial diarrhoea
   (c) Infection of the urinary & respiratory tract, bacterial diarrhoea
   (d) Respiratory tract infections

629. Drug of choice of Syphilis treatment?
   (a) Gentamycin
   (b) Penicillin
   (c) Chloramphenicol
   (d) Doxycycline

630. Drug used for malaria chemoprophylaxis and treatment?
   (a) Chlorazepam
   (b) Quinidine
   (c) Quinine
   (d) Sulphonamides

631. Drug used for treatment of amoebiasis?
   (a) Nitrofurantoin
   (b) Iodoquinol
   (c) Pyrazinamide
   (d) Mefloquine

632. Drug used for toxoplasmosis treatment?
    (a) Chloroquine
    (b) Tetracycline
    (c) Suramin
    (d) Pyrimethamine

633. All of the following antimalarial drugs are 4-quinoline derivatives except?
    (a) Chloroquine
    (b) Mefloquine
    (c) Primaquine
    (d) Amodiaquine

634. All of the following antimalarial drugs influence schizonts except?
    (a) Chloroquine
    (b) Mefloquine
    (c) Primaquine
    (d) Quinidine

635. Antimalarial drug influencing tissue schizonts?
    (a) Mefloquine
    (b) Chloroquine
    (c) Quinidine
    (d) Primaquine

636. Group of antibiotics having antimalarial effect?
    (a) Mefloquine
    (b) Tetracycline
    (c) Carbapenems
    (d) Penicillins

637. Amebicide drug for the treatment of an asymptomatic intestinal form of amoebiasis?
    (a) Chloroquine
    (b) Diloxanide
    (c) Emetine
    (d) Doxycycline

638. Drugs used for the treatment of intestinal amoebiasis?
    (a) Metraonidazole & diloxanide
    (b) Diloxanide & streptomycin
    (c) Diloxanide & iodoquinol
    (d) Emetine & metraonidazole

639. Drug for the treatment of hepatic amoebiasis
    (a) Diloxanide or iodoquinol
    (b) Tetracycline or Doxycycline
    (c) Metraonidazole
    (d) Erythromycin

640. Anthelmintic drug which block Ach transmission at myoneural junction?
    (a) Piperazine
    (b) Pirenzepine
    (c) Niclosamide
    (d) Praziquantel

641. Drug inhibits the oxidative phosphorylation in some species of helminths?
    (a) Niclosamide
    (b) Praziquantel
    (c) Mebendazole
    (d) Piperazine

642. Drug used for the treatment of ascaridosis &enterobiosis?
    (a) Pyrantel
    (b) Praziquantel
    (c) Niclosamide
    (d) Bithionol

643. Anti-helminthic drug which acts by increasing cell membrane permeability for calcium, resulting in paralysis, dislodgement and death of helminths?
    (a) Niclosamide
    (b) Pyrantel
    (c) Praziquantel
    (d) Diloxanide

644. Mebendazole act by
    (a) Inhibit the oxidative phosphorylation
    (b) Increasing cell membrane permeability to ions
    (c) Inhibit microtubule synthesis
    (d) All the above

645. Luminal amoebicide drug?
    (a) Metranidazole
    (b) Emetine
    (c) Diloxanide
    (d) Tetracycline

646. Drug of choice for round warm infections?
    (a) Niclosamide
    (b) Praziquantel
    (c) Bithionol
    (d) Pyrantel

647. Gonadotropin releasing hormone agonist?
    (a) Octreotide
    (b) Tamoxifen
    (c) Leuprolide
    (d) Anastrozole

648. Drugs belong to aromatase inhibitors?
    (a) Octreotide
    (b) Anastrozole
    (c) Flutamide
    (d) Tamoxifen

649. Estrogen inhibitor?
    (a) Tamoxifen
    (b) Flutamide
    (c) Anastrozole
    (d) Leuprolide

650. Mechanism of methotrexate?
    (a) Inhibition of DHFR
    (b) Activation of cell differentiation
    (c) Catabolic depletion of serum arginine
    (d) All the above

651. Group of drugs used as subsidiary medicines in cancer treatment?
    (a) Cytoprotectors
    (b) Bone marrow growth factors
    (c) Antimetastatic agents
    (d) All the above

652. Contraindications for anticancer drugs are
    (a) Depression of bone marrow
    (b) Acute infections
    (c) Severe hepatic or renal insufficiency
    (d) All the above

653. All of the following drugs are derivatives of nitrosoureas except?
    (a) Carmustine
    (b) Vincristine
    (c) Lomustine
    (d) Semustine

654. Mechanism of anticancer drugs belonging to plant alkaloids?
    (a) Inhibition of DNA dependent RNA synthesis
    (b) Cross linking of DNA
    (c) Mitotic arrest at a metaphase
    (d) Nonselective inhibition of aromatases

655. Enzyme drug used for acute leukaemia treatment?
    (a) DHFR
    (b) Asparginase
    (c) Aromatase
    (d) DNA Gyrase

656. Clinical use of oestrogen in oncology?
    (a) Leukaemia
    (b) Prostate cancer
    (c) Endometiral cancer
    (d) Brain tumours

657. Anticancer drug belongs to inorganic metal complexes?
    (a) Dacarbazine
    (b) Cisplatin
    (c) Methotrexate
    (d) Vincristine

658. Fluorouracil belongs to
    (a) Antibiotics
    (b) Antimetabolites
    (c) Plant alkaloids
    (d) Bone marrow growth factors

659. Antibiotic for cancer chemotherapy?
    (a) Cytarabine
    (b) Doxorubicin
    (c) Gentamycin
    (d) Etoposide

660. Methotrexate is
    (a) Purine antagonist
    (b) Folic acid antagonist
    (c) Antibiotic
    (d) Alkylating agent

661. Anticancer drug belongs to pyrimidine antagonist?
    (a) Fluorouracil
    (b) Mercaptopurine
    (c) Thioguanine
    (d) Methotrexate

662. Mechanism of alkylating agent?
    (a) Producing carbonium ions altering protein structure
    (b) Producing carbonium ions altering DNA structure
    (c) Structural antagonism against purine & pyrimidine
    (d) Inhibition of DNA dependent RNA polymerase

663. Anticancer drug of plant origin?
    (a) Dactinomycin
    (b) Vincristine
    (c) Methotrexate
    (d) Procarbazine

664. Anticancer alkylating drug a derivative of alkylsulphonate?
    (a) Fluorouracil
    (b) Carboplatin
    (c) Vinblastine
    (d) Busulphan

665. Group of hormonal drugs used for the cancer treatment?
    (a) Mineralocorticoids & glucocorticoids
    (b) Glucocorticoids & gonadal hormones
    (c) Gonadal hormones & somatostatin
    (d) Insulin

666. Anticancer alkylating drug derivative of ethylenimine?
    (a) Mercaptopurine
    (b) Thiotepa
    (c) Chlorambucil
    (d) Procarbazine

667. All of the following anticancer drugs are the analogs of nucleosides except?
    (a) Acyclovir
    (b) Zidovudine
    (c) Saquinavir
    (d) Didanosine

668. Drug derivative of adamantine?
    (a) Didanosine
    (b) Rimantadine
    (c) Gancyclovir
    (d) Foscarnet

669. Anticancer alkylating drug a derivative of chloroethylamine?
    (a) Methotrexate
    (b) Cisplatin
    (c) Cyclophosphamide
    (d) Carmustine

670. Which of the following are adverse effect of anticancer drugs except?
    (a) Low selectivity to cancer cells
    (b) Bone marrow depression
    (c) Depression of angiogenesis
    (d) Depression of immune system

671. Antiviral drug derivative of pyrophosphate?
    (a) Foscarnet
    (b) Didanosine
    (c) Zidovudine
    (d) Vidarabine

672. Which of the following antiviral drug inhibits the viral DNA synthesis?
    (a) Interferon
    (b) Saquinavir
    (c) Amantidine
    (d) Acyclovir

673. Antiviral drug saquinavir has which of the following adverse effect?
    (a) Nausea
    (b) Rhinitis
    (c) Abdominal pain
    (d) All the above

674. Antiviral drug inhibiting uncoating of viral RNA?
    (a) Vidarabine
    (b) Rimantadine
    (c) Acyclovir
    (d) Didanosine

675. Drug of choice for herpes and cytomegalo virus   infection treatment?
    (a) Saquinavir
    (b) Interferon alpha
    (c) Didanosine
    (d) Acyclovir

676. Drug inhibiting viral proteases?
    (a) Rimantadine
    (b) Acyclovir
    (c) Saquinavir
    (d) Zalcitabine

677. Mechanism of alkylating agents?
    (a) Intrastrand cross-linking of DNA
    (b) Blocking of Synthesis of DNA or RNA
    (c) Inhibition of topoisomerase
    (d) None of the above

678. Anticancer drugs which inhibit the spindle formation and microtubule?
    (a) Alkylating agent
    (b) Antimetabolites
    (c) Plant alkaloids
    (d) All the above

679. Toxic metabolite one anticancer drug causes bladder damage?
    (a) Lomustine
    (b) Cyclophosphamide
    (c) Melphalan
    (d) Cisplatin

680. Effect of acrolein is terminated by
    (a) Mesna
    (b) Melphalan
    (c) Estramustine
    (d) Busulphan

681. Cytarabine inhibits?
    (a) DHFR
    (b) Dihydro pteroate synthetase
    (c) DNA polymerase
    (d) THFR

682. Doxorubicin Inhibits?
    (a) Topoisomerase I
    (b) Topoisomerase II
    (c) Both a & b
    (d) None

683. Irinotecan is the inhibitor of
    (a) Topoisomerase II
    (b) Topoisomerase I
    (c) Microtubules
    (d) Spindle formation

684. Drug belongs to the class of non-nucleoside reverse transcriptase inhibitors?
    (a) Zidovudine
    (b) Vidarabine
    (c) Nevirapine
    (d) Gancyclovir

685. All of the following drugs are antiretroviral agents except?
    (a) Acyclovir
    (b) Zidovudine
    (c) Zalcitabine
    (d) Didanosine

686. Drug used for influenza A treatment?
    (a) Acyclovir
    (b) Rimantadine
    (c) Saquinavir
    (d) Foscarnet

687. Drug derivative of nucleosides used in the treatment of HIV infection?
    (a) Acyclovir
    (b) Zidovudine
    (c) Interferon-α
    (d) Pencyclovir

688. Antiviral drug which belongs to endogenous proteins?
     (a) Amantidine
     (b) Saquinavir
     (c) Interferon-α
     (d) Pencyclovir

689. Drug belongs to the class of nucleoside reverse transcriptase inhibitors?
     (a) Didanosine
     (b) Gancyclovir
     (c) Nevirapine
     (d) Vidarabine

690. All of the following drugs are anti-influenza agents except?
     (a) Acyclovir
     (b) Amantidine
     (c) Interferons
     (d) Rimantadine

691. Unwanted effect of zidovudine
     (a) Hallucinations, dizziness
     (b) Anaemia, neutropenia
     (c) Hypertension, vomiting
     (d) Peripheral neuropathy

692. Unwanted effect of IV infusion of acyclovir?
     (a) Renal insufficiency, tremors, delirium
     (b) Rashes, diarrhoea & nausea
     (c) Neuropathy, abdominal pain
     (d) Anemia, neutropenia, nausea, insomnia

693. Drug induces peripheral neuropathy & oral ulceration?
     (a) Acyclovir
     (b) Zalcitabine
     (c) Zidovudine
     (d) Saquinavir

694. Which of the following drug is penicillinase resistant penicillin?
     (a) Oxacillin
     (b) Amoxicillin
     (c) Penicillin G
     (d) Penicillin V

695. Minimal duration of antibacterial treatment is?
     (a) Not less than one day
     (b) Not less than 5 days
     (c) Not less than 10-14 days
     (d) Not less than 3 weeks

696. combination of antimicrobial drugs used to
     (a) Provide synergism
     (b) Provide broad spectrum
     (c) Prevent the emergence of resistance
     (d) All the above

KEY

1. (c)	2. (d)	3. (d)	4. (d)	5. (d)
6. (b)	7. (b)	8. (d)	9. (b)	10. (d)
11. (d)	12. (d)	13. (d)	14. (d)	15. (b)
16. (d)	17. (a)	18. (b)	19. (d)	20. (d)
21. (d)	22. (d)	23. (b)	24. (c)	25. (b)
26. (a)	27. (b)	28. (b)	29. (b)	30. (a)
31. (b)	32. (b)	33. (b)	34. (b)	35. (b)
36. (c)	37. (b)	38. (b)	39. (b)	40. (d)
41. (c)	42. (a)	43. (a)	44. (d)	45. (a)
46. (a)	47. (a)	48. (a)	49. (b)	50. (b)
51. (d)	52. (d)	53. (c)	54. (b)	55. (b)
56. (a)	57. (c)	58. (a)	59. (b)	60. (a)
61. (a)	62. (a)	63. (c)	64. (d)	65. (a)
66. (b)	67. (a)	68. (c)	69. (c)	70. (d)
71. (b)	72. (b)	73. (b)	74. (a)	75. (c)
76. (a)	77. (a)	78. (a)	79. (c)	80. (c)
81. (d)	82. (d)	83. (d)	84. (d)	85. (d)
86. (c)	87. (b)	88. (a)	89. (b)	90. (d)
91. (a)	92. (c)	93. (a)	94. (b)	95. (b)
96. (c)	97. (c)	98. (c)	99. (b)	100. (c)
101. (a)	102. (c)	103. (a)	104. (d)	105. (b)
106. (b)	107. (c)	108. (a)	109. (b)	110. (b)
111. (d)	112. (a)	113. (a)	114. (a)	115. (b)

116. (a)	117. (d)	118. (b)	119. (c)	120. (d)
121. (c)	122. (a)	123. (b)	124. (d)	125. (d)
126. (b)	127. (d)	128. (b)	129. (d)	130. (d)
131. (c)	132. (a)	133. (b)	134. (d)	135. (d)
136. (a)	137. (c)	138. (c)	139. (a)	140. (a)
141. (c)	142. (c)	143. (a)	145. (a)	145. (a)
146. (a)	147. (c)	148. (a)	149. (a)	150. (a)
151. (c)	152. (d)	153. (c)	154. (c)	155. (a)
156. (c)	157. (c)	158. (a)	159. (a)	160. (b)
161. (a)	162. (d)	163. (c)	164. (a)	165. (b)
166. (d)	167. (c)	168. (b)	169. (d)	170. (d)
171. (b)	172. (d)	173. (c)	174. (a)	175. (b)
176. (d)	177. (a)	178. (c)	179. (d)	180. (b)
181. (b)	182. (d)	183. (b)	184. (c)	185. (a)
186. (a)	187. (d)	188. (a)	187. (c)	188. (c)
189. (a)	190. (b)	191. (c)	192. (d)	193. (d)
194. (d)	195. (a)	196. (d)	197. (a)	198. (d)
199. (b)	200. (c)	201. (c)	202. (b)	203. (c)
204. (b)	206. (c)	207. (c)	208. (d)	209. (c)
210. (c)	211. (d)	212. (a)	213. (d)	214. (b)
215. (d)	216. (c)	217. (c)	218. (d)	219. (d)
220. (a)	221. (b)	222. (c)	223. (b)	225. (b)
226. (c)	227. (d)	228. (c)	229. (b)	230. (c)
231. (c)	232. (d)	233. (b)	234. (a)	235. (d)

236. (b)	237. (c)	238. (d)	239. (a)	240. (b)
241. (b)	242. (c)	243. (d)	244. (d)	245. (d)
246. (d)	247. (a)	248. (a)	249. (b)	250. (c)
251. (c)	252. (d)	253. (d)	254. (c)	255. (d)
256. (d)	257. (c)	258. (c)	259. (b)	260. (c)
261. (b)	262. (a)	263. (a)	264. (b)	265. (b)
266. (c)	267. (b)	268. (a)	269. (b)	270. (b)
271. (b)	272. (a)	273. (b)	274. (b)	275. (b)
276. (b)	277. (c)	278. (b)	279. (b)	280. (d)
281. (d)	282. (d)	283. (b)	284. (d)	285. (c)
286. (a)	287. (a)	288. (a)	289. (c)	290. (d)
291. (d)	292. (b)	293. (c)	294. (a)	295. (c)
296. (a)	297. (a)	298. (a)	299. (c)	300. (a)
301. (d)	302. (a)	303. (a)	304. (c)	305. (d)
306. (c)	307. (d)	308. (d)	309. (d)	310. (d)
311. (d)	312. (c)	313. (d)	314. (a)	315. (c)
316. (b)	317. (c)	318. (a)	319. (d)	320. (d)
321. (c)	322. (c)	323. (d)	324. (d)	325. (d)
326. (c)	327. (d)	328. (b)	329. (a)	330. (a)
331. (b)	332. (b)	333. (a)	334. (d)	335. (d)
336. (a)	337. (a)	338. (a)	339. (a)	340. (c)
341. (a)	342. (b)	343. (b)	344. (c)	345. (b)
346. (c)	347. (b)	348. (c)	349. (c)	350. (b)
351. (b)	352. (a)	353. (a)	354. (b)	355. (b)

356. (d)	357. (a)	358. (b)	359. (b)	360. (d)
361. (c)	362. (c)	363. (d)	364. (b)	365. (a)
366. (d)	367. (b)	368. (d)	369. (a)	370. (c)
371. (d)	372. (c)	373. (a)	374. (d)	375. (b)
376. (d)	377. (d)	378. (a)	379. (c)	380. (b)
381. (d)	382. (d)	383. (b)	384. (d)	385. (c)
386. (c)	387. (b)	388. (c)	389. (a)	390. (d)
391. (b)	392. (a)	393. (c)	394. (c)	395. (c)
396. (a)	397. (c)	398. (d)	399. (b)	400. (b)
401. (b)	402. (c)	403. (c)	404. (d)	405. (b)
406. (d)	407. (b)	408. (a)	409. (b)	410. (a)
411. (c)	412. (c)	413. (a)	414. (c)	415. (b)
416. (a)	417. (c)	418. (a)	419. (d)	420. (c)
421. (b)	422. (b)	423. (b)	424. (c)	425. (d)
426. (a)	427. (d)	428. (b)	429. (d)	430. (b)
431. (b)	432. (a)	433. (a)	434. (b)	435. (c)
436. (a)	437. (b)	438. (c)	439. (b)	440. (d)
441. (a)	442. (a)	443. (c)	444. (a)	445. (c)
446. (b)	447. (b)	448. (c)	449. (b)	450. (d)
451. (b)	452. (a)	453. (b)	454. (a)	455. (c)
456. (d)	457. (b)	458. (b)	459. (b)	460. (c)
461. (a)	462. (c)	463. (b)	464. (d)	465. (d)
466. (c)	467. (d)	468. (c)	469. (c)	470. (b)
471. (a)	472. (b)	473. (a)	474. (a)	475. (a)

476. (a)	477 (b)	478. (c)	479. (b)	480. (a)
481. (d)	482. (d)	483. (a)	484. (a)	485. (c)
486. (a)	487. (a)	488. (c)	489. (a)	490. (d)
491. (d)	492. (a)	493. (d)	494. (b)	495. (c)
496. (b)	497. (d)	498. (a)	499. (a)	500. (d)
501. (c)	502. (d)	503. (a)	504. (c)	505. (c)
506. (c)	507. (d)	508. (b)	509. (d)	510. (d)
511. (a)	512. (d)	513. (b)	514. (a)	515. (c)
516. (a)	517. (b)	518. (c)	519. (b)	520. (c)
521. (b)	522. (d)	523. (a)	524. (a)	525. (d)
526. (c)	527. (c)	528. (b)	529. (d)	530. (a)
531. (d)	532. (d)	533. (d)	534. (a)	535. (a)
536. (a)	537. (b)	538. (c)	539. (d)	540. (a)
541. (b)	542. (a)	543. (a)	544 (a)	545. (a)
546. (c)	547. (b)	548. (a)	549. (d)	550. (b)
551. (c)	552. (b)	553. (d)	554. (d)	555. (a)
556. (b)	557. (c)	558. (d)	559. (d)	560. (d)
561. (b)	562. (a)	563. (b)	564. (b)	565. (d)
566. (b)	567. (d)	568. (a)	569. (b)	570. (a)
571. (c)	572. (d)	573. (a)	574. (c)	575. (d)
576. (a)	577. (c)	578. (d)	579. (d)	580. (d)
581. (d)	582. (c)	583. (a)	584. (a)	585. (b)
586. (d)	587. (a)	588. (a)	589. (c)	590. (a)
591. (d)	592. (c)	593. (d)	594. (c)	595. (d)

596. (a)	597. (a)	598. (d)	599. (d)	600. (c)
601. (c)	602. (c)	603. (d)	604. (a)	605. (a)
606. (b)	607. (b)	608. (c)	609. (b)	610. (d)
611. (b)	612. (a)	613. (d)	614. (c)	615. (c)
616. (b)	617. (b)	618. (b)	619. (b)	620. (b)
621. (d)	622. (c)	623. (d)	624. (c)	625. (b)
626. (c)	627. (d)	628. (c)	629. (b)	630. (a)
631. (a)	632. (d)	633. (c)	634. (c)	635. (d)
636. (b)	637. (b)	638. (a)	639. (c)	640. (a)
641. (a)	642. (a)	643. (c)	644. (c)	645. (c)
646. (d)	647. (c)	648. (c)	649. (a)	650. (a)
651. (d)	652. (d)	653. (b)	654 (c)	655. (a)
656. (b)	657. (b)	658. (b)	659. (b)	660. (b)
661. (a)	662. (b)	663. (b)	664. (d)	665. (b)
666. (b)	667. (c)	668. (b)	669. (c)	670. (c)
671. (b)	672. (d)	673. (d)	674. (b)	675. (d)
676. (c)	677. (a)	678. (c)	679. (b)	680. (a)
681. (c)	682. (b)	683. (b)	684. (c)	685. (a)
686. (b)	687. (b)	688. (c)	689. (a)	690. (a)
691. (a)	692. (a)	693. (b)	694. (a)	695. (b)
696. (d)				

1. Nitrogenous organic molecule that has a pharmacological effect on humans & animals are?
   - (a) Glycosides
   - (b) Alkaloids
   - (c) Tannins
   - (d) Resins

2. Alkaloids are classified into true, proto & pseudo alkaloids based on
   - (a) Biological pathway used to construct the molecule
   - (b) Number of 'N' atoms
   - (c) Both a & b
   - (d) Their alkalinity

3. True alkaloids are derived from
   - (a) Amino acids & they share a heterocyclic ring with N
   - (b) Amino acids & is not a part of heterocyclic ring
   - (c) Not derived from amino acids
   - (d) None

4. Proto alkaloids are derived from
   - (a) Amino acids & they share a heterocyclic ring with N
   - (b) Amino acids & is not a part of heterocyclic ring
   - (c) Not derived from amino acids
   - (d) None

5. Pseudo alkaloids are derived from
   - (a) Amino acids & they share a heterocyclic ring with N
   - (b) Amino acids & is not a part of heterocyclic ring
   - (c) Not derived from amino acids
   - (d) None

6. High reactive substances with biological activity even in lower doses are?
   - (a) True alkaloids
   - (b) Pseudo alkaloids
   - (c) Proto alkaloids
   - (d) Atypical alkaloids

7. Nicotine is a
   - (a) Yellow solid alkaloid & volatile in nature
   - (b) Brown liquid alkaloid &volatile in nature
   - (c) Brown liquid glycoside & non-volatile in nature
   - (d) Yellow solid glycoside & non-volatile in nature

8. Which of the following is true?
   - (a) Coniine & sparteine are liquid alkaloids
   - (b) Betanidine & berberine are solid alkaloids
   - (c) Sanguinarine salts are copper red in color
   - (d) All the above

9. Tree bases of alkaloids are?
   - (a) Soluble in organic solvents
   - (b) Insoluble in organic solvents
   - (c) Insoluble in water
   - (d) Both a & c

10. Which of the following is highly soluble in water?
    (a) Quinine hydrochloride
    (b) Quinine sulphate
    (c) Both a & b
    (d) None

11. The alkaloids may occur in plants as
    (a) In Free from   (b) In Salts form
    (c) As N-Oxides   (d) All the above

12. An example for true alkaloids is?
    (a) Dopamine
    (b) Caffeine
    (c) Mescaline
    (d) All of the above

13. An example for isoquinoline alkaloids are?
    (a) Cocaine   (b) Morphine
    (c) Quinine   (d) Vasaka

14. L-ornithine, L-lysine, L-phenylalanine, L-tyrosine, L-tryptophan, & L-histidine amino acids are the precursors for?
    (a) True alkaloids
    (b) Pseudo alkaloids
    (c) Both a & b
    (d) None

15. Proto alkaloids are derived from?
    (a) Amino acid L-tryptophan
    (b) Amino acid L-tyrosine
    (c) Both a & b
    (d) Non amino acid precursors

16. Hordenine, mescaline, & yohimbine are examples for?
    (a) True alkaloids
    (b) Pseudo alkaloids
    (c) Proto alkaloids
    (d) None

17. An example of pseudo alkaloid is
    (a) Coniine   (b) Hygrine
    (c) Tropine   (d) Harmine

18. An example of pseudo alkaloid is
    (a) Capsaicin   (b) Ephedrine
    (c) Solanidine   (d) All

19. An example of pseudo alkaloid is
    (a) Theobromine
    (b) Codeine
    (c) Lycorine
    (d) Serotonin

20. Typical alkaloids are
    (a) Heterocyclic alkaloids & contain 'N' in hetero cyclic ring
    (b) Non-heterocyclic alkaloids
    (c) Non-heterocyclic alkaloids & contain 'N' in hetero cyclic ring
    (d) Heterocyclic alkaloids

21. Atypical alkaloids are?
    (a) Heterocyclic alkaloids & contain 'N' in hetero cyclic ring
    (b) Non-heterocyclic alkaloids
    (c) Non-heterocyclic alkaloids & contain 'N' in hetero cyclic ring
    (d) Heterocyclic alkaloids

22. Nicotine is obtained from?
    (a) Dried leaves of nicotiana a bacum
    (b) Dried entire plant of nicotiana tabacum
    (c) Dried young leaves of nicotiana tabacum
    (d) Dried leaves and flowers of nicotiana tabacum

23. Tobacco contains
    (a) Pyrrolidine & piperidine
    (b) Pyrrolidine & pyridine ring or pyridine & piperidine
    (c) Pyrrolidine & pyrrole ring
    (d) Pyrrolizidine ring

24. The poisonous effect of tobacco smoke is due to decomposition of nicotine to
    (a) Pyridine & furfural
    (b) Collidine
    (c) Hydrocyanic acid & carbon monoxide
    (d) All the above

25. Boscia angustifolia belongs to which family?
    (a) Scrophularaceae
    (b) Leguminoseae
    (c) Capparidaceae
    (d) Polygonaceae

26. Nicotine is sprayed in the form of
    (a) Nicotin hydrochloride
    (b) Nicotine chloride
    (c) Nicotine sulphate
    (d) All the above

27. Nicotine has advantage over synthetic insecticide is?
    (a) It is safe
    (b) Much less toxic to warm blooded animals
    (c) Easy to handle
    (d) All the above

28. Betal nuts are obtained from?
    (a) Seeds of areca catechu belonging to palmaceae
    (b) Fruits of areca catechu belonging to palmaceae
    (c) Seeds of areca caliso belonging to meliaceae
    (d) Fruits of areca caliso belonging to meliaceae

29. The amount of arecoline in areca is
    (a) 0.1% to 2 %
    (b) 0.1% to 0.5 %
    (c) Less than 0.1 %
    (d) 2%-2.5 %

30. Areca nut contains a number of alkaloids of?
    (a) Pyrrolizidine series
    (b) Piperidine series
    (c) Pyrrolidine & piperidine
    (d) Pyrrolidine series

31. Areca contains arecoline, chemically it is?
    (a) Methyl ester of arecanine
    (b) Ethyl ester of arecanine
    (c) N-Methyl Guvacine
    (d) Tetrahydronicotine

32. Areca contains arecaine, chemically it is?
    (a) Methyl ester of arcanine
    (b) Ethyl ester of arcanine
    (c) N-Methyl guvacine
    (d) Tetrahydronicotinic

33. Areca contains guvacine, chemically it is?
    (a) Methyl ester of arcanine
    (b) Ethyl ester of arcanine
    (c) N-Methyl guvacin
    (d) Tetrahydronicotin

34. Areca nut contains Fats and tannins in the ratio?
    (a) 14% & 15 % respectively
    (b) 24% & 25 % respectively
    (c) 4% & 5 % respectively
    (d) 10% & 12 % respectively

35. Areca is used as
    (a) Anthelmintic
    (b) Nerve tonic
    (c) Urinary disorders
    (d) All the above

36. Areca chewing may cause
    (a) Mouth cancer
    (b) Tooth coloration
    (c) Mouth ulcers
    (d) Dental decay

37. Areca caliso, A. concima, A. ipot, A. laxa, A. nagensis & A. triandra are
    (a) Substituents of areca nuts
    (b) Adulterants of areca nuts
    (c) Allied species of areca nuts
    (d) Source of areca nuts

38. Sago palm nuts (metroxylon species), dried tapioca (manihot esculenta) & species of sweet potato are
    (a) Substituents of areca nuts
    (b) Adulterants of areca nuts
    (c) Allied species of areca nuts
    (d) Source of areca nuts

39. Caryota curningii & hetero spathe elata are?
    (a) Substituents of areca nuts
    (b) Adulterants of areca nuts
    (c) Allied species of areca nuts
    (d) Source of areca nuts

40. Caryota urens resembling genuine areca nuts & coated with concentrated areca nut (Kali)?
    (a) Form the principal substituent
    (b) Form the principal adulterant
    (c) Both a & b
    (d) None

41. Adulteration in areca can be identified by
    (a) Decrease of 10% fibre content of the sample
    (b) Increase of 10% fibre content of the sample
    (c) Decrease of 10% fat content of the sample
    (d) Increase of 10% fat content of the sample

42. Areca nuts also called as?
    (a) Panag
    (b) Pannach
    (c) Pinang
    (d) Plnanghana

43. Grown of areca plants require?
    (a) Heavy rainfAll of the above&temperature between 15°C -38°C
    (b) Light rainfAll of the above&temperature between 25°C -40°C
    (c) Does not require rainfAll of the above& tolerate to 25°C
    (d) Heavy rainfAll of the above& temperature between 10°C -18°C

44. Lobelia is called as?
    (a) Indian tobacco
    (b) Asthama weeds
    (c) Puke weed
    (d) All the above

45. Lobelia consists of?
    (a) Dried leaves of lobelia inflate belonging to lobeliaceae
    (b) Dried aerial parts of lobelia nicotianifolia
    (c) Dried leaves of lobelia inflate belonging to solanaceae
    (d) Dried aerial parts of lobelia inflate belonging to solanaceae

46. The lobelia content in lobelia should not less than
    (a) 0.55%   (b) 0.65%
    (c) 0.75%   (d) 045%

47. The arecoline content is areca shout not less than
    (a) 0.15%   (b) 0.25%
    (c) 0.35%   (d) 0.45%

48. The ash content in areca nuts?
    (a) NMT 3%   (b) NMT 4%
    (c) NMT 5%   (d) NMT 6%

49. Which part of the lobelia contains high percentage of lobeline?
    (a) Leaves   (b) Flower
    (c) Seed   (d) Stem

50. $C_{22}H_{27}O_2N$ is?
    (a) Lobelanine   (b) Lobeline
    (c) Lobelanidine   (d) Lobelidine

51. Lobeline forms
    (a) Hydrobromide   (b) Methiodide
    (c) Hydrochloride (d) All the above

52. Lobelia is used as a?
    (a) Respiratory stimulant
    (b) Nervine stimulant
    (c) Cardiac stimulant
    (d) Both a & b

53. C_5H_5N is?
    (a) Pyridine
    (b) Azabenzene & azine
    (c) Both a & b
    (d) Piperidine

54. Alkaloids are not precipitated by?
    (a) Millon's reagent
    (b) Hager's reagent
    (c) Wagner's reagent
    (d) Dragendroff's reagent

55. Modified diterpenes are active constituents of
    (a) Colchicum
    (b) Ephedra
    (c) Taxus
    (d) All the above

56. Phenyl ethyl amines are active constituents of?
    (a) Ephedrine
    (b) Hordenine

(c) Mescaline

(d) All the above

57. Precursor compound for pyrrolidine alkaloids is
    (a) L-Tyrosine   (b) L-Ornithine
    (c) L-Tryptophan   (d) L-Lysine

58. Precursor compound for piperidine alkaloids is?
    (a) L-Tyrosine   (b) L-Ornithine
    (c) L-Tryptophan   (d) L-Lysine

59. Precursor compound for phenyl ethyl amino alkaloids is?
    (a) L-Tyrosine   (b) L-Ornithine
    (c) L-Tryptophan   (d) L-Lysine

60. Precursor compound for Indole alkaloids is?
    (a) L-Tyrosine   (b) L-Ornithine
    (c) L-Tryptophan   (d) L-Lysine

61. Precursor compound for Phenethylisoquinoline alkaloids is?
    (a) L-Tyrosine
    (b) L-Phenylalanine
    (c) Both a and b
    (d) None

62. Nicotinic acid is the precursor for the?
    (a) Pyrrolizidine
    (b) Pyridine alkaloids
    (c) Indole alkaloids
    (d) Pyrrolidine & piperidine

63. Precursor compound for imidazoline alkaloids is?
    (a) L-Histidine
    (b) L-arginine

(c) Anthranilic acid

(d) L-Ornithine

64. Precursor compound for marine alkaloids is?
    (a) L-Histidine
    (b) L-arginine
    (c) Anthranilic acid
    (d) L-Ornithine

65. Precursor compound for quinazoline alkaloids is?
    (a) L-Histidine
    (b) L-arginine
    (c) Anthranilic acid
    (d) L-Ornithine

66. Precursor compound for pyrrolizidine alkaloids is?
    (a) L-Histidine
    (b) L-arginine
    (c) Anthranilic acid
    (d) L-Ornithine

67. Lobeline solution in sulphuric acid with formaldehyde gives
    (a) Green color
    (b) Pale green color
    (c) Red color
    (d) Pink color

68. Lobeline solution on boiling products smell of
    (a) Acetophenone
    (b) Benzophenone
    (c) Benzaldehyde
    (d) Acetaldehyde

69. Dragendroff' reagent is
    (a) Potassium Bismuth Iodide
    (b) Potassium Mercuric iodide
    (c) Saturated picric acid solution
    (d) Dilute iodine solution

70. Mayer's Reagent is
    (a) Potassium Bismuth Iodide
    (b) Potassium Mercuric iodide
    (c) Saturated picric acid solution
    (d) Dilute iodine solution

71. Hager's reagent is
    (a) Potassium Bismuth Iodide
    (b) Potassium Mercuric iodide
    (c) Saturated picric acid solution
    (d) Dilute iodine solution

72. Wagner's Reagent is
    (a) Potassium Bismuth Iodide
    (b) Potassium Mercuric iodide
    (c) Saturated picric acid solution
    (d) Dilute iodine solution

73. To alkaloid solution added few drops of tannic acid
    (a) Formation of buff colored precipitate was observed
    (b) Formation of red colored precipitate was observed
    (c) No change was observed
    (d) Formation of yellow colored precipitate was observed

74. Alkaloidal solution is acidified & then added NH_3 (Ammonium solution)
    (a) Formation of pink colored precipitate was observed
    (b) Formation of yellow colored precipitate was observed
    (c) Formation of pale yellow colored precipitate was observed
    (d) No precipitate was observed

75. Formation of orange red color precipitate was observed with?
    (a) Dragendroff's reagent
    (b) Hager's Reagent
    (c) Mayer's Reagent
    (d) Wagner's reagent

76. Formation of creamy-white precipitate was observed with
    (a) Dragendroff's reagent
    (b) Hager's Reagent
    (c) Mayer's Reagent
    (d) Wagner's reagent

77. Formation of crystalline-yellow precipitate was observed with
    (a) Dragendroff's reagent
    (b) Hager's Reagent
    (c) Mayer's Reagent
    (d) Wagner's reagent

78. Formation of reddish brown precipitate was observed with
    (a) Dragendroff's reagent
    (b) Hager's Reagent
    (c) Mayer's Reagent
    (d) Wagner's reagent

79. Which of the following statement is false?
    (a) Two stereo isomers of tropene are tropine & pseudotropine
    (b) Tropane ring is composed of pyrrolidine & piperidine ring
    (c) Tropane is 3-hydroxy tropene
    (d) Tropane alkaloids have 7-azabicycloheptane nucleus

80. Tropane alkaloids have
    (a) 7-Azabicyclo heptanes nucleus
    (b) 8-Azabicyclo octane nucleus
    (c) 6-Azabicyclo heptanes nucleus
    (d) 8-Azatricyclo octane nucleus

81. Tropane alkaloids are used as a
    (a) Anticholinergic drugs
    (b) Preanaesthetic drugs in surgery
    (c) To treat motion sickness
    (d) All the above

82. Hydrohyoscinine is the main alkaloid in
    (a) Datura stramonium
    (b) Atropa belladonna & A. acuminata
    (c) Dubosia myoporoides
    (d) All the above

83. Belladonna is also called as
    (a) Woolly fox glove leaves
    (b) Fox glove leaves
    (c) Deadly night shade leaves
    (d) Shaded leaves

84. Belladonna contains 0.3% alkaloids calculated as
    (a) L-Hyoscine   (b) Tropane
    (c) L-Hyoscyanine (d) Tropene

85. Cultivation of belladonna is satisfactory at an altitude of
    (a) 1000 m from sea level
    (b) 1400 m from sea level
    (c) 1200 m from sea level
    (d) 1800 m from sea level

86. The chief habitat of belladonna is
    (a) Andhra Pradesh
    (b) Jammu & in forest of sindh & chinab valley
    (c) Himachal Pradesh
    (d) Madhya Pradesh

87. Atropine is a
    (a) Tropine (-)-tropate
    (b) Tropine (-)-tropane

    (c) Tropine (±)-tropate
    (d) Tropine (±)-tropane

88. Hyoscyanine is a
    (a) Tropine (±)-tropate
    (b) Tropine (-)-tropate
    (c) Tropene (±)-tropane
    (d) Tropene (-)-tropane

89. Vitalis-morin test is positive for
    (a) Quinine   (b) Ergot
    (c) Belladonna   (d) Ephedrine

90. Drug is treated with nitric acid, & then methanolic KOH soln. is added, it gives violet coloration. This indicates the presence of
    (a) Indole alkaloids
    (b) Tropane alkaloids
    (c) Cardiac Glycosides
    (d) Resins

91. Parasitic stomata is also called as?
    (a) Rupacious
    (b) Solanaeous
    (c) Labiatae
    (d) Ranunculaceous

92. Which drug is used as an antidote in opium & chloralhydrate poisoning?
    (a) Belladonna   (b) Rauwolfia
    (c) Kurchi   (d) Colchicum

93. Datura metal contains?
    (a) NLT 0.02% of L-Hyoscyamine
    (b) NLT 0.20% of L-Hyoscyamine
    (c) NLT 0.02% of L-Hyoscine
    (d) NLT 0.20% of L-Hyoscine

94. Ailanthus glandulosa is distinct from the belladonna by
    - (a) The presence of cluster crystals of calcium oxalate near the veins
    - (b) Presence of idioblast cells
    - (c) Presence of needle shaped crystals
    - (d) All the above

95. $C_{17}H_{21}O_4N$ (Hyoscine) is an?
    - (a) Ester of tropic acid & scopine
    - (b) Ester of tropic acid & tropine
    - (c) Ester of tropene & mandelic acid
    - (d) Ester of tropene & tropic acid

96. $C_{17}H_{23}NO_3$ (Hyoscyamine) is an?
    - (a) Ester of tropic acid & scopine
    - (b) Ester of tropic acid & tropine
    - (c) Ester of tropene & mandelic acid
    - (d) Ester of tropene & tropic acid

97. Homatropine is an
    - (a) Ester of tropic acid & scopine
    - (b) Ester of tropic acid & tropine
    - (c) Ester of tropene & mandelic acid
    - (d) Ester of tropene & tropic acid

98. Anisocytic stomata is present in
    - (a) Vasaka
    - (b) Lobelia
    - (c) Datura
    - (d) Senna

99. Diacytic or caryophyllaceous or cross celled stomata is present in?
    - (a) Vasaka & Tulsi
    - (b) Spearmint
    - (c) Peppermint
    - (d) All the above

100. Anisocytic or cruciferous or unequal celled stoma is present in?
    - (a) Belladonna
    - (b) Tobacco & datura
    - (c) Hyoscyamus & stramonium
    - (d) All the above

101. Anisocytic stoma is also called as?
    - (a) Solanacious stomata
    - (b) Labitae stomata
    - (c) Ranunculacrous stomata
    - (d) Rubiaceae

102. Diacytic stomata is also called as
    - (a) Solanaceous stomata
    - (b) Labitae stomata
    - (c) Ranunculacious stomata
    - (d) Rubiaceae

103. Anoamocytic (Ranunculaceous or Irregular) celled stoma is present in
    - (a) Digitalis
    - (b) Eucalyptus & senna
    - (c) Lobelia & neem
    - (d) All the above

104. Duboisia consists of
    - (a) Dried entire plant of duboisia myoporoides belonging to the family solanaceae
    - (b) Dried leaves of duboisia myoporoides belonging to the family solanaceae
    - (c) Dried entire plant of duboisia myoporoides belonging to the family campanulaceae
    - (d) Dried leaves of duboisia myoporoides belonging to the family campanulaceae

105. The chief constituent of duboisia hopwoodii was found to be
    - (a) Nicotine & non-nicotine
    - (b) Scopolamine & atropine

(c) Tropane & hyoscine
(d) Tropic acid & tropane

106. Atropine on treating with gold chloride & HCl gives
(a) Lemon green precipitate
(b) Pale pink precipitate
(c) Lemon yellow precipitate
(d) Pale green precipitate

107. Erythroxylon coca & erythroxylon truxillense commercially known as
(a) Truxillo & bolivian respectively
(b) Bolivian & peruvian coca respectively
(c) Peruvian & truxillo coca respectively
(d) Bolivian & huánuco coca respectively

108. Which form of alkaloids are pharmacologically more active?
(a) Dextro isomer
(b) Leavo isomer
(c) Racemic form
(d) All the above

109. Aconite belongs to the group of
(a) Terpenoidal alkaloid
(b) Triterpenoid glycoside
(c) Steroidal alkaloid
(d) Tetraterpenoid glycoside

110. Opium factory is situated at?
(a) Ghazipur (U.P.)
(b) Assam (Kashia & Jaintia wills)
(c) Mungapoo (West Bengal)
(d) Kelara (Andhra Pradesh)

111. Morphine, codeine & theabine belongs to
(a) Quinaline ring system
(b) Benzyl Isoquinoline ring system
(c) Phenanthrene ring system
(d) Naphthalene ring system

112. Papaverine, narcotine & narceine belong to
(a) Quinoline ring system
(b) Benzyl isoquinoline ring system
(c) Phenanthrene ring system
(d) Naphthalene ring system

113. Which of the following are absent in opium
(a) Mucilage, sugar, & wax
(b) Salts of Potassium, magnesium & calcium
(c) Starch, tannins, calcium oxalate, crystals
(d) Narceine, codanine, lanthopine

114. Alkaloids of opium are present in the form of?
(a) Sulphates   (b) Oxalic acid
(c) Meconic acid   (d) Tartaric acid

115. Heroin is
(a) Diacetyl morphine
(b) Methyl morphine
(c) Ethyl morphine
(d) Butyl morphine

116. Rio or brazilian ipecac is obtained from?
(a) Cephaelis acuminata belongs to apocynaceae
(b) Cephaelis acuminata belongs to rubiaciae

(c) Cephaelis ipecacauanha belongs to apocyanaceae

(d) Cephaelis ipecacauanha belongs to rubiaceae

117. Cartagena or panama Ipecac is obtained from
   (a) Cephaelis acuminata contain NLT 2% ether soluble alkaloids
   (b) Cephaelis ipecacuanha contain NLT 0.2% alcohol soluble alkaloids
   (c) Cephaelis acuminata contain NLT 0.2% ether soluble alkaloids
   (d) Cephaelis ipecacuanha contain NLT 2% alcohol soluble alkaloids

118. Italian belladonna leaves are obtained from
   (a) Atropa belladonna
   (b) Atropa acuminata
   (c) Solanum nigrum
   (d) Ailanthus glandulosa

119. Hyoscyamine an alkaloid obtained from atropa belladonna
   (a) Readily recemises to atropine with ethanolic alkali, atropine (±) Hyoscyamine
   (b) Readily disintegrates into atropine with acid solution atropine is (-) Hyoscyamine
   (c) Readily rearranges into atropine with alkali solution atropine is (+) Hyoscyamine

   (d) Readily rearranges to atropine with ethanolic alkali, atropine is (+) Hyoscyamine

120. Choose the correct description for ergot?
   (a) Loosely arranged or in smAll of the abovemore or less agglutinated angular masses
   (b) A pseudo parenchyma formed by the interwoven closely appressed compact septate hyphae
   (c) The crystocarps have fallen out leaving corresponding oval perforation in the ramuli
   (d) Colourless septate hyphae about one quarter the width of a cotton trichome and they became twisted

121. Rescinnamine is derived from
   (a) Trimethoxy cinnamic acid
   (b) Triethoxy cinnamic acid
   (c) Trimethoxy propionic acid
   (d) Trimethoxy reserpic acid

122. Reserpine is derived from
   (a) Tryptophan & tryptamine
   (b) L-arginine & asparagine
   (c) L-Histidine
   (d) L-Ornithine

123. Ailanthus glandulosa is identified by presence of
   (a) Idioblasts of acicular crystals
   (b) Palisade ratio of 2 to 4
   (c) Cluster crystals of calcium oxalate near the veins & unicellular thick walled trichomes
   (d) All the above

124. Rauwolfia serpentine can be distinguished from other adulterants of rauwolfia species by
 (a) Presence of starch grains
 (b) Presence of calcium oxalate crystals
 (c) Presence of trichomes
 (d) Presence of sclereids

125. Precursor for the biosynthesis of tropane group alkaloid is
 (a) Leucine   (b) Lysine
 (c) Ornithine   (d) Tyrosine

126. Imidazole alkaloids are derived from?
 (a) Anthranilic acid
 (b) L-Histidine
 (c) Nicotinic acid
 (d) L-Tyrosine

127. Alkaloids derived from ornithine are
 (a) Atropine
 (b) Cocaine
 (c) Hyoscyamine
 (d) All the above

128. Water soluble of ergot contains
 (a) Ergometrine group
 (b) Ergocornine group
 (c) Ergotamine group
 (d) Ergotoxine group

129. Cocaine, an alkaloid derived from coca leaves acts by
 (a) Increasing nor-adrenaline synthesis
 (b) Inhibiting monoamine oxidase
 (c) Inhibiting catechol-O-methyl transferase
 (d) Inhibiting noradrenaline reuptake

130. Crow fig is
 (a) Castor   (b) Nux Vomica
 (c) Nutmeg   (d) Linseed

131. Jesuits Bark is
 (a) Kurchi   (b) Cinchona
 (c) Arjuna   (d) Cascara

132. Maximum alkaloidal content in the cinchona bark is found in plants of age
 (a) 3 to 5 years old
 (b) 4 to 6 years old
 (c) 6 to 9 years old
 (d) 9 to 12 years old

133. Government factories extracting cinchona alkaloids are situated at?
 (a) Mungapoo (West Bengal)
 (b) Annamallais (Tamilnadu)
 (c) Both a & b
 (d) Ghazipur (U.P)

134. Cinchona grows satisfactorily at the altitude of
 (a) 1000 to 3000 mts
 (b) 2000 to 4000 mts
 (c) 700 to 1000 mts
 (d) 1000 to 1500 mts

135. Quinidine is
 (a) Cardiac depressant
 (b) Antispasmodic
 (c) Antimalarial
 (d) Antiaemobic

136. Van-Urk's test is positive for the
 (a) Ergot   (b) Atropine
 (c) Caffeine   (d) Cinchona

137. Vitali-Morin test is positive for
 (a) Ergot   (b) Atropine
 (c) Caffeine   (d) Cinchona

138. Murexide test is positive for
    (a) Ergot   (b) Atropine
    (c) Caffeine   (d) Cinchona

139. Thalleioquin test is positive for
    (a) Ergot   (b) Atropine
    (c) Caffeine   (d) Cinchona

140. Ergot gives
    (a) Red fluorescence in UV light
    (b) Blue fluorescence in water
    (c) Strong odor of trimethylamine when treated with NaOH
    (d) All the above

141. Which of the following statement is correct?
    (a) Ergotamine is used in migraine
    (b) Ergometrine is used as oxytocic
    (c) Ergocryptine and ergocriystine are used in treatment of mammary tumors
    (d) All the above

142. Cocaine on treating with sulphuric acid heated followed by addition of water gives characteristic smell of
    (a) Acetaldehyde
    (b) Methyl benzoate
    (c) Trimethylamine
    (d) Benzaldehyde

143. Quinidine gives white precipitate on treating with
    (a) AgNO$_3$ solution which is soluble in HNO$_3$
    (b) AgNO$_3$ solution which is insoluble in HNO$_3$
    (c) AgNO$_3$ solution which is soluble in HCl
    (d) AgNO$_3$ solution which is insoluble in HCl

144. Coca seeds are derived from?
    (a) Erythroxylum coca var spruceanum
    (b) Theobroma CoCao
    (c) Erythroxylum truxillense
    (d) Erythroxylum monogynum

145. Tea plants are cultivated in
    (a) Assam
    (b) Japan and java
    (c) West Bengal
    (d) All the above

146. Color of the leaves changes during fermentation is due to the presence of an enzyme?
    (a) Thease   (b) Diastase
    (c) Oxidase   (d) Amylase

147. Tea is obtained from
    (a) Leaves of leaf buds of Thea sinensis
    (b) Seeds & Leaf buds of Thea sinensis
    (c) Fruits of young leaves of Thea sinensis
    (d) All the above

148. Coca is used as
    (a) An ingredients in ointments
    (b) Nutritive and diuretic
    (c) Both a & b
    (d) Local anaesthetic

149. Coffee is the valuable remedy in the case of
    (a) Poisoning caused due to opium & alcohol
    (b) Snake bite

(c) Both a & b

(d) None of the above

150. Myristica fragrans has two of the following characteristics

(a) An in deciduous tree, which produces drupaceous, pale yellow fruits

(b) Each fruit has several round seeds with smooth surface and ligneous tegument, and the orange red fleshy aril, the mace is present inside the seed

(c) A deciduous tAll of the abovetree, which produces ligneous capsules

(d) Each fruit has a unique ovoid seed, with ligneous legument surrounded by orange red laciniate fleshy aril the mace

(a) b & c   (b) a & c

(c) a & d   (d) b & d

151. Ephedra is used in the treatment of?

(a) Asthmatic conditions

(b) Tuberculosis

(c) Hypertension

(d) Cough

152. Diagnostic character for the microscopical identification of Kurchi bark is?

(a) Fibre with Y-shaped fits

(b) Horse shoe shaped stone cells

(c) Scleerides containing calcium oxalate crystals

(d) Stratified cork

153. Meadow saffron seed is

(a) Colchicum seed

(b) Crocus sativus seed

(c) Nutmeg seed

(d) Linseed

154. Biological source of colchicum seed is?

(a) Colchicum autumnale

(b) Colchicum speciosum

(c) Colchicum Luteum

(d) All the above

155. Alkaloid which inhibits the cholinesterase undergoes hydrolysis is solution to give methyl carbamic acid & seroline?

(a) Scopolamine

(b) Pyridostigmine

(c) Neostigmine

(d) Physostigmine

156. Precursor for the ergot alkaloids

(a) Phenylalanine (b) Tryptophan

(c) Tryptamine   (d) Lysergic acid

157. The alkaloidal concentration in coca leaves vary from

(a) 3%-4%   (b) 0.7%-1.5%

(c) 0.01%-0.02%   (d) 6%-11%

158. The Shape of tinnaevelly senna is

(a) Ovate   (b) Lanceolate

(c) Elliptical   (d) Linear

159. Following is an example for pyridine alkaloid?

(a) Datura   (b) Kurchi

(c) Lobelia   (d) Pilocarpus

160. Colchicine seen is biogenetically derived from

(a) Tyrosineand & phenylalanine

(b) Tryptophan & phenylalanine

(c) Ornithine & tryptophan

(d) Ornithine & phenylalanine

161. Main constituent in the dried ripe seeds of Colchicum luteum and colchicum autumnale is derived from?

(a) Tyrosine, phenylalanine & di hydroxy phenylalanine

(b) Tryptophan & tryptamine

(c) Ornithine

(d) Lysine

162. Colchicine is used clinically for

(a) Gout

(b) Asthama

(c) Analgesic

(d) Anti-inflammatory

163. Indian ginseng is?

(a) Ginseng   (b) Turmeric

(c) Withania   (d) Saffron

164. Ma-huang is

(a) Cinchona   (b) Ephedra

(c) Kurchi   (d) Saffron

165. Ephedra sinica & ephedra equisetina can be distinguished by type of

(a) Branching   (b) Stomata

(c) Scaly leaves   (d) Alkaloids

166. Withanolides are present in

(a) Ashwagandha (b) Kurchi

(c) Yam   (d) Veratrum

167. American hellebore is

(a) Veratrum

(b) Kurchi

(c) Atropa

(d) Ashwagandha

168. Veratrum belongs to

(a) Apocynaceae

(b) Solanaceae

(c) Papaveraceae

(d) Liliaceae

169. American veratrum is obtained form

(a) Veratrum viride

(b) Veratrum sativum

(c) Veratrum album

(d) Veratrum fragrans

170. European Veratrum is obtained from

(a) Veratrum viride

(b) Veratrum sativum

(c) Veratrum album

(d) Veratrum fragrans

171. Veratrum is used as

(a) Antihypertensive

(b) Cardiac depressant

(c) Sedative & insecticide

(d) All the above

172. Solasodine is obtained from

(a) Dried berries of solanum khasianum

(b) Dried tubers of solanum tuberosum

(c) Dried fruits of solanum esculatum

(d) All the above

173. Solasodine is used as precursor for?

(a) Corticosteroids

(b) Sex hormones

(c) Oral contraceptives

(d) All the above

174. Following is a glycoalkaloid?
    (a) Ephedrine   (b) Solasodine
    (c) Conessine   (d) Vasicinone

175. Carbohydrates are the
    (a) Polyhydroxy aldoses or aldehydes
    (b) Polyhydroxy ketones
    (c) Both a and b
    (d) Non-nitrogenous polyphenols

176. The general formula of carbohydrates is
    (a) (C_2H_2O) (b) $(CH_2O)_n$
    (c) $(CHO_2)_n$ (d) All the above

177. Monosaccharide are the sugars which
    (a) Cannot be hydrolysed further to simple compounds
    (b) Yields two molecules on hydrolysis
    (c) Yields three molecules on hydrolysis
    (d) Yields indefinite molecules on hydrolysis

178. Carbohydrates are identified by?
    (a) Mayer's test
    (b) Millon's test
    (c) Molisch' test
    (d) Match stick test

179. Gums are
    (a) Physiological products
    (b) Pathological products
    (c) Nitrogenous products
    (d) Polyphenolic products

180. Acacia contains
    (a) Oxidase enzyme
    (b) Calcium, magnesium & potassium salts of arabic acid
    (c) Peroxidases & pectinases
    (d) All the above

181. Gum on heating with dil. acids yields
    (a) Sugars   (b) Proteins
    (c) Amino acids   (d) All the above

182. Mucilages are
    (a) Physiological products
    (b) Esters of complex polysaccharides
    (c) Both a and b
    (d) Pathological products

183. Agar is known as
    (a) Japanese isinglass
    (b) Bengal quince
    (c) Jaguar gum
    (d) Irish mass extract

184. Agar contains
    (a) Galactose polymer
    (b) Agarose & agaropectin
    (c) Sulphonated polysaccharide
    (d) All the above

185. Find out the wrong statement?
    (a) Agaropectin is responsible for the viscosity of the solution
    (b) Agarose is responsible for gel strength
    (c) Acid insoluble ash of agar is not more than 2.0%
    (d) Agar contain cellulose and nitrogen containing substance

186. Agar is used as
    (a) An emulsifier
    (b) Laxative

(c) Preparation of jellies, confectionary items & in microbiology

(d) All the above

187. Agar substituted with
    (a) Gelatin
    (b) Danish agar
    (c) Both a & b
    (d) None

188. Agar is distinguished from danish agar, which
    (a) Has half of its gel strength of japanese agar
    (b) Has gel strength double than japanese agar
    (c) Has gel strength triple than japanese agar
    (d) None

189. The presence of gelatin in agar can be detected by?
    (a) The gel strength which is half of its gel strength of agar
    (b) Addition of equal volume of 1% of agar solution, the solution produces turbidity or precipitation
    (c) Both a & b
    (d) None

190. Loss on drying for agar will not be more than
    (a) 5%
    (b) 9%
    (c) 16%
    (d) 18%

191. Agar has swelling index of
    (a) NLT 6
    (b) NLT 10
    (c) NLT 12
    (d) NLT 16

192. Jaguar gum is
    (a) Karaya gum
    (b) Acacia gum
    (c) Gum tragacanth
    (d) Guar gum

193. Indian tragacanth is
    (a) Karaya gum
    (b) Acacia gum
    (c) Gum tragacanth
    (d) Guar gum

194. Guar gum obtained from
    (a) Powder of endosperm of the seeds of cyamopsis tetragonolobus
    (b) Gummy exudation from stems and branches of astragalus gummifer
    (c) Gummy exudate from the anogeissus latifolia
    (d) All the above

195. Guar gum contains
    (a) Guaran
    (b) 65% of galactose & 35% of mannose
    (c) Proteins (5%-7%)
    (d) All the above

196. Water soluble protein of guar gum is called as?
    (a) Galactomannan or guaran
    (b) Bassorin
    (c) Tragacanth
    (d) All the above

197. Guaran consists of linear chains of D-galactose & D-mannose in the ratio of
    (a) 1:1
    (b) 1:2
    (c) 1:3
    (d) 1:4

198. The Gum solution when mixed with 0.5 mL of benzidine & 0.5 mL of H_2O_2 produces blue color is?
    (a) Acacia
    (b) Guar gum
    (c) Both a & b
    (d) None

199. The gum solution when mixed with 0.5 mL of benzidine & 0.5 mL of H_2O_2 produces no blue color is?
    (a) Acacia
    (b) Guar gum
    (c) Both a and b
    (d) None

200. The gum will not produce pink color when treated with ruthenium red solution is
    (a) Guar gum, tragacanth & acacia
    (b) Sterculia gum & karaya
    (c) Agar
    (d) All the above

201. The aqueous solution of gum is converted to a gel by the addition of smAll of the aboveamount of borax is
    (a) Karaya
    (b) Tragacanth
    (c) Guar gum
    (d) All the above

202. The 2% solution of lead acetate gives a white precipitate with?
    (a) Guar gum
    (b) Sterculia gum
    (c) Acacia
    (d) All the above

203. Guar gum is used
    (a) As a protective colloid, a binding & disintegrating & emulsifying agent
    (b) To decrease serum total cholesterol levels
    (c) To affect gastrointestinal transit may contribute to its hypoglycin activity
    (d) All the above

204. Acacia should not contain?
    (a) More than 15% of moisture & 5% ash
    (b) Tannin & starch
    (c) Dextrin
    (d) All the above

205. Indian gum is
    (a) Gum acacia
    (b) Gum tragacanth
    (c) Guar gum
    (d) Karaya gum

206. Acacia is used as
    (a) As demulcent and also administered intravenously in haemolysis
    (b) Suspending agent
    (c) Good emulsifying agent
    (d) All the above

207. Mel is
    (a) Honey
    (b) Male fern
    (c) Myrrh
    (d) Mustard

208. Taste of honey is
    (a) Sweet
    (b) Sweet & faintly acid
    (c) Sweet & faintly bitter
    (d) All the above

209. Test is used to distinguish honey from its adulterant is
    (a) Frihe' test
    (b) Frohde's test
    (c) Fehling's test

(d) Both a & c

210. Specific rotation of honey is
  (a) $+3^{\circ}C$ to $-6^{\circ}C$
  (b) $+3^{\circ}C$ to $-10^{\circ}C$
  (c) $+3^{\circ}C$ to $-3^{\circ}C$
  (d) $+1^{\circ}C$ to $-3^{\circ}C$

211. Honey which contains crystallised dextrose is called as
  (a) Saturated honey
  (b) Granulated honey
  (c) Crystallised Honey
  (d) All the above

212. Artificial invert sugar gives
  (a) Instant red color with resorcinol in HCl
  (b) Transient red color with resorcinol in HCl
  (c) Pink color with resorcinol in HCl
  (d) None

213. Natural honey gives
  (a) Instant red color with resorcinol in HCl
  (b) Transient red color with resorcinol in HCl
  (c) Pink colour with resorcinol in HCl
  (d) None

214. The density of honey is
  (a) 1.498   (b) 1.472
  (c) 1.463   (d) 1.456

215. Indian Psyllium is
  (a) Isapghol seeds
  (b) Castor seeds
  (c) Psyllium seeds

(d) Psorolea seeds

216. Swelling factor for isapghol seed is
  (a) 9-12   (b) 10-14
  (c) 12-17   (d) 14-19

217. The andhra pradesh plantago ovate seeds are substituted with
  (a) Plantago rhodosperma
  (b) Plantago asiatica
  (c) Plantago purshii
  (d) All the above

218. Find the wrong statement?
  (a) Isapghol mucilage consists of two complex polysaccharides of which one is soluble in hot water & the other is soluble in cold water
  (b) Pentosan on hydrolysis yields xylose, arabinose
  (c) Aldobionic acid on hydrolysis galactoronic acid & rhamnose
  (d) Proteins and fixed oils are absent in isabghol

219. Rheutinium red on treatment with ispaghula?
  (a) Shows red color
  (b) Does not shoe red color
  (c) Shows faint pink color
  (d) None

220. Ispaghula seeds are used
  (a) As bulk laxative
  (b) As excellent demulcent
  (c) In dysentery, chronic diarrhea
  (d) All the above

221. Isabghol is used in cosmetics because?
    (a) It is an excellent demulcent
    (b) Mucilage of isapghol has a property of gloriness or stringiness
    (c) Both a & b
    (d) None

222. Isapghol seeds are adulterated with seeds of plantago lanceolate & identified by
    (a) Oblong, elliptical shape of seed
    (b) Yellowish-brown color of seed
    (c) Swelling factor of seed is 5
    (d) All the above

223. The product formed by removing cations from the isabghol mucilage by treatment with cation exchange resins followed by spray drying is an acid form of polysaccharide. This finds special application as
    (a) Enteric coating material
    (b) Tablet disintegration
    (c) Sustained release drug formulations
    (d) All the above

224. Aldobionic acid present in Isabghol seeds on hydrolysis yields?
    (a) Galactoronic acid & rhamnose
    (b) Xylose & arabinose
    (c) Both a & b
    (d) None

225. Pentosan present in isabghol husk on hydrolysis yields
    (a) Xylose & arabinose
    (b) Galacturonic acid & rhamnose
    (c) Both a & b
    (d) None

226. Spogel or flea seeds are
    (a) Isabghl seeds   (b) Castor seeds
    (c) Linseeds   (d) None

227. Which of the following statement in wrong
    (a) Pectin is a protective colloid which assists absorption of toxin in the gastro-intestinal tract
    (b) Pectin is used as thickening agent
    (c) Pectin is used as an emulsifier, gelling agent
    (d) Pectin is used as tablet disintegrator

228. Pectin is incompatible with
    (a) Calcium
    (b) Gelatin
    (c) Both a & b
    (d) Hydrochloric acid

229. Amylum is
    (a) Starch   (b) Agarose
    (c) Acacia   (d) Asafoetida

230. Maize starch is obtained from
    (a) Zea mays
    (b) Triticum aestivum
    (c) Oryza sativa
    (d) Solanum tuberosum

231. Rice starch is obtained from
    (a) Zea mays
    (b) Triticum aestivum
    (c) Oryza sativa
    (d) Solanum tuberosum

232. Potato starch is obtained from
    (a) Solanum lycopersicum
    (b) Solanum nelongana
    (c) Oryza sativa
    (d) Solanum tuberosum

233. Wheal starch is obtained from
    (a) Solanum lycopersicum
    (b) Solanum melongana
    (c) Oryza sativa
    (d) Solanum tuberosum

234. Gluten is absent in the
    (a) Potato   (b) Rice
    (c) Wheat   (d) Maize

235. The specific gravity of starch is
    (a) Less than 1
    (b) Greater than 1
    (c) Less than 2
    (d) Greater than 2

236. The starch grains exhibit no concentric striations are
    (a) Maize   (b) Potato
    (c) Wheat   (d) Rice

237. In starch amylase and amylopectin are present in the proportion of
    (a) 1: 1   (b) 1: 2
    (c) 2: 1   (d) 1: 3

238. Which of the following gives blue colour with iodine?
    (a) Amylose
    (b) Amylopectin
    (c) Agarose
    (d) All the above

239. Which of the following gives bluish black color with iodine?
    (a) Amylose
    (b) Amylopectin
    (c) Agarose
    (d) All the above

240. Which of the following statement is false?
    (a) Amylose is water soluble
    (b) Amylopectin is water insoluble
    (c) Swells in water & α–amylose is responsible for gelatinising property of the starch
    (d) Beta amylose swells in water

241. Potato starch on treating with dilute HCl, forms
    (a) Hydrolysed starch
    (b) Soluble starch
    (c) Oxidised starch
    (d) Insoluble starch

242. Starch on boiling with water form stiff jelly, on addition of iodine to that solution it appears
    (a) Deep brown color
    (b) Black color
    (c) Blue color & color disappears on warming & reappears on cooling
    (d) None

243. Starch is used as an
    (a) Antidote for calcium poisoning
    (b) Antidote for iodine poisoning
    (c) Antidote for iron poisoning
    (d) Antidote for magnesium poisoning

244. Gum arabic is adulterated with
    (a) Karaya   (b) Tragacanth
    (c) Agar   (d) All the above

245. Sterculia gum is
    (a) Gum Karaya   (b) Guar gum
    (c) Tragacanth   (d) Agar

246. Sterculia gum is mainly substituted with
  (a) Gum Tragacanth
  (b) Guar gum
  (c) Agar
  (d) Sodium alginate

247. Gum Karaya swells upto
  (a) 10-30
  (b) 30-50
  (c) 50-70
  (d) 60-100 times in water

248. The acid insoluble ash is in gum karaya is
  (a) NMT 0.5%   (b) NMT 1.0%
  (c) NMT 1.5%   (d) NMT 2%

249. 1% solution of tragacanth has a viscosity of not less than
  (a) 150 centipoises
  (b) 200 centipoises
  (c) 250 centipoises
  (d) 300 centipoises

250. Water insoluble portion of tragacanth is known as
  (a) Tragacanthin
  (b) Bassorin
  (c) Tragacantha
  (d) None

251. Water soluble portion is known as
  (a) Tragacanthin   (b) Bassorin
  (c) Tragacantha   (d) None

252. Honey is called as invert sugar because
  (a) Its optical rotation is opposite to sugar
  (b) It contain glucose, fructose &sucrose

  (c) Both a & b
  (d) None

253. Bassorin present in tragacanth is responsible for
  (a) Oxidizing property of the drug
  (b) Hydrolyzing property of the drug
  (c) Gelatinizing property
  (d) Reducing property of the drug

254. Tannins are
  (a) Complex, organic, non nitrogenous, polyphenolic substances of higher molecular weight compounds
  (b) Non-organic non-nitrogenous, products of plant origin
  (c) Organic nitrogenous substances with high molecular weight
  (d) None of the above

255. If tannins are hydrolysed by mineral acid or enzymes such as tannase, they are called as
  (a) Condensed tannins
  (b) Nonhydrolysed tannins
  (c) Hydrolysed tannins
  (d) Phlobaphenes

256. Condensed tannins on treatment with enzymes or mineral acids, they are polymerised or decomposed into red colored substance called as
  (a) Condensed tannins
  (b) Nonhydrolysed tannins
  (c) Hydrolysed tannins
  (d) Phlobaphenes

257. On drug distillation of hydrolysed tannins are converted into
    (a) Catechol derivatives
    (b) Pyrogallol derivatives
    (c) Gallic acid derivatives
    (d) Anthocyanin derivatives

258. On drug distillation of hydrolysed tannins are converted into
    (a) Catechol derivatives
    (b) Pyrogallol derivatives
    (c) Gallic acid derivatives
    (d) Anthocyanin derivatives

259. Hydrolysed tannins produce?
    (a) Green color with ferric chloride
    (b) Blue color with ferric chloride
    (c) Violet color with ferric chloride
    (d) Brown color with ferric chloride

260. Condensed tannins produce?
    (a) Green color with ferric chloride
    (b) Blue color with ferric chloride
    (c) Violet color with ferric chloride
    (d) Brown color with ferric chloride

261. Hydrolysed tannins are quickly hydrolysed & the products of hydrolysis are
    (a) Gallic acid or ellagic acid
    (b) Phlobaphenes
    (c) Catechol
    (d) All the above

262. Examples of hydrolysed tannins are
    (a) NutgAll of the above& rhubarb
    (b) Oak & myrobalan
    (c) Clove & chestror
    (d) All the above

263. Tannins are soluble in
    (a) Water   (b) Alcohol
    (c) Ether   (d) Benzene

264. When a matchstick is dipped in dilute extract of drug, dried moistened it with concentrated HCl & warm it near a flame. It gives pink or red color. This indicates the solution contains
    (a) Alkaloids   (b) Resins
    (c) Tannins   (d) Glycosides

265. A solution on addition of gelatin, cause precipitation. The solution is identified as
    (a) Resins   (b) Alkaloids
    (c) Tannins   (d) Glycosides

266. Vanillin HCl test is used for identification of
    (a) Alkaloids   (b) Tannins
    (c) Resins   (d) Volatile oils

267. Phenazone test is used for identification of
    (a) Alkaloids   (b) Tannins
    (c) Resins   (d) Volatile oils

268. Tannins are highly soluble in
    (a) Water
    (b) Alcohol
    (c) Water &alcohol
    (d) organic solvents

269. Examples of condensed tannins are
    (a) Green tea
    (b) Wild cherry bark
    (c) Cinnamon & cola
    (d) All the above

270. Pseudo tannins are
   (a) Does not obey the goldbeater's skin test
   (b) Low molecular weight compounds
   (c) Both a & b
   (d) None

271. Haritaki is
   (a) Myrobalan
   (b) Bahera
   (c) Arjuna
   (d) Black catechu

272. Myrobalan contains
   (a) Chebulonic acid
   (b) Free tannic acid, gallic acid & ellagic acid
   (c) Anthraquinone glycosides
   (d) All the above

273. Which of the following is not a constituent of triphala?
   (a) Bahera
   (b) Myrobalan
   (c) Amla
   (d) Arjuna

274. Galls are
   (a) Barks
   (b) Leaves
   (c) Insects
   (d) Pathological outgrowths

275. Myrobalan is
   (a) Dried, ripe & fully matured fruits of terminalia chebula
   (b) Dried, ripe & fully matured fruits of terminalia belerica
   (c) Both a & b
   (d) None of the above

276. Cutch or kattha is
   (a) Blue catechu
   (b) Pale catechu
   (c) Myrobalan
   (d) All the above

277. Gambier or gambir is
   (a) Blue catechu
   (b) Pale catechu
   (c) Myrobalan
   (d) All the above

278. Pale catechu is the
   (a) Dried aqueous extract prepared from heart wood of acacia catechu
   (b) Dried aqueous extract of leaves and young shoots of uncaria gambir
   (c) Dried alcoholic extract prepared from wood of acacia catechu
   (d) Dried alcoholic extract of leaves and young shoots of uncaria gambir

279. Black catechu is the
   (a) Dried aqueous extract prepared from heart wood of acacia catechu
   (b) Dried aqueous extract of leaves & young shoots of uncaria gambir
   (c) Dried alcoholic extract prepared from wood of acacia catechu
   (d) Dried alcoholic extract of leaves & young shoots of uncaria gambir

280. Gambier fluorescein test is positive
   (a) Pale catechu
   (b) Black catechu
   (c) Both a & b
   (d) none of the above

281. Chlorophyll is present in
  (a) Pale catechu
  (b) Black catechu
  (c) Both a & b
  (d) None of the above

282. Pale catechu is
  (a) Reddish brown color with first bitter and then sweet in taste
  (b) Light brown to black color with astringent taste
  (c) Orange to brown color with astringent taste
  (d) None of the above

283. When lime water is added to aqueous extract of black catechu of shows
  (a) Brown color
  (b) Brown color which turns to red precipitate on standing for some time
  (c) Black color, which turns to red precipitate on standing for some time
  (d) Black color

284. The complex amorphous products or compounds of more or less solid characteristics which on heating first sets softened and then melt are
  (a) Lipids   (b) Resins
  (c) Tannins   (d) Waxes

285. Resins dissolve completely in
  (a) Alcohols
  (b) Benzene
  (c) Solvent ether
  (d) All the above

286. Resin acids are
  (a) The carboxylic acid group containing resinous substances which may or may not have association with phenolic compounds
  (b) Complex alcoholic compounds of high molecular weight compounds
  (c) Phenolic compounds of high molecular weight
  (d) Inert resin products

287. Resin alcohols are
  (a) The carboxylic acid group containing resinous substances which may or may not have association with phenolic compounds
  (b) Complex alcoholic compounds of high molecular weight compounds
  (c) Phenolic compounds of high molecular weight
  (d) Inert resin products

288. Resinotannols or resin phenols are
  (a) The carboxylic acid group containing resinous substances which may or may not have association with phenolic compounds
  (b) Complex alcoholic compounds of high molecular weight compounds
  (c) Phenolic compounds of high molecular weight
  (d) Inert resin products

289. Resenes are
   (a) The carboxylic acid group containing resinous substances which may or may not have association with phenolic compounds
   (b) Complex alcoholic compounds of high molecular weight compounds
   (c) Phenolic compounds of high molecular weight
   (d) Inert resin products

290. Esters of the resin acids or the other aromatic acids are called as
   (a) Gum resins
   (b) Resenes
   (c) Gluco esters
   (d) None of the above

291. Resins combined with sugars by glycosylation are called as
   (a) Gum resins
   (b) Resenes
   (c) Gluco esters
   (d) None of the above

292. Homogenous mixture of resin with volatile oil is
   (a) Oleoresin
   (b) Gum resin
   (c) Oleo gum resin
   (d) Balsams

293. The resinous mixtures which contain a high proportion of aromatic balsamic acids such as benzoic acid, cinnamic acid & their esters are
   (a) Oleoresin
   (b) Gum resin
   (c) Oleo gum resin
   (d) Balsams

294. Copaiba & ginger is an example for
   (a) Gum resin
   (b) Oleo gum resin
   (c) Oleoresin
   (d) Balsam

295. Asafoetida is an example for
   (a) Gum resin
   (b) Oleo gum resin
   (c) Oleoresin
   (d) Balsam

296. Colophonium or yellow resin is
   (a) Colophony
   (b) Colocynth
   (c) Capsicum
   (d) Ginger

297. Abetic anhydric or amber resin is
   (a) Colophony   (b) Colocynth
   (c) Capsicum   (d) Ginger

298. The solid residue left after distilling off the volatile oil from the oleoresin obtained from pinus palustris is
   (a) Colophony   (b) Colocynth
   (c) Capsicum   (d) Ginger

299. The major contributor or producer of colophony is
   (a) New Zealand
   (b) India
   (c) U.S.A
   (d) European countries

300. Which of the following is not the character of colophony?
   (a) Pale yellow to amber fragments
   (b) Burns with smoky flame
   (c) Acid number is not less than 150
   (d) Soluble in water

301. Colophony contains
    (a) α, β & γ-abetic acids
    (b) Resenes
    (c) Sipinic acid
    (d) All the above

302. During distillation of colophony
    (a) (-) Pinaric acid is converted into abetic acid
    (b) (+) Pinaric acid is converted into abetic acid
    (c) (±) Pinaric acid is converted into abetic acid
    (d) None of the above

303. On addition of acetic acid & a drop of concentrated sulphuric acid, a drug shows the purple color readily changing to violet, identify the drug
    (a) Colophony   (b) Asafoetida
    (c) Benzoin   (d) All the above

304. Colophony on treating with petroleum ether & double the volume of dilute solution of copper acetate won added petroleum ether layer shows
    (a) Green color
    (b) Pale green color
    (c) Pink
    (d) pale pink color

305. Colophony is mainly used as
    (a) Anticancer agent
    (b) Stimulant & diuretic
    (c) Anti-inflammatory
    (d) Anti arthritic

306. The members of burseraceae are characterised in having
    (a) Volatile oil
    (b) Oleo gum resin
    (c) Oleo resins
    (d) None of the above

307. The adulteration of colophony with black resin or apic resin can be confirmed by their
    (a) Melting point   (b) Acid value
    (c) Ash value   (d) Solubility

308. Himalayan may apple is
    (a) Podophylldum (b) Colophony
    (c) Asafoetida   (d) Capsicum

309. American podophyllum consists of
    (a) Dried rhizomes and roots of podophyllium emodi
    (b) Dried rhizomes of podophyllium hexandrum
    (c) Dried rhizomes & roots of podophyllum peltatum
    (d) All the above

310. α & β peltatins are present in
    (a) Indian podophyllum
    (b) American Podophyllum
    (c) Both a & b
    (d) Balsams

311. The active principle in podophyllium resin is
    (a) Podophyllotoxin
    (b) Podophyllin
    (c) Podophyllum
    (d) Podophyllotoxon

312. Resins containing high percentage of cinnamic acid are called as
    (a) Gummy resins (b) Balsams
    (c) Resenes   (d) Resinols

313. Etoposide is mainly used in
   (a) Treatment of testicular & lung cancer
   (b) Treatment of veneral & other warts
   (c) Both a & b
   (d) None of the above

314. Podophyllotoxin is ter-anhydronapthalene derivative with OH & lactone group in trans position which are essential for
   (a) Anti-mitotic activity
   (b) Purgative activity
   (c) Both a & b
   (d) None of the above

315. Podophyllotoxin is teranhydronapthalene derivative with OH & lactone group in cis position which are essential for
   (a) Anti-mitotic activity
   (b) Purgative activity
   (c) Both a & b
   (d) None of the above

316. Podophyllum on treating with alcohol & strong copper acetate solution, it shows brown colour it indicates the presence of
   (a) Indian podophyllum
   (b) American podophyllum
   (c) Both a & b
   (d) None of the above

317. Podophyllum on treating with alcohol and strong copper acetate solution, it shows green colour without precipitate, it indicates the presence of
   (a) Indian podophyllum
   (b) American podophyllum
   (c) Both a & b
   (d) None of the above

318. Jalap consists of
   (a) Dried tubercles of ipomoea purge
   (b) Dried stems of ipomoea batatus
   (c) Dried tubercles of ipomoea batatus
   (d) Dried stems of ipomoea purge

319. Ether soluble portion of jalap resin is called as
   (a) Jalapin   (b) Tiglic acid
   (c) Convolvulin   (d) All the above

320. Ether insoluble portion of jalap resin is called as
   (a) Jalapin
   (b) Tiglic acid
   (c) Convolvulin
   (d) All the above

321. Convolvulin on hydrolysis gives
   (a) Rhamnoconvolvulic acid
   (b) Tiglic acid
   (c) Exogenic acid
   (d) All the above

322. The main active constituents of jalap are
   (a) Ether soluble part
   (b) Ipurganol
   (c) Ether insoluble part
   (d) Aesculetin

323. Jalap is used
   (a) As a powerful cathartic
   (b) As a cytotoxic agent
   (c) As a carminative
   (d) As a nervine stimulant

324. Indian hemp or marihuana is
 (a) Jalap   (b) Benzoin
 (c) Asafoetida   (d) Cannabis

325. Cannabis consist of
 (a) Dried flowering tops of plants cannabis sativa belonging to moraceae
 (b) Dried flowering tops of female plants of cannabis sativa belonging to moraceae
 (c) Dried leaves of plants cannabis sativa belonging to cananabdaceae
 (d) Dried leaves and stems of plants cannabis sativa belonging to cananabinaceae

326. The resinous exudation collected from the leaves of hemp plants is called as
 (a) Bhang or Siddhi
 (b) Ganja
 (c) Charas
 (d) All of the above

327. The active europic principle present in Indian hemp
 (a) Tetrahydrocannabinol
 (b) Cannabidiolic acid
 (c) Cannabinol
 (d) Cannabichromene

328. Cannabis used as
 (a) Sedative
 (b) Analgesic
 (c) Antispasmodic & anticonvulsant
 (d) All the above

329. The pungent principle of capsicum is known as
 (a) Capsanthin   (b) Capasaisin

 (c) Carolene   (d) Capsine

330. Capsicum is
 (a) Oleogum resin
 (b) Oleo resin
 (c) Resin
 (d) Resene

331. Jalap belongs to
 (a) Berberidaceae
 (b) Convolvulaceae
 (c) Burseraceae
 (d) Umbelliferae

332. Myrrh is
 (a) Oleo resin
 (b) Oleo gum resin
 (c) Gum resin
 (d) Resene

333. Myrrh belonging to the family
 (a) Burseraceae
 (b) Conoulvulaceae
 (c) Berberidaceae
 (d) Umbelliferae

334. Which of the following is true in case of myrrh?
 (a) It contains ether soluble resin acids
 (b) It contains ether insoluble acids are α & β heerabomyerholic acid
 (c) It contains oxidase enzyme
 (d) All the above

335. In India myrrh is substituted by
 (a) Commiphora erythraea
 (b) Balsamodendron mukul
 (c) Yemen myrrh
 (d) All the above

336. Myrrh yields not more than
    (a) 70% of alcohol insoluble matter
    (b) 60% of alcohol insoluble matter
    (c) 50% of alcohol insoluble matter
    (d) 40% alcohol insoluble matter

337. Devil's dung is
    (a) Asafoetida   (b) Myrrh
    (c) Benzoin   (d) Jalap

338. Galbanum contains
    (a) Umbelliferone
    (b) Free umbelliferone
    (c) Both a & b
    (d) None

339. Asafoetida is a
    (a) Gum resin
    (b) Oleo gum resin
    (c) Oleoresin
    (d) Resene

340. Which of the following statement is false in case of asafoetida?
    (a) Asaresinoltannol is present in the free or combined from b
    (b) Free umbelliferone is present
    (c) Ferulic acid is present &on treatment with HCl is converted to umbellic acid
    (d) On treating it with 50% nitric acid, the drug gives green color

341. Asafoetida is adulterated with
    (a) Gum arabic
    (b) Gypsum
    (c) Chalk & Baraly or wheat flour
    (d) All the above

342. The specific odour of asafoetida is due to
    (a) Sulphur compounds
    (b) Calcium compounds
    (c) Magnesium compounds
    (d) Ammonium compounds

343. On treatment of ferulic acid with hydrochloric acid, it is converted into umbelliferone
    (a) Which gives green fluorescence with ammonia
    (b) Which gives blue fluorescence with ammonia
    (c) Which gives green fluorescence with nitric acid
    (d) Which gives blue fluorescence with nitric acid

344. Alcoholic solution of tolu balsam gives green color with ferric chloride due to
    (a) Cinnamic & benzoic acid
    (b) Toluresinotannols
    (c) Oxidation of cinnamic acid
    (d) Benzyl benzoate

345. Balsam of tolu is mainly adulterated with
    (a) Fictitious tolu balsam
    (b) Colophony
    (c) Both a & b
    (d) Gypsum

346. Tolu balsam is adulterated with colophony and is identified by dissolving the drug in petroleum ether and added double the volume of dilute solution of copper acetate
    (a) Petroleum ether layer gives pale pink color

(b) Petroleum ether layer gives blue color

(c) Petroleum ether layer gives green color

(d) Petroleum ether layer gives green color

347. When balsams are treated warmed with potassium permanganate the odor of
(a) Acetaldehyde is produced
(b) Benzaldehyde is produced
(c) Strong penetrating odour is produced
(d) None of the above

348. Peru balsam is obtained from
(a) Trunk of the tree myroxylon balsamum after the kark has been beaten and scorched
(b) Roots of the tree myroxylon balsamum
(c) Flowering tops of the tree myroxylon balsamum
(d) All of the above

349. Sumatra benzoin is obtained from
(a) Balsamic resin from styrax tonkinhsis
(b) Balsamic resin from styrax paralleloneurus
(c) Balsamic resin from styrax Benzoin
(d) Both b & c

350. Benzoin is
(a) Oleo resin
(b) Balsamic resin
(c) Resene
(d) Oleogum resin

351. Siam benzoin differs from sumatra benzoin
(a) In that it contains insufficient benzoic acid to give an odor of benzaldehyde
(b) In that it contains insufficient cinnamic acid to give an odor of cinnamaldehyde
(c) In that it contains insufficient cinnamic acid to give an odor of benzaldehyde
(d) None of the above

352. Siam benzoin is obtained from
(a) Stem of styrax benzoin
(b) Stem of styrax paralleloneurus
(c) Stem of styrax tonkinesis
(d) All the above

353. Indian saffron is
(a) Benzoin   (b) Turmeric
(c) Asafoetida   (d) Zinger

354. Zinger is used as
(a) Emetic   (b) Antiemetic
(c) Spasmolytic (d) Both b & c

355. When turmeric powder treated with sulphuric acid it gives
(a) Green color
(b) Crimson color
(c) Pale pink color
(d) Violet color

356. Bol is
(a) Myrrh
(b) Podophyllum
(c) Colophony
(d) Coloynth

357. 0.5 gm of asafoetida is boiled with dil. HCl & it is filtered in to ammonia solution. A blue fluorescence is produced due to presence of
(a)   Volatile oil
(b)   Umbelliferone
(c)   Asaresinotannol
(d)   Sulphate compounds

358. The pungency of ginger is due to
(a)   Gingerol   (b)   Starch
(c)   Camphene   (d)   Shagol

359. The pungency of gingerol can be destroyed by boiling with
(a)   10% sulphuric acid
(b)   2% potassium hydroxide
(c)   1% mercuric chloride
(d)   5% acetic anhydride

360. The red colouring matter present in capsicum is
(a)   Capsanthin
(b)   Capsorubin
(c)   Both a & b
(d)   None of the above

361. Terpenoids include
(a)   Hydrocarbons
(b)   Hydrocarbons & their oxygenated derivatives
(c)   Polyuronides
(d)   None

362. Terpenes include
(a)   Hydrocarbons
(b)   Hydrocarbons and their oxygenated derivatives
(c)   Polyuronides
(d)   None

363. Volatile oils are also termed as ethereal oils because
(a)   They are essences or active constituents of plants
(b)   They evaporate when exposed to air at an ordinary temperature
(c)   They are obtained from ethers
(d)   None of the above

364. Volatile oils are also termed as essential oils because
(a)   They are essences or active constituents of plants
(b)   They evaporate when exposed to air at an ordinary temperature
(c)   They are obtained from ethers
(d)   None of the above

365. Chemically volatile oils are derived from
(a)   Fixed oils
(b)   Hydrocarbons
(c)   Hydrocarbons & their oxygenated derivatives
(d)   None of the above

366. Which compounds fetch more prices in perfumery?
(a)   Terpene volatile oil
(b)   Terpeneless volatile oil
(c)   Terpene volatile oil with gums
(d)   None of the above

367. Terpeneless volatile oil fetches more prices in perfumery because?
(a)   Of their specificity
(b)   Of their stability
(c)   Both a & b
(d)   None of the above

368. Volatile oils are insoluble in
    (a) Water   (b) Alcohol
    (c) Chloroform   (d) All the above

369. The drug which contain hydrocarbon volatile oil is
    (a) Peppermint oil
    (b) Turpentine oil
    (c) Sandal wood oil
    (d) Chenopodium oil

370. Drug which contain aldehyde volatile oil
    (a) Lemon grass oil
    (b) Cinnamon oil
    (c) Saffron
    (d) All the above

371. The drug which contain ketone volatile oil is
    (a) Fennel
    (b) Lemongrass oil
    (c) Chenopodium
    (d) All the above

372. The drug which contain ester group in volatile oil is
    (a) Gaultheria oil
    (b) Leamon gross oil
    (c) Tulsi
    (d) Nutmeg

373. The common method used for extraction of volatile oil is
    (a) Distillation
    (b) Expression
    (c) Extraction with non-volatile solvents
    (d) All the above

374. Volatile oils can be identified by
    (a) Alcoholic solution of sudan III reagent
    (b) A drop of tincture alkane
    (c) Both a & b
    (d) Using sodium hydrogen sulphate

375. The following drug is used as diuretic
    (a) Eucalyptus
    (b) Jatamansi
    (c) Juniper
    (d) Clove

376. The following drug is used as sedative
    (a) Citronella
    (b) Jatamansi
    (c) Lemongrass
    (d) Chenopodium

377. The following drug is used as local irritant
    (a) Clove   (b) Citronella
    (c) Turpentine   (d) Juniper

378. Clove is used as
    (a) Local anaesthetic
    (d) Local irritant
    (c) Counter irritant
    (d) Anthelmintic

379. Spearmint or pudina consist of
    (a) Dried leaves & flowering tops of spicata menthe
    (b) Dried leaves & flowering tops of ocinum species
    (c) Dried leaves & flowering tops of eucalyptus glabra
    (d) Dried leaves & flowering tops of mentha piperita

380. Cassia bark is the
    (a) Dried stem bark of cinnamomnum cassia
    (b) Dried inner stem bark of cinnamomum zeylanicum
    (c) Dried inner stem bark of cinnamomum burmarin
    (d) All of the above

381. Cinnamon bark consist of
    (a) Dried stem bark of cinnamomum cassia
    (b) Dried inner stem bark of cinnamomum zeylanicum
    (c) Dried inner stem bark of cinnamomum burmarin
    (d) All the above

382. Cinnamon is used as
    (a) Antirheumatic
    (b) Antispasmodic
    (c) Diaphoretic
    (d) All the above

383. Coriander consists of
    (a) Coriandrol
    (b) Umbelliferone
    (c) Borneol & camphor
    (d) All the above

384. The main ingredient of the preparation of woodward's gripe water is?
    (a) Coriander   (b) Dill
    (c) Caraway   (d) Fennel

385. The colorless pungent liquid with aromatic odor in fennel is
    (a) Anethole   (b) Fenchone
    (c) Phellandrene   (d) Limonene

386. The adulteration of fennel with exhausted fennel fruits can be distinguished by
    (a) Having apical adore
    (b) Absence of fenchone and fruits sink in water
    (c) They look dark greenish-brown color
    (d) All the above

387. The Indian variety of fennel taslesis
    (a) Sweet
    (b) Very sweet
    (c) Camphoraceous
    (d) Aromatic

388. Cuminum cyminum is substituted by
    (a) Fennel
    (b) Dill
    (c) Jeera
    (d) All the above

389. The largest producer of cardamom is
    (a) India
    (b) Sri Lanka
    (c) Guatemala
    (d) All the above

390. Which of the following is the larger cardamom?
    (a) Allepy variety (b) Malabar
    (c) Mysore variety (d) Mangalore

391. The bitter substances present in the orange peel are
    (a) Hesperedin
    (b) Neohesperidin
    (c) Isohesperidin
    (d) Aurantiamarin & aurantimaric acid

392. The fat & volatile oil of nutmeg are used in the treatment of?
   (a) Tuberculosis
   (b) Leprosy
   (c) Rheumatism
   (d) Ulcer

393. Banda soap is obtained from
   (a) Lemon   (b) Nutmeg
   (c) Rasna   (d) Tulsi

394. When potassium hydroxide (50%) is added to thick section of drug it produces needle shaped crystals of potassium euginate & identify the drug?
   (a) Clove   (b) Fennel
   (c) Dill   (d) Caraway

395. Which of the following drug is a dental analgesic?
   (a) Clove   (b) Fennel
   (c) Dill   (d) Caraway

396. When clove is adulterated with clove stalks they can be identified by
   (a) Floating on freshly & boiled & cooled water
   (b) Presence of thick-walled stone cells
   (c) Decreased volatile oil content
   (d) All the above

397. Stringy bark tree is
   (a) Chenopodium (b) Eucalyptus
   (c) Palmarosa   (d) Cardamom

398. Jesuit's tea or mexican tea is
   (a) Chenopodium ambrosioides
   (b) Cinnamoaum camphore
   (c) Valeriana wallichi
   (d) Cymbopogon nardus

399. Valerian is used in the treatment of
   (a) Insomnia & hysteria
   (b) Cholera
   (c) Epilepsy
   (d) All the above

400. Nord grass is
   (a) Cymbopogon camphora
   (b) Chenopodium ambrosioides
   (c) Cinnamomum camphora
   (d) Cymbopogon citrates

401. Citronella oil is used as
   (a) Insect repellent
   (b) Bactericidal
   (c) Stimulant
   (d) All the above

402. The main odorous and medicinal constituent of sandalwood is
   (a) Santalol
   (b) Santalenes
   (c) Santene
   (d) Nor-tricyclo ekasantalene

403. β-ionone is the starting material for the synthesis of
   (a) Vitamin C   (b) Vitamin B
   (c) Vitamin A   (d) Vitamin D

404. Chenopodium oil is used against
   (a) Intestinal Amoebae
   (b) Hook warms
   (c) Dwarf-tape warms
   (d) All the above

405. Which of the following is false in case of cinnamon chips?
   (a) These are pieces of untrimmed bark
   (b) They show abundant cork cells

    (c) They are slightly bitter and dark in colour
    (d) It is the substituent or adulterant for cinnamon

406. Oil of winter green is
    (a) Gaultheria procumbens
    (b) Eucalyptus glabra
    (c) Cymbopogon citrates
    (d) Chenopodium ambrosioidis

407. Palmarosa is obtained from
    (a) Leaves and tops of cymbopogon martini
    (b) Leaves and tops of cymbopogon citratus
    (c) Leaves and tops of cymbopogon nardus
    (d) All the above

408. Musk is adulterated with plant
    (a) Fiber zibethicus (American musk)
    (b) Beaver (Castor fiber)
    (c) Civet (Viverra zibetha)
    (d) Musk mallow

409. The elongated thick walled sclerenchymatous cells with tapering ends and narrow lumen are
    (a) Vegetable fibres
    (b) Animal fibres
    (c) Mineral fibres
    (d) Synthetic fibres

410. Example for vegetable fibre is
    (a) Flax, hemp, jute
    (b) Silk & wool
    (c) Glass & asbestos
    (d) Nylon, & orlon

411. Example for animal fibre is
    (a) Flax, hemp, jute
    (b) Silk & wool
    (c) Glass & asbestos
    (d) Nylon & Orlon

412. Example for mineral fibre is
    (a) Flax, hemp, jute
    (b) Silk & wool
    (c) Glass & asbestos
    (d) Nylon & Orlon

413. Example for synthetic fibre is
    (a) Flax, hemp, jute
    (b) Silk & wool
    (c) Glass & asbestos
    (d) Nylon & Orlon

414. Synthetic fibres are prepared from
    (a) Ether cellulose or proteins
    (b) Organic molecules by polycondensation
    (c) Sand & oxides of aluminium
    (d) All the above

415. Regenerated fibres are prepared from
    (a) Ether cellulose or proteins
    (b) Organic molecules by polycondensation
    (c) Sand & oxides of aluminium
    (d) All the above

416. Which of the following is false for cotton?
    (a) Cotton is soluble with ballooning with cuoxam reagent
    (b) Cotton is insoluble in 5% KOH and 6% H_2SO_4
    (c) Cotton is soluble in 80% H_2SO_4
    (d) When moisten with iodine followed by a drop of 8% w/w H_2SO_4 cotton does not show blue color

417. On heating silk in crucible or adulance slowly towards flame
    (a) It gives foul odour and burns slowly giving bead followed by white ash
    (b) It melts leaving hard bead
    (c) It does not melt
    (d) It form a soft bead

418. On heating wool in crucible or advance slowly towards flame
    (a) It gives foul odor & burns slowly giving bead followed by white ash
    (b) It melts leaving hard bead
    (c) It does not melt
    (d) It form a soft bead

419. Wool on treating with Cuoxam reagent
    (a) It is insoluble but swells and scales separates separate
    (b) It is partially soluble
    (c) It is insoluble
    (d) None of the above

420. Silk on treating with Cuoxam reagent?
    (a) It is insoluble but swells & scales separates separate
    (b) It is partially soluble
    (c) It is insoluble
    (d) None of the above

421. Nylon on treating with Cuoxam reagent?
    (a) It is insoluble but swells & scales separates separate
    (b) It is partially soluble
    (c) It is insoluble
    (d) None of the above

422. When nylon is moisten with iodine, followed by a drop of H_2SO_4 it gives?
    (a) Yellow color
    (b) No blue color
    (c) Blue color
    (d) Brown color

423. When silk & wool are moisten with iodine, followed by a drop of H_2SO_4 it gives?
    (a) Yellow color
    (b) No blue color
    (c) Blue color
    (d) Brown color

424. When treating carbohydrate fibres with iodine & sulphuric acid
    (a) They show blue colour or brownish red color
    (b) They show yellow stain
    (c) They show red stain
    (d) None of the above

425. On treating carbohydrates with millon's reagent it
    (a) Does not shows red color
    (b) Shows red color
    (c) Shows yellow color
    (d) Does not yellow color

426. Polyester on treating with cuoxam reagent
    (a) It is insoluble
    (b) It is insoluble and scales separates
    (c) It is soluble
    (d) None of the above

427. The raw cotton discarded by the textile industry is called
    (a) Linters
    (b) Staple
    (c) Combers waste
    (d) None

428. Wagner's reagent is
    (a) Iodine-potassium iodide solution
    (b) Potassium mercuric iodide solution
    (c) Picric acid solution
    (d) Potassium bismuth iodide solution

429. Mayer's reagent is
    (a) Iodine-potassium iodide solution
    (b) Potassium mercuric iodide solution
    (c) Picric acid solution
    (d) Potassium bismuth iodide solution

430. Hager's reagent is
    (a) Iodine-potassium iodide solution
    (b) Potassium mercuric iodide solution
    (c) Picric acid solution
    (d) Potassium bismuth iodide solution

431. Dragendroff's reagent is
    (a) Iodine-potassium iodide solution
    (b) Potassium mercuric iodide solution
    (c) Picric acid solution
    (d) Potassium bismuth iodide solution

432. Vitalis-morin test is used for identification of
    (a) Purine alkaloids
    (b) Tropane alkaloids
    (c) Indole alkaloids
    (d) Quinoline alkaloids

433. Thalleioquin test is used for identification of
    (a) Purine alkaloids
    (b) Tropane alkaloids
    (c) Indole alkaloids
    (d) Quinoline alkaloids

434. Indole alkaloids are identified by treating with
    (a) Sulphuric acid & P-dimethyl amino benzaldehyde
    (b) Acetic acid & potassium dichromate
    (c) Nitric acid & sodium picrate
    (d) All the above

435. Van-Urk's test is used for identification of
    (a) Purine alkaloids
    (b) Tropane alkaloids
    (c) Indole alkaloids
    (d) Imidazole alkaloids

436. Terpenoids are identified by
    (a) Salkoawski test
    (b) Liebermann Burchard test
    (c) Rochan test
    (d) All the above

437. Murexide test is used for the identification of
    (a) Indole alkaloids
    (b) Tropane alkaloids
    (c) Purine alkaloids
    (d) Glycoalkaloid

438. Sugar part of cardenolides are identified by
    (a) Keller-kiliani test
    (b) Legal test
    (c) Baljet test
    (d) All the above

439. Foam test is used for the identification of
    (a) Saponin
    (b) Cyanogentic glycosides
    (c) Anthraquinone glycosides
    (d) Flavonoid glycosides

440. Haemolytic test is used for identification of
    (a) Saponin
    (b) Cyanogeneic glycosides
    (c) Anthraquinone glycosides
    (d) Flavonoid glycosides

441. Shinoda test is used for identification of
    (a) Saponin
    (b) Cyanogenetic glycosides
    (c) Anthraquinone glycosides
    (d) Flavanoid glycosides

442. Flavonoids give yellow colour with
    (a) Addition of alkali
    (b) Addition of Conc. H_2SO_4
    (c) Both a & b
    (d) Gelatin

443. Vanillin-hydrochloric acid test is used for identification of
    (a) Resins   (b) Glycosides
    (c) Tannins   (d) Alkaloids

444. Gold beater's skin test is used for the identification of
    (a) Resins   (b) Glycosides
    (c) Tannins   (d) Alkaloids

445. Ninhydrin test is used for identification of
    (a) Amino acids   (b) Tannins
    (c) Sterols   (d) Volatile oils

446. Borntrager test is used for identification of
    (a) Anthraquinone glycosides
    (b) Cyanogenic glycosides
    (c) Flavonoid glycosides
    (d) Leucoanthocyanidin glycoside

447. Cyanogenic glycosides give brick red colour by treating with
    (a) HCl & sodium picrate
    (b) HCl & NH_3
    (c) HNO_3 & picric acid
    (d) Acetic anhydride & HCl

448. Adulteration means
    (a) Addition of completely different substance in place of original drug
    (b) Addition of impure, cheap, filthy or putrid substances to genuine drug
    (c) Addition of one type of drug with other type of drug
    (d) All the above

449. Substitution means
    (a) Addition of completely different substance in place of original drug
    (b) Addition of impure, cheap, filthy or putrid substances to genuine drug

(c) Addition of one type of drug with other type of drug

(d) All the above

450. Admixture means
   (a) Addition of completely different substance in place of original drug
   (b) Addition of impure, cheap, filthy or putrid substances to genuine drug
   (c) Addition of one type of drug with other type of drug
   (d) All the above

451. Stomatal index of indian senna is
   (a) 17 to 20   (b) 18 to 23
   (c) 15 to 18   (d) 16 to 24

452. The moisture content in digitalis purpurea is not more than
   (a) 3%   (b) 4%
   (c) 5%   (d) 6%

453. Coca is identified by
   (a) Paracytic stomata
   (b) Actinocytic
   (c) Anisocytic
   (d) Diacytic stomata

454. Eucalyptus is identified by its
   (a) Pleasant odor
   (b) Aromatic odor
   (c) Camphoraceous odor
   (d) Unpleasant odor

455. Cape aloes are identified by its
   (a) Greenish brown color
   (b) Brownish black color
   (c) Liver brown
   (d) Brownish yellow

456. Lobelia is identified by
   (a) Lignified trichome unicellular
   (b) Sharp, short, pointed curved unicellular
   (c) Large, conical, strongly shrunken unicellular
   (d) Short, conical, unicellular

457. Optical rotation of honey is
   (a) $+3°$ to $-15°$ (b) $+10°$ to -15^0
   (c) $+8°$ to $-18°$ (d) $+12°$ to $-18°$

458. Water insoluble extractive components indicate the presence of
   (a) Tannins, sugars, mucilage and presence of
   (b) Carbonates, oxides, phosphates, silicates & silica
   (c) Both and & b
   (d) None

459. Ash content of drugs indicate the presence of
   (a) Tannins, sugars, mucilage and presence of
   (b) Carbonates, oxides, phosphates, silicates & silica
   (c) Both a & b
   (d) None

460. The kinematic viscosity of liquid paraffin is
   (a) Not more than 64 centistokes at $37.8°$
   (b) Not less than 46 centistokes at $37.8°$
   (c) Not less than 64 centistokes at $37.8°$
   (d) Not more than 46 centistokes at $37.8°$

461. The melting point of bees wax is
   (a) 60°C-66°C   (b) 63°C-68°C
   (c) 62°C-65°C   (d) 65°C-69°C

462. The quantitative values determined for the identification of leaf drugs remain constant throughout the age of plant except
   (a) Stomatal number
   (b) Veinlet termination number
   (c) Vein islet number
   (d) Stomatal number

463. Asafoetida is soluble in
   (a) Chloral hydrate solution
   (b) Carbon disulphide
   (c) Both a & b
   (d) Alcohol & water

464. The acid insoluble ash value of cardamom
   (a) 6% w/w   (b) 3.5% w/w
   (c) 0.75% w/w   (d) 5% w/w

465. Which of the following is wrong statement?
   (a) Stomata number is the average number of stomata present per square in the leaf epidermis
   (b) Stomatal index is the number of stomata form to the total number of epidermal cells
   (c) Vein islet number is the number of vein islet present per square number of leaf surface midway between the midrib & margin
   (d) Vein termination is the number of Veinlet termination present per mm2 of leaf surface

466. Senna shows calcium oxalate crystals in the form of?
   (a) Prisms
   (b) Acicular
   (c) Cluster crystals
   (d) Rosette crystals

467. Which of the following is a channel bark?
   (a) Cascara   (b) Cinnamon
   (c) Kurchi   (d) Cinchona

468. Which of the following is recurved bark?
   (a) Cascara   (b) Cinnamon
   (c) Kurchi   (d) Cinchona

469. While performing the chemo microscopy of a drug lignified trichomes were observed. Probable drug is?
   (a) Buchu   (b) Lobelia
   (c) Nux-Vomica   (d) Mint leaves

470. Total ash value in case of crude drug signifies
   (a) Organic content of the drug
   (b) Mineral matter in the drug
   (c) Addition of extraneous matter such as sand, stone etc
   (d) Woody matter present in the drug

   (a) c & d   (b) b &c
   (c) a & b   (d) a & d

471. The enzyme present in human saliva is
   (a) Amylase   (b) Papain
   (c) Pepsin   (d) All

472. The non protein part of an active enzyme is
    (a) Apoenzyme
    (b) Holoenzyme
    (c) Co-factor
    (d) All the above

473. The enzyme posses amylase, lipase & protease activity is
    (a) Amylase   (b) Pancreatin
    (c) Pepsin   (d) Papain

474. Pancreatin is precipitated by
    (a) Strong alcoholic solutions
    (b) Metallic salts
    (c) Both a & b
    (d) Water

475. Cangored dye test is used to know the
    (a) Amylase activity of an enzyme
    (b) Proteolytic activity of an enzyme
    (c) Lipolytic activity of an enzyme
    (d) All the above

476. The enzyme shows relieving symptoms of episiotomy is
    (a) Amylase   (b) Papain
    (c) Pancreatin   (d) Diastase

477. Decolorisation of potassium permanganate solution takes place when it added to a solution of
    (a) Amylase
    (b) Papain
    (c) Pancreatin
    (d) All the above

478. Pepsin (proteolytic enzyme) is obtained from
    (a) Mucous membrane of fresh stomach of sus scrofa
    (b) Pancreas of the bos taurus.

    (c) Latex of the unripe fruit of tropical melon tree, carica papaya.
    (d) All the above

479. Trypsinogen (inactive enzyme) converted to trypsin (active form) by the action of
    (a) Amylase
    (b) Enterokinase
    (c) Pepsin
    (d) All the above

480. Trypsin when added to a solution of milk powder
    (a) Translucent mass was observed
    (b) Breakdown of casein was observed
    (c) This test is employed to determine the rate of reaction.
    (d) All of the above are correct.

481. In dicotyledons
    (a) The primary root persists & gives rise to the tap root.
    (b) The primary root soon perishes and is replaced by a cluster of fibrous roots.
    (c) The primary root persists and gives rise to taproot and fibrous roots.
    (d) None

482. in monocotyledons,
    (a) Veins or veinlets do not end freely
    (b) Veins or veinlets do not end freely in mesophyll
    (c) Veins or veinlets may or may not do not end freely in mesophyll
    (d) None

483. The vascular bundles are arranged in a ring and are collateral & open
   (a) In all ngiosperms plants
   (b) In all dicotyledon plants
   (c) In all monocotyledon plants
   (d) In gymnospermae plants

484. Strophanthus kombe a cardioactive drug belongs to the family
   (a) Compositae
   (b) Liliaceace
   (c) Apocyanaceae
   (d) Leguminosae

485. The characteristic fruit of asteraceae or compositae is
   (a) Beery or drupe
   (b) Capsule
   (c) One-seeded
   (d) Cypscla

486. The central ones (disc florets) are tubular, and the marginal ones ray florets are ligulate are found in the flowers of
   (a) Convoivulaceae
   (b) Compositae
   (c) Umbelliferae
   (d) Leguminosae

487. The embryo is curved & the seed remain attached to a wiry frame work, called replum, which surrounds the fruit is present in
   (a) Labiatae
   (b) Umbelliferae
   (c) Cruciferae
   (d) Leguminosae

488. The examples of gramineae are
   (a) Rice
   (b) Bamboo
   (c) Maize
   (d) All of the above

489. The verticellaster inflorescence (often cyme) is seen in
   (a) Labiatae
   (b) Leguminosae
   (c) Lilliaceae
   (d) Papaveraceae

490. The leaves are simple, radical or cauline in
   (a) Rubiaceae
   (b) Liliaceae
   (c) Rutaceae
   (d) All the above

491. Cinchona, ipecac., belongs to
   (a) Rutaceae
   (b) Papaveraceae
   (c) Rubiaceae
   (d) Umbelliferae

492. Mericarp showing five longitudinal ridges, oil canals (vitae) in the furrows is the characteristic of
   (a) Umbelliferae (b) Solanaceae
   (c) Cruciferae   (d) Labiatae

493. Digitalis belongs to the family
   (a) Scrophularaceae
   (b) Papaveraceae
   (c) Solanaceae
   (d) None

494. Poppy belongs to
   (a) Rutaceae
   (b) Apocyanaceae
   (c) Papaveraceae
   (d) Solanaceae

495. Tulsi belongs to
    (a) Labiatae
    (b) Umbelliferae
    (c) Graminae
    (d) Cruciferae

496. Anisocytic or crucifetous or unequal celled stomata present in
    (a) Digitalis   (b) Datura
    (c) Ephedra   (d) Vasaka

497. Pod or lomentum is the characteristic feature of
    (a) Graminae   (b) Ruiaceae
    (c) Leguminosae   (d) Solanaceae

498. The number of xylem bundles in dicotyledons & monocotyledons respectively,
    (a) 2 to 6 &5 to 8
    (b) 5 to 8& 2to6
    (c) 4 to 8 &2 to 6
    (d) 3 to 7 &6 to 9

499. In dicotyledons
    (a) Embryo bears 2 cotyledons
    (b) Embryo bears 1 cotyledon
    (c) Embryo bear1 or 2 cotyledons
    (d) None

500. Hutchinson's system of classification is advanced then Bentham & hooker system because
    (a) Concept of genetic classification
    (b) Concept of phylogenetic classifcation
    (c) Both a& b
    (d) None

501. The cellulose based or vegetable fibre is
    (a) Jute   (b) Silk
    (c) Nylon   (d) Asbestos

502. The protein based or animal fibre is
    (a) Jute   (b) Silk
    (c) Nylon   (d) Asbestos

503. An example for regenerated or synthetic fibre is
    (a) Nylon   (b) Terylene
    (c) Asbestos   (d) Both a & b

504. The fibre burns with a flame, gives very little odor or fumes, but does not produce a bead & leaves a smAll of the abovewhite ash is
    (a) Cotton   (b) Silk
    (c) Nylon   (d) Asbestos

505. The fibre on treating with iodine and sulphuric acid shows blue colour is
    (a) Asbestos   (b) Silk
    (c) Nylon   (d) Cotton

506. With cuoxam reagent, the fibre dissolves with ballooning, leaving a few fragments of cuticle is
    (a) Asbestos   (b) Silk
    (c) Cotton   (d) Nylon

507. The fibre does not give red stain with phloroglucinol and hydrochloric acid is
    (a) Asbestos   (b) Silk
    (c) Cotton   (d) Nylon

508. Jute is obtained from
    (a) Phloem fibres from the stems of various species of corchorus
    (b) Trichomes from the seeds of various species of gossypium
    (c) Pericyclic fibres from the stems of various species of cannabis
    (d) Pericyclic fibres from the stems of various species of linum

509. Cotton is obtained from
    (a) Phloem fibres from the stems of various species of corchorus
    (b) Trichomes from the seeds of various species of gossypium
    (c) Pericyclic fibres from the stems of various species of cannabis
    (d) Pericyclic fibres from the stems of various species of linum

510. Flax is obtained from
    (a) Phloem fibres from the stems of various species of corchorus
    (b) Trichomes from the seeds of various species of gossypium
    (c) Pericyclic fibres from the stems of various species of cannabis
    (d) Pericyclic fibres from the stems of various species of linum

511. Hemp is obtained from
    (a) Phloem fibres from the stems of various species of corchorus
    (b) Trichomes from the seeds of various species of gossypium
    (c) Pericyclic fibres from the stems of various species of cannabis
    (d) Pericyclic fibres from the stems of various species of linum

512. Flax belongs to the family
    (a) Tiliaceae   (b) Linaceae
    (c) Cannabinaceae (d) Malvaceae

513. Cotton belongs to the family
    (a) Tiliaceae   (b) Linaceae
    (c) Cannabinaceae (d) Malvaceae

514. Jute belongs to the family
    (a) Tiliaceae   (b) Linaceae
    (c) Cannabinaceae (d) Malvaceae

515. Hemp belongs to the family
    (a) Tiliaceae
    (b) Linaceae
    (c) Cannabinaceae
    (d) Malvaceae

516. The fibre insoluble in 5%KOH solution is
    (a) Wool
    (b) Silk
    (c) Cotton
    (d) All of the above

517. Jute & hemp mainly composed of
    (a) Cellulose
    (b) Cellulose, hemicelluloses & lignin
    (c) Pectocellulose
    (d) None

518. The process in which hairs & seeds of cotton are separated is called as
    (a) Retting process
    (b) Ginning process
    (c) Both a & b
    (d) None

519. Silk is mainly composed of
    (a) Fibion
    (b) Gluten
    (c) Keratin
    (d) All the above

520. Wool mainly consist of protein
    (a) Fibrion
    (b) Gluten
    (c) Keratin
    (d) All the above

521. Gelatin mainly consist of protein
    (a) Fibrion
    (b) Glutein
    (c) Keratin
    (d) All the above

522. The fibre soluble in warm alkaline solution is
    (a) Wool   (b) Cotton
    (c) Both a & b   (d) None

523. The fibre formed by condensation copolymers formed by reaction of equal parts of a diamine &dicarboxylic acid is
    (a) Nylon   (b) Orlon
    (c) Both a & b   (d) None

524. Asbestos is a
    (a) Double silicate of calcium & magnesium
    (b) Aluminium silicate
    (c) Magnesium silicate
    (d) Calcium silicate

525. Purified absorbent cotton is almost made up of
    (a) Cellulose   (b) Chitin
    (c) Sodium alginate (d) Talc

526. Raw cotton consists of
    (a) 91%Cellulose   (b) Chitin
    (c) Sodium alginate (d) Talc

527. For sterilization of sutures, the technique followed is
    (a) Moist heat sterilization
    (b) Dry heat sterilization
    (c) X-ray sterilization
    (d) Gamma ray sterilization.

528. According to I.P surgical dressing should be stored at a temperature not exceeding
    (a) 25°C   (b) 30°C
    (c) 40°C   (d) 60°C

529. Wilkinite is
    (a) Kaolin   (b) chitin
    (c) Bentonite   (d) Talc

530. When bentonite mounted wit safranin, it acquires
    (a) Black color
    (b) Pink or red color
    (c) Green color
    (d) White color

531. The hormone oxytocin is obtained from
    (a) Pregnant human urine
    (b) Posterior pituitary glands of cattles & pigs
    (c) Anterior pituitary glands of man, horse & sheep
    (d) Adrenal medulla of man

532. Oestrogen is obtained from
    (a) Pregnant human urine
    (b) Posterior pituitary glands of cattles & pigs
    (c) Anterior pituitary glands of man, horse & sheep
    (d) Adrenal medulla of man.

533. Gonadotropin hormone is obtained from
    (a) Pregnant human urine
    (b) Posterior pituitary glands of cattles & pigs
    (c) Anterior pituitary glands of man, horse & sheep
    (d) Adrenal medulla of man.

534. Adrenaline or ephedrine is obtained from
    (a) Pregnant human urine
    (b) Posterior pituitary glands of cattles & pigs
    (c) Anterior pituitary glands of man, horse & sheep.
    (d) Adrenal medulla of man.

535. Enzyme fibrinolysin is obtined from
    (a) Human plasminogen
    (b) Pancrease of ox
    (c) Glandular layer of hog stomach
    (d) All the above

536. Pancreatin is obtained from
    (a) Human plasminogen
    (b) Pancrease of ox
    (c) Glandular layer of hog stomach
    (d) All the above

537. Pepsin is obtained from
    (a) Human plasminogen
    (b) Pancrease of ox
    (c) Glandular layer of hog stomach
    (d) All the above

538. Talc consists of
    (a) Double silicate of aluminium & magnesium
    (b) Hydrated magnesium silicate
    (c) Hydrated aluminium silicate
    (d) None

539. Fuller's earth (multanimatti) consists
    (a) Double silicate of aluminium & magnesium
    (b) Hydrated magnesium silicate
    (c) Hydrated aluminium silicate
    (d) None

540. Kaolin consists of
    (a) Double silicate of aluminium & magnesium
    (b) Hydrated magnesium silicate
    (c) Hydrated aluminium silicate
    (d) None

541. Talc is obtained from
    (a) Finest variety of soap stone
    (b) Weathering &decomposition of feldspar of granite
    (c) Siliceous skeletons of fossil diatoms
    (d) Mining (in open query)

542. Kaolin is obtained from
    (a) Finest variety of soap stone.
    (b) Weathering &decomposition of feldspar of granite
    (c) Siliceous skeletons of fossil diatoms
    (d) Mining (in open query)

543. Diatomite or kieselguhr is obtained from
    (a) Finest variety of soap stone
    (b) Weathering &decomposition of feldspar of granite
    (c) Siliceous skeletons of fossil diatoms.
    (d) Mining (in open query)

544. Antibiotic cephalosporin is obtained from
    (a) Fungi Cephalosporin
    (b) Actinomyces species
    (c) Streptomyces species
    (d) Penicillin species

545. Erythromycin is obtained from
    (a) Streptomycetes erythreus
    (b) Fungi cephalosporium
    (c) Pencillin chrysogenum
    (d) All the above

546. The crude drugs derived from parts of plant or animal by some process of extraction & followed by purification are termed as
    (a) Organised crude drugs
    (b) Unorganised crude drugs
    (c) Identical crude drugs
    (d) None.

547. The crude drugs derived from parts of plant or animal & are made up of cells or have definite structure are termed as
    (a) Organised crude drugs
    (b) Unorganised crude drugs
    (c) Identical crude drugs
    (d) None

548. Alphabetical classification has the following merit(s)
    (a) It is easy & quick to use
    (b) Tracing & addition of drug is easy devoid of confusion
    (c) Both a & b
    (d) Plant & animal drugs are easily identified

549. The classification system fails to take in to an account chemical of active constituents and therapeutic significance of crude drugs is
    (a) Taxonomical classification
    (b) Chemical classification
    (c) Biological classification
    (d) All

550. The classification system is more convenient for practical study is
    (a) Morphological classification system
    (b) Chemical classification system
    (c) Chemotaxonomical classification system
    (d) Pharmacological classification system

551. The classification system is more popular & convenient for phytochemical studies is
    (a) Morphological classification system
    (b) Chemical classification system
    (c) Chemotaxonomical classification system
    (d) Pharmacological classification system

552. The classification estabilishes a relationship between position of the plant & attempts to utilise chemical facts for more exact understanding of the biological evolution & relationships is
    (a) Morphological classification system
    (b) Chemical classification system
    (c) Chemotaxonomical classification system
    (d) Pharmacological classification system

553. The following drug is classified as local anaesthetic is
    (a) Coca   (b) Vinca
    (c) Cannabis   (d) Opium

554. Opium is used as
    (a) Smooth muscle relaxants
    (b) Skeletal muscle relaxants
    (c) Central analgesic
    (d) Both a & c.

555. Aloe, opium & myrrh are examples for
    (a) Organised crude drugs
    (b) Unorganised crude drugs
    (c) Both a & b
    (d) None.

556. Vinca, belladonna &clove are examples for
    (a) Organised crude drugs
    (b) Unorganised crude drugs
    (c) Both a & b
    (d) None

557. Quassia is an example for
    (a) Barks   (b) Woods
    (c) Flowers   (d) Seeds.

558. Gelatin & caesin are examples for
    (a) Protein   (b) enzyme
    (c) Hormone   (d) Vitamin

559. Benzoin is
    (a) Oleoresin
    (b) Balasmic resin
    (c) Resene
    (d) Oleogum resin

560. Cinchona is an example for
    (a) Alkaloidal drug
    (b) Glycosidal drug
    (c) Tannin drug
    (d) Resin

561. The following drug is an example for anthelmintic activity
    (a) Quassia   (b) Vidange
    (c) Male fern   (d) All the above

562. Myrobalan is an example for
    (a) Tannin   (b) Resin
    (c) Volatile oil   (d) Alkaloid

563. Bees wax is an example for
    (a) Carbohydrate   (b) Lipid
    (c) Resin   (d) Protein

564. Kurchi posses
    (a) Anti amoebic activity
    (b) Antimalarial activity
    (c) Anthelmintic activity
    (d) All the above

565. Quinidine is used to treat
    (a) Malaria   (b) Arrhythmias
    (c) Anticancer   (d) All the above

566. The aminoacids produced through shikimic acid pathway
    (a) Phenylalanine (b) Tyrosine
    (c) Tryptophan   (d) All the above

567. _______ is the key intermediate from carbohydrate for the biosynthesis of C6-C3units (phenyl propane derivatives)
    (a) Shikimic acid pathway
    (b) Embden-meyerhof pathway
    (c) Clavin cycle
    (d) None

568. The precursor, that is D-erythrose 4-phosphate & phosphoenol pyruvate combine to form 3-deoxy-D-arabino-heptulosonic acid -7-phosphate (DAHP), a reaction catalyzed by
(a) Phospho-2-oxo-3-deoxyheptonate aldolase
(b) Phospho-2-oxo-3-deoxyheptonate oxidase
(c) Phospho-2-oxo-3-deoxyhexonate aldolase
(d) Phospho-2-oxo-3-deoxyhexonate oxidase

569. Anthranilic acid is the precursor for
(a) Tryptophan
(b) Tyrosine
(c) Phenylalanine
(d) All the above

570. The tropane alkaloids are derived from the
(a) L-Ornithine   (b) Tryptophan
(c) Phenylalanine (d) Tryrosine

571. Ornithine is a precursor of the cyclic pyrrolidine that occur in the alkaloiod
(a) Nicotine
(b) Nornicotine
(c) Nicotinic acid
(d) All the above

572. The starting material for the synthesis of tropane alkaloids
(a) Ornithine
(b) Methylornithine
(c) Both a & b
(d) None

573. Lysine is precursor for
(a) Pyrrolidine ring
(b) Piperidine
(c) Both a & b
(d) None

574. Tropinone on
(a) Reduction , it converts to tropine
(b) Oxidation ,it converts to tropine
(c) Reduction, it converts to tropic acid
(d) Oxidation it converts to tropic acid

575. Tryptophan & its decarboxylated products (tryptamine) are precursors for the biosynthesis of
(a) Tropane alkaloids
(b) Indole alkaloids
(c) Quinoline alkaloids
(d) Isoquinoline alkaoiods.

576. Codeinone,codeine & morphine are derived from the aminoacid
(a) Tryptophan   (b) Tyrosine
(c) Tropic acid   (d) None

577. Precursor for the synthesis of ephedrine is
(a) L-phenylalanine
(b) Tryptamine
(c) Tryptophan
(d) None

578. Precursor for the biosynthesis of Lysergic acid are
(a) Tryptophan
(b) An isoprene unit
(c) Both a & b
(d) None

579. Indian gooseberry is
 (a) Myrobalan
 (b) Amla
 (c) Pale catechu
 (d) Gall

580. Emblica officinalis belongs to the family
 (a) Euphorbiaceae
 (b) Acanthaceae
 (c) Combretaceae
 (d) Amaranthaceae

581. Amla contain
 (a) Vitamin c, minerals & aminoacids
 (b) Edible tissue contain protein concentration 3-fold and ascorbic acid concentration 160 fold compared to that of the apple.
 (c) Contain mixture of gallic acid, ellagic acid & phyllembillin
 (d) All the above

582. Triphala, a famous ayurvedic preparation contain
 (a) Amla, behera & Arjuna
 (b) Chebula, amla & adusa
 (c) Behera, chebula & amla
 (d) Chebula, behera and gall.

583. The acid insoluble ash present in amla is
 (a) Not More Than 2%
 (b) Not More Than 3%
 (c) Not More Than 4%
 (d) Not More Than 6%.

584. Adusa consists of
 (a) Fresh or dried leaves of adhatoda vasica
 (b) Fresh or dried leaves of achyranthes aspera
 (c) Fresh or dried bark of terminalia arjuna
 (d) None.

585. Vasaka belongs to
 (a) Amaranthaceae
 (b) Acanthaceae
 (c) Euphorbiaceae
 (d) Zygophyllaceae.

586. Vasaka is uesd as
 (a) Antitussive   (b) Antiseptic
 (c) Oxytocic   (d) Both a & c.

587. Prickiy chaff flower is called as
 (a) Achyranthes aspera
 (b) Adhatoda vasica
 (c) Emblica officinalis
 (d) All the above

588. Achyranthes aspera belongs to family
 (a) Amaranthaceae
 (b) Acanthaceae
 (c) Euphorbiaceae
 (d) Zygophyllaceae

589. Triterpeniod saponins in apamarga yield
 (a) Glycyrrhizinic acid as an aglycone
 (b) Oleanolic acid as an aglycone
 (c) Glycyrrhetinic acid as an aglycone
 (d) All the above

590. Terminalia Arjuna belongs to family
 (a) Combretaceae
 (b) Zygophyllaceae
 (c) Burseraceae
 (d) Solanaceae

591. Kantakari belongs to family
    (a) Combretaceae
    (b) Zygophyllaceae
    (c) Burseraceae
    (d) Solanaceae

592. Gokhru belongs to family
    (a) Combretaceae
    (b) Zygophyllaceae
    (c) Burseraceae
    (d) Solanaceae

593. Guggul belongs to family
    (a) Combretaceae
    (b) Zygophyllaceae
    (c) Burseraceae
    (d) Solanaceae

594. The diuretic property of terminalia arjuna is due to
    (a) Triterpenoids   (b) Saponins
    (c) Glycosides   (d) None

595. Ashoka consists of
    (a) Dried bark of Saraca indica belongs to leguminoseae
    (b) Dried bark of terminalia indica belongs to Combretaceae
    (c) Dried leaves of Saraca indica belongs to leguminoseae
    (d) Dried leaves of terminalia indica belong to combretaceae.

596. Bhilama consists of
    (a) Semecarpus anacardium tree
    (b) Terminalia belerica fruits
    (c) Tribulus terrestris plant
    (d) Adhatoda vasica leaves

597. Brahmi consists of
    (a) Dried or fresh herd of centella asiatica
    (b) Dried herb of swertia chirata
    (c) Dried stems of tinospora cordifolia
    (d) Whole plant of pluchea lanceolata

598. Rasana belongs to
    (a) Anacardiaceae
    (b) Asteraceae
    (c) Zygophyllaceae
    (d) Ranunculaceae

599. Chirak consists of
    (a) Dried mature root of plumbago zeylanica
    (b) Dried entire herb of swertia chirata
    (c) Dried entire whole plant of achryranthes aspera
    (d) None

600. Guggul is
    (a) Oleo-gum-resin
    (b) Oleo resin
    (c) Gum resin
    (d) Oleo gum

601. Guggul acts as
    (a) Inhibits platelet aggregation
    (b) Antirheumatic
    (c) Antiseptic
    (d) All the above

602. Salai-gogil is the synonym of
    (a) Gymnema   (b) Guggul
    (c) Garlic   (d) None

603. Greek hay is called as
    (a) Fenugreek
    (b) Methi
    (c) Menti
    (d) All the above

604. Trigonella-foenum graecum is used as
    (a) Anticholestelemic
    (b) Anti-inflammatory
    (c) Antitumor & antidiabetic
    (d) All the above

605. Punarnava is called as
    (a) Sanadika
    (b) Gophaghni
    (c) Kommeberu
    (d) All the above

606. Punarnava consists of
    (a) Fresh as well as dried whole plant of boerhaavia diffusa
    (b) Fresh as well as dried whole plant of butea monosperma
    (c) Fresh as well as dried whole stembark of symplocos racemosa
    (d) None

607. Punarnava belongs to family
    (a) Nyctaginaceae
    (b) Pipilionaceae
    (c) Symplocaceae
    (d) None

608. Dabur (dabur vatika antidandruff shampoo) contain one of the ingredient as
    (a) Trigonella –foenum-graecum
    (b) Palas
    (c) Tylophora
    (d) All the above

609. The father of plant tissue culture is
    (a) Gautheret
    (b) Gottlieb Haberlandt
    (c) Laibach
    (d) Hannig

610. The regulation of organ formation by changing the ratio of auxin:cytokinin is first attempted by
    (a) Skoog & Miller
    (b) Morel & Martin
    (c) Carlson
    (d) Guha & Mahethwari.

611. The ability of the callus cells to differentiate into a plant organ or a whole plant is
    (a) Redifferentiation
    (b) Dedifferentiation
    (c) Totipotency
    (d) None

612. The phenomenon of mature cells reverting to meristematic state to produce callus is
    (a) Dedifferentiation
    (b) Redifferentiation
    (c) Totipotent ability
    (d) None

613. The unorganised & undifferentiated mass of plant cell is reffered as
    (a) Explant
    (b) Callus
    (c) Totipotency
    (d) None

614. The ability of the plant cell to reproduce is called
   (a) Totipotency
   (b) Dedifferentiation
   (c) Redifferentiation
   (d) None

615. Plant cell devoid of cell wAll of the aboveis called
   (a) Protoplast   (b) Cytoplasts
   (c) Cybrids   (d) Hybrids

616. In suspension culture the Lag phase is characterised by
   (a) Preparation of cells to divide
   (b) Highest rate of multiplication
   (c) Decrease in cell division
   (d) A constant number of cells and their size

617. In suspension culture the Log phase is characterised by
   (a) Preparation of cells to divide
   (b) Highest rate of multiplication
   (c) Decrease in cell division
   (d) A constant number of cells and their size

618. The cytoplasmic hybrids where the nucleus is derived from only one parent and the cytoplasm is derived from both the parents are called as
   (a) Hybrids   (b) Cybrids
   (c) Heterokaryon   (d) None

619. The inorganic cation, regulates osmotic potential is
   (a) Potassium
   (b) Molybdenum
   (c) Zinc
   (d) All the above

620. The hormone responsible for stimulation of closing of stomata is due to
   (a) Abscisic
   (b) Cytokinin
   (c) Ethylene
   (d) All the above

621. The hormone responsible for stimulation of opening of stomata is due to
   (a) Abscisic
   (b) Cytokinin
   (c) Ethylene
   (d) All the above

622. In plant tissue culture the leaf surface can be sterilized by
   (a) 0.1% w/v Mercuric chloride
   (b) 2% Hypochloride
   (c) 10% Calcium hypochloride
   (d) All tha above

623. The micronutrient essential in the medium is
   (a) Nacl   (b) $Cocl_2$
   (c) Kcl   (d) $Cacl_2$

624. The P^H of the medium is
   (a) 6.6   (b) 6.0
   (c) 5.6   (d) 5.0

625. The tissue growth observed is
   (a) Undifferentiated cells suspended in the medium
   (b) Undifferentiated cells suspended in the medium
   (c) Differentiated mass of cells
   (d) Surface growth of undifferentiated mass of cells

626. The phytohormone shows triple response growth is
    (a) Ethylene
    (b) Abscissic acid
    (c) Cytokinin
    (d) Auxins

627. The PH suitable for the growth of explant in plant tissue culture is
    (a) 5.0 to 6.0   (b) 6.0 to 7.0
    (c) Above 7   (d) Below 4.5

628. The vitamins essential in plant tissue culture media is
    (a) Nicotinic acid (b) Pyridoxin
    (c) Thiamine   (d) Myoinositol

629. In ayurvedic preparations the first word may indicate the
    (a) Disease for which preparation is used
    (b) Name of some god or saint
    (c) Property of the preparation
    (d) All the above

630. In ayurvedic preparations the second word may indicate the
    (a) Disease for which preparation is used
    (b) Name of some god or saint
    (c) Property of the preparation
    (d) All the above

631. Avaleha is the
    (a) Solid dosage form of drug in ayurveda
    (b) liquid dosage form of drug in ayurveda
    (c) Semi Solid dosage form of drug in ayurveda
    (d) Powder dosage form of drug in ayurveda.

632. Bhasma is the
    (a) Solid dosage form of drug in ayurveda
    (b) Liquid dosage form of drug in ayurveda
    (c) Semi Solid dosage form of drug in ayurveda
    (d) Powder dosage form of drug in ayurveda

633. The preparation of asava & arista are
    (a) Should be clear with out any froth
    (b) Should show aromatic alcoholic odour
    (c) Should not become sour
    (d) All the above

634. The semisolid preparation of drugs prepared with the addiction of jaggery, sugar or sugar candy & boiled with prescribed drug juice or decoction is
    (a) Leha or avaleha
    (b) Arka
    (c) Asava or Aristha
    (d) Taila

635. The preparation in which fixed oil is boiled with prescribed kasayas (decoction) & kalkas (pastes) of drugs are
    (a) Tailas   (b) Leha
    (c) Asavas   (d) Arka

636. In preparation of bhasma, the processes involved are
    (a) Sodana   (b) Marana
    (c) Both a & b   (d) None

637. Churna is a
    (a) Powder form of drug obtained by calcination
    (b) Fine powder of drug or drugs.
    (c) Semisolid preparation of drug
    (d) None

638. Medicines prepared in the form of tablet or pills are known as
    (a) Vati and Gutika
    (b) Asava and Arista
    (c) Avaleha or leha
    (d) All.

639. The addition of one article to another through accident, ignorance or carelessness is called as
    (a) Admixture
    (b) Deterioration
    (c) Substitution
    (d) Sophistication

640. The addition of completely different substance in the place of original drug is called as
    (a) Admixture
    (b) Deterioration
    (c) Substitution
    (d) Sophistication

641. The following is an example for intentional adulteration
    (a) Coriander seeds collected when their are unripe
    (b) Ginger rhizomes are collected along with cork
    (c) Mother cloves with clove stalks
    (d) Pyrethrum flowers heads with stems & flowers

642. The following is an examples for substitution with artifically manufactured substances
    (a) Compressed chicory in place of coffee
    (b) Properly cut & shaped baswood for nutmeg
    (c) Paraffin wax made yellow colored & substituted for bees wax
    (d) All the above

643. Addition of citral to citrus oils is an example of
    (a) Substitution of synthetic principles to original drug
    (b) Substitution of drug with exhausted drug
    (c) Substitution of drug with superficially similar inferior drug
    (d) All the above

644. Kurchi bark is example for
    (a) Chanelled bark
    (b) Compound bark
    (c) Recurved bark
    (d) Quill

645. An example of paracytic or rubiaceous or parallel celled stomata is
    (a) Senna & Coca
    (b) Spearmint & peppermint
    (c) Datura &Stramonium
    (d) Digitalis & Lobelia.

646. An example of Anomocytic or ranunculaceous or irregular-celled stomata is
    (a) Senna & Coca
    (b) Spearmint & peppermint

(c) Datura &Stramonium

(d) Digitalis & Lobelia

647. An example ofAnisocytic or cruciferous or unequal stomata is
(a) Senna & Coca
(b) Spearmint & peppermint
(c) Datura &Stramonium
(d) Digitalis & Lobelia

648. An example of Diacytic or Caryophyllaceous or cross celled stomata is
(a) Senna & Coca
(b) Spearmint & peppermint
(c) Datura &Stramonium
(d) Digitalis & Lobelia

649. Nux-vomica contains
(a) Large conical, strong shrunken unicellular covering trichomes
(b) Lignified trichomes
(c) Short, sharply pointed curved unicellular covering trichomes
(d) Short,conical, unicellular covering trichomes

650. Digitalis purpurea contains
(a) Unicellular head & unicellular stalk trichome
(b) Unicellular stalk & biseriate head trichome
(c) Both a & b
(d) All.

651. Unicellular glandular trichomes are present in
(a) Piper   (b) Vasaka
(c) Both   (d) None

652. Tobacco contains
(a) Multicellular head, multicellular biseriate stalk
(b) Unicellular stalk & biseriate head
(c) Multicellular multiseriate head, multicellular uniseriate stalk
(d) Unicellular glandular trichomes.

653. Melting point of bees wax is
(a) 62-65   (b) 75-85
(c) 34-44   (d) 50-56

654. Moisture content of ergot should not more than
(a) 5   (b) 8
(c) 10   (d) 15

655. Carbon tetrachloride is used to induce
(a) Diabetic condition in animal
(b) Liver toxicity in animal
(c) Cancer in animal
(d) All the above

656. Senna shows calcium oxalate crystals in the form of
(a) Solitary (single) crystals
(b) Crystals fibres
(c) Rosette aggregates
(d) All the above

657. Drug evaluation means
(a) Determination of purity &quality
(b) Debasement of an article
(c) Confirmation of identity
(d) All the above

658. Adulteration means
(a) Determination of purity &quality
(b) Debasement of an article
(c) Confirmation of identity
(d) All the above

659. The taste of liquorice is
    (a) Sweet   (b) pungent
    (c) Allieous   (d) Acrid

660. Crude fibre value of a drug is a measure of
    (a) Soft tissue matter
    (b) Woody matter
    (c) Mineral matter
    (d) Organic matter.

661. In gel permeation chromatography molecules are separated on the basis of their
    (a) Chemical nature
    (b) Size &shape
    (c) Adsorptive matter
    (d) Partitioncoefficient.

662. Derivatization is done in GC
    (a) To convert a less polar compound to a more polar compound
    (b) To convert volatile compound to non-volatile
    (c) To convert a polar compound to less polar compound
    (d) To liquefy a solid

663. Derivatization techniques in HPLC are intended to enhance
    (a) Molecular weight
    (b) Detectability
    (c) Reversibility
    (d) Reproducibility

664. The pressure used in HPLC is
    (a) 1000-3000psi
    (b) 1000-6000psi
    (c) 1000-5000psi
    (d) 2000-6000psi

665. Solvent programming, also called gradient elution involves
    (a) Changing the column length
    (b) Changing the mobile phase composition
    (c) Using the mobile phase composition
    (d) Solubility of the ion exchange resin

666. Partition chromatography is known as
    (a) Solid-liquid
    (b) liquid –liquid
    (c) Gas –liquid
    (d) None

667. What is the nature of the mobile phase the reverse phase chromatography
    (a) Polar
    (b) Non-polar
    (c) Mixture of both
    (d) Can be any it depends on the nature of analyte.

668. What is the diameter of silica particle in HPTLC
    (a) $\leq 5\ \mu m$ (b) $\geq 20 \mu m$
    (c) $\leq 50\ \mu m$ (d) None

669. In size exclusion chromatography the stationary phases used are
    (a) Alumina   (b) Dextran
    (c) Phosphate   (d) Styrene
    (a) a, d   (b) b, c
    (c) b, d   (d) a, c

670. Choose the correct semirigid gel used for exclusion chromatography
    (a) Sephadex   (b) Gelatin
    (c) Cellulose   (d) Alumina

671. In quantitative T.L.C radioactive material can be studied by
    (a) Visual comparison
    (b) Densiometer
    (c) Gravimetry
    (d) Geiger muller counters

672. Bitters are used as
    (a) Digestive
    (b) Stomachic
    (c) Febrifuge
    (d) All

673. Bitterness value is obtained organoleptically by comparison with a solution (which act as a standar (d)
    (a) Quinine HCl
    (b) Quinidine HCl
    (c) Quinine sulphate
    (d) Quinidine sulphate

674. Which of the following is an example for coumarin bitter principles?
    (a) Angelicin
    (b) Santonin
    (c) Lupilon
    (d) All the above

675. Gentiopicrin is obtained from?
    (a) Gentiana lutea
    (b) Gelidium amansii
    (c) Gymnema Sylvester
    (d) All the above

676. Kutkoside is obtained from
    (a) Picrorrhiza kurroa
    (b) It is a bitter principle
    (c) It is used in the treatment of jaundice
    (d) All the above

677. Sweetners are used
    (a) To mask the bitter taste
    (b) As a preservative
    (c) Impact sweet taste
    (d) All the above

678. Sweetness potency is compared with...
    (a) 100 gm/L solution of sucrose
    (b) 1000 gm/L solution of sucrose
    (c) 10 gm/L solution of sucrose
    (d) None

679. The disadvantage of using liquorice as sweeting agent is
    (a) Cause oedema
    (b) Cause hypertension
    (c) Both
    (d) None

680. Thaumatin is (sweetness is)
    (a) (350x) >> Sucrose
    (b) (3500x) >> Sucrose
    (c) (35x) >> Sucrose
    (d) None

681. Coloring pigment present in beet root is
    (a) Betanidine
    (b) Betanin
    (c) Betain
    (d) None

682. Crocsin is obtained from
    (a) Styles and stigmas of the plant crocus sativa
    (b) Flowers of the plant crocus sativa
    (c) Calyx and corolla of the crocus sativus
    (d) None

683. Curcumin impact yellow color is
    (a) Good in acid
    (b) Poor in alkali
    (c) Poor in acid
    (d) both a & b

684. Crassin acetate is a anticancer agent obtained from
    (a) Euncoea asperula
    (b) Pseudoplexaura porosa
    (c) Haliclona viridis
    (d) Merecenaria mercenaria

685. Ara-c is a potent
    (a) Anticancer agent
    (b) Antibiotic agent
    (c) Cardiovascular agent
    (d) Antimicrobial

686. Asperitol is obtained from
    (a) Euncoea asperula
    (b) Pseudoplexaura porosa
    (c) Haliclona viridis
    (d) Merecenaria mercenaria

687. Autonomium from Verongia fistularis posses
    (a) Adrenergic effects
    (b) Cholinergic effects
    (c) Both a & b
    (d) Antibiotic activity

688. Holothurians
    (a) Triterpeniod aglycone moiety
    (b) Obtained from asterosaponins & holothurians
    (c) Posses cariotonic & haemolytic activity
    (d) All the above

689. Simularin posses
    (a) Cytotoxic compound
    (b) Antimicrobial compound
    (c) Antibiotic compound
    (d) Cardiovascular compound

690. Holotoxin is
    (a) Cytotoxic compound
    (b) Antimicrobial compound
    (c) Antibiotic compound
    (d) Cardiovascular compound

691. Eptatretin & laminine posses
    (a) Cytotoxic compound
    (b) Antimicrobial compound
    (c) Antibiotic compound
    (d) Cardiovascular compound

692. Anthopleurins posses
    (a) + ve inotropic effect
    (b) + ve chronotropic effects
    (c) Both a& b
    (d) None

693. Dandalone is
    (a) Cytotoxic compound
    (b) Antimicrobial compound
    (c) Anti-inflammatory compound
    (d) All the above

694. Holotoxins A, B & C from sea cucumber acts as
    (a) Antimicrobial agent
    (b) Potent cardioactive agent
    (c) Anti-inflammatory agent
    (d) None

695. Debromolaurenterol is obtain from
    (a) Sea hare aplysia californica
    (b) Red algae laurencia pacifica
    (c) Red algae asparogopsis taxiformis
    (d) All.

696. Acanthelin posses
    (a) Antimycobacterium activity
    (b) Cardiovascular activity

(c) Anticancer activity
(d) None

697. Which of the following statement is true for sphingosine?
(a) Methoxy derivative of adenosine
(b) Obtained from cryptotethya crypta
(c) Reduces both rate & force of contraction of heart
(d) All the above

698. Spongosine
(a) Acts by reducing heart rate
(b) Acts by reducing force of contraction of heart
(c) Both a & b
(d) None

699. Which of the following is correct for asperitol
(a) Obtained from gorgonian coral
(b) A non-lactonic cembranoid
(c) Cytotoxic agent
(d) All the above

700. Cardiac glycosides are example for
(a) O-glycoside
(b) N-glycoside
(c) S-glycoside
(d) C-glycosides

701. Sinigrin is an example for
(a) O-glycosides
(b) N-glycosides
(c) S-glycoside
(d) C-glycosides

702. Cascara is an example for
(a) O-glycosides
(b) N-glycosides

(c) S-glycoside
(d) C-glycosides

703. Bearberry is an example for
(a) Phenol glycosides
(b) Aldehyde glycosides
(c) Flavone glycosides
(d) Saponin glycoside

704. Vanilla is an example for
(a) Phenol glycosides
(b) Aldehyde glycosides
(c) Flavone glycosides
(d) Saponin glycosides

705. Solanum is an example for
(a) Phenol glycosides
(b) Aldehyde glycosides
(c) Steroidal glycoside
(d) Flavone glycosides

706. Almond is an example for
(a) Bitter glycoside
(b) Cyanogetic&cyanophora glycoside
(c) Steriodal glycoside
(d) Sterol glycoside

707. Glycosides are easily hydrolysed by
(a) Water
(b) Mineral acids
(c) Enzymes
(d) All the above

708. Modified borntrager's test or Modified anthraquinone test is used for identification of
(a) O-glycosides
(b) N-glycosides
(c) S-glycoside
(d) C-glycosides

709. Griping action of senna is due to
     (a) its resin or emodin content
     (b) Salicylic acid content
     (c) 6-hydroxymusizin content
     (d) Kaempferol

710. Foam test is used for the identification of
     (a) Cardiac glycoside
     (b) Anthraquinone glycoside
     (c) Saponin glycoside
     (d) Bitter glycoside

711. The type of stoma present in cassia angustifolia is
     (a) Paracytic stomata
     (b) Diacytic stomata
     (c) Anisocytic stomata
     (d) Anomocytic stomata

712. The type of stoma present in digitalis purpurea is
     (a) Paracytic stomata
     (b) Diacytic stomata
     (c) Anisocytic stomata
     (d) Anomocytic stomata

713. The type of stoma present in vasaka is
     (a) Paracytic stomata
     (b) Diacytic stomata
     (c) Anisocytic stomata
     (d) Anomocytic stomata

714. Stomatal index of Indian senna is
     (a) 17-20   (b) 11.4-13.3
     (c) 12.5-17.5   (d) 15-18

715. Stomatal index of alexandrian senna is
     (a) 17-20   (b) 11.4-13.3
     (c) 12.5-17.5   (d) 15-18.

716. Chittem bark is
     (a) Cinchona calisaya
     (b) Rhamnus purshiana
     (c) Saraca indica
     (d) Cinnamomum zeylanicum

717. The bark of cascara is collected at least 1 year before use because
     (a) Freshly collected cascara bark contain anthranol derivatives, which causes gripping action
     (b) Freshly collected cascara bark posses emetic effects
     (c) Both a & b
     (d) None

718. Cascara contain
     (a) O-glycosides
     (b) C-glycosides
     (c) S-glycoside
     (d) Both O&C glycoside

719. Which of the following is correct in case of anthrone
     (a) Pale yellow substance & without any solubility in alkali
     (b) Brownish yellow substances & soluble in alkali
     (c) It shows strong florescence
     (d) Both A & C

720. Which of the following is wrong in case of Anthronal
     (a) Pale yellow substance & without any solubility in alkali
     (b) Brownish yellow substances & soluble in alkali
     (c) It shows strong florescence
     (d) Both A & C

721. Palmidin B on hydrolysis produces
    (a) Aloe-emodin-anthrone + chrysophanol anthrone
    (b) Aloe-emodin-anthrone + emodin anthrone
    (c) Emodin-anthrone + chrysophanol anthrone
    (d) All the above

722. Rhubard on addition of alkalies shows
    (a) Red color due to the presence of anthraquinone glycosides
    (b) Pink color due to the presence of saponin glycosides
    (c) Deepiolet color florescence due to anthraquinones
    (d) Red color due to the presence of hydrolysed tannins

723. Rhapontic rhubarb
    (a) Does not contain rhein
    (b) Does not contain emodin or aloe-emodin
    (c) It contain rhaponticin & posses estrogenic action
    (d) All the above

724. Monkey–skin aloe is also called as
    (a) Cape aloe
    (b) Socotrine aloe
    (c) Zanziber aloes
    (d) Curacao aloe

725. Cape aloes are collected &packed in
    (a) Wooden boxes (b) Goat skin
    (c) Monkey skin (d) None

726. Aloe which is characterized by fragments consists of quite large prisms present in group or in dispersed form are
    (a) Curacao aloe
    (b) Cape aloe
    (c) Socotrine aloe
    (d) Zanziber aloes

727. The color obtained in schoenteten's reaction or borax test with aloes is
    (a) Pink color
    (b) Green florescence
    (c) Pale green color
    (d) Pale yellow florescence

728. Klunge's isobarbalion test gives wine red color with
    (a) Curacao aloe
    (b) Cape aloe
    (c) Socotrine aloe & zanziber aloes
    (d) All the above

729. Cardenolides posses
    (a) Five membered lactone ring with one double bond
    (b) Six membered lactone ring with one double bond
    (c) Both a & b
    (d) None

730. The sugar (glycone) part of the cardiac glycosides
    (a) Is responsible for therapeutical activity
    (b) To potentiate the medicinal activity of aglycone part
    (c) Useful in solubilization of aglycone there by, beneficial in absortion & distribution in the body
    (d) None

731. Digitoxin on hydrolysis yields
    (a) Gitoxigenin &3digitoxose molecules
    (b) Digitoxigenin &3digitoxose molecules
    (c) Gitoxigenin &3digitalose molecules
    (d) Digitoxigenin & 3gitoxigenin molecules

732. Verbascum thapsus can be identified by
    (a) Presence of large woolly branched candelabra trichomes
    (b) Presence of uniseriate covering trichomes
    (c) Presence of multiseriste trichomes forming hook at the top
    (d) Straight lateral veins

733. Comfrey leaves are identified by
    (a) Presence of large woolly branched candelabra trichomes
    (b) Presence of uniseriate covering trichomes
    (c) Presence of multiseriste trichomes forming hook at the top
    (d) Straight lateral veins

734. Primrose (primula vulgaris) leaves are identified a by
    (a) Presence of large woolly branched candelabra trichomes
    (b) Presence of uniseriate covering trichomes
    (c) Straight lateral veins
    (d) Both b & c

735. The a glycone part of peruvoside is
    (a) Cannogenin
    (b) Cannogenol
    (c) Cannogenic acid
    (d) Digitoxigenin

736. European squill is
    (a) Dried slices of the bulbs of urginea indica
    (b) Dried slices & Scaly leaves of urginea maritima
    (c) Both a & b
    (d) None

737. The cardiac glycosides (glucosillaren) on hydrolysis gives
    (a) glucose + glucose + rhamnose + scillarenin
    (b) proscillaridin A + glucose
    (c) glucose + fructose + rhamnose + proscillaridin
    (d) None

738. Liquorice consists of
    (a) Triterpenoid glycyrrhizin which is a potassium & calcium salt of glycyrrhizinic acid
    (b) Triterpenoid glycyrrhizin which is a magnesium & calcium salt of glycyrrhizinic acid
    (c) Triterpend glycyrrhizin which is a potassium & magnesium salt of glycyrrhizinic acid
    (d) None

739. Mineralocorticoid activity of liquorice is due to
    (a) Carbenoxolone
    (b) Glycyrrhizin
    (c) Glycyrrhetinic acid
    (d) Both a & c

740. Chinese ginseng is
 (a) Panax ginseng
 (b) Panax notoginseng
 (c) Panax quinquefolium
 (d) Panax Japanese

741. Which of the following root is called as manroot
 (a) Rauwolfia
 (b) Ipeacacuanha
 (c) Ginseng
 (d) Jalap

742. Panax belongs to
 (a) Leguminosae (b) Araliaceae
 (c) Apocynaceae (d) Liliaceae

743. The aglycone part of panaxosides is
 (a) Dammarol
 (b) Oleanolic acid
 (c) Panaxytriol
 (d) Panaxadiol

744. Which of the following drug posses immunomodulatory activity
 (a) Ginseng
 (b) Liquorice
 (c) Ashwagandha
 (d) All the above

745. Which of the following is called Rattle snake root
 (a) Senega   (b) Rauwolfia
 (c) Ashwagandha (d) All

746. Senega consists of
 (a) Dried roots &stolons of polygala senega belongs to rosaceae
 (b) Dried roots & root stock of polygala senega belongs to polygalaceae
 (c) Dried leaves &twigs of polygala senega belongs to rosaceae
 (d) None

747. White senega is
 (a) Polygala alba root
 (b) Glinus oppositifolia
 (c) Polygala chinensis
 (d) All the above

748. Sweet taste of senega is due to
 (a) Senegenin
 (b) Presenegenin
 (c) Methyl salicylate
 (d) Polygalitol

749. Psoralea belong to
 (a) Araliaceae
 (b) Leguminosae
 (c) Apocyanaceae
 (d) Liliaceae

750. The drug psoralea when dissolved in alcohol & little sodium hydroxide it shows
 (a) Yellow florescence
 (b) Blue florescence
 (c) Green florescence
 (d) Pink florescence.

751. Dioscorea does not contain
 (a) Diosgenin
 (b) Smilagenin & epismilagenin
 (c) Yammogenin
 (d) Edible starch

752. The following drug is substitute for dioscorea
 (a) Dioscorea flouibunda
 (b) Dioscorea deltoidea
 (c) Costus speciosus
 (d) Dioscorea villosa

753. Deglycyrrhized liquorice (DGL) Shows
    (a) Antigastric effects
    (b) Reduced mineralocorticoid activity
    (c) Healing activity
    (d) All the above

754. Khellin present in ammivisnaga shows
    (a) Bitter taste
    (b) Smooth muscle relaxant activity
    (c) Both a & b
    (d) None

755. Khellin, visnagin & khelloside are present in
    (a) Ammi majus
    (b) Ammi visnaga
    (c) Psoralea corylifolia
    (d) Both b & c

756. Gentiopicroside from gentian luteal
    (a) Is water soluble, crystalline compound
    (b) Has bitter value of 12000
    (c) Breakdown to gentiogenin & glucose.
    (d) All the above

757. Sertia chirata is substituted with
    (a) Swertia densifolia
    (b) Swertia ciliate
    (c) Swertia paniculata
    (d) All the above

758. Which of the following drug is called as bitter wood
    (a) Sandal wood
    (b) Red sanders wood
    (c) Quassia wood
    (d) Sassafras

759. Picrasma excels belong to
    (a) Gentianaceae
    (b) Scrophulariaceae
    (c) Simaroubaceae
    (d) Zygophyllaceae

760. Which of the following country can be recognised as the medicinal garden of the world
    (a) China   (b) Egypt
    (c) South America (d) India

761. India has the major supplier of medicinal plants in the world market until, 1977, when it was kept to second position by
    (a) South korea   (b) China
    (c) Eygpt   (d) Japan

762. One of the important items of export, covering approximately 80% of the world requirement, is a proteolytic enzyme, papain mainly manufactured in
    (a) Andhra Pradesh
    (b) Maharastra
    (c) Arunachal Pradesh
    (d) Japan

763. The commercial production of pectin from thalamus of sunflower is also carried out at
    (a) Andhra Pradesh
    (b) Maharashhtra
    (c) Arunachal Pradesh
    (d) Japan

764. __________is a leader in the production &export of high value perfumes (attars) for the world market
    (a) China   (b) Egypt
    (c) South America (d) India

765. India has adopted restrictive export policy in respect of those crude drugs, which were indiscriminately exploited in the forest such as
    (a) Atropa belladonna
    (b) Artemisia brevifolia
    (c) Swertia chirata
    (d) All the above

766. The country which occupies 26th rank in import &14th in respect of export in world in the trade of essential oils
    (a) India   (b) Japan
    (c) China   (d) None

767. As a general rule, the acute toxicity of essential oils by the oral route is
    (a) Low or very low
    (b) Medium
    (c) High or very high
    (d) None

768. A specific immunologic reaction to an immunogen is called
    (a) Allergy
    (b) Hypersensitivity
    (c) Both a & b
    (d) None

769. The different types of allergens are
    (a) Inhalant allergens
    (b) Ingestant &Injectant allergens
    (c) Contact & infectant allergens
    (d) None

KEY

1. (c)	2. (a)	3. (a)	4. (b)	5. (c)
6. (a)	7. (b)	8. (d)	9. (d)	10. (a)
11. (d)	12. (a)	13. (b)	14. (a)	15. (c)
16. (b)	17. (a)	18. (d)	19. (a)	20. (a)
21. (c)	22. (a)	23. (b)	24. (d)	25. (c)
26. (b)	27. (d)	28. (a)	29. (b)	30. (b)
31. (a)	32. (c)	33. (d)	34. (a)	35. (d)
36. (a)	37. (a)	38. (b)	39. (a)	40. (b)
41. (b)	42. (c)	43. (a)	44. (d)	45. (b)
46. (a)	47. (b)	48. (c)	49. (c)	50. (c)
51. (d)	52. (d)	53. (c)	54. (a)	55. (b)
56. (d)	57. (b)	58. (d)	59. (a)	60. (c)
61. (c)	62. (b)	63. (a)	64. (b)	65. (c)
66. (d)	67. (c)	68. (a)	69. (a)	70. (b)
71. (c)	72. (d)	73. (a)	74. (a)	75. (a)
76. (b)	77. (c)	78. (d)	79. (d)	80. (b)
81. (d)	82. (d)	83. (c)	84. (b)	85. (b)
86. (b)	87. (c)	88. (b)	89. (c)	90. (c)
91. (a)	92. (a)	93. (b)	94. (d)	95. (a)
96. (b)	97. (c)	98. (b)	99. (d)	100. (d)
101. (a)	102. (b)	103. (d)	104. (b)	105. (a)
106. (c)	107. (b)	108. (b)	109. (a)	110. (a)
111. (c)	112. (b)	113. (c)	114. (c)	115. (a)

116. (d)	117. (a)	118. (d)	119. (a)	120. (b)
121. (a)	122. (a)	123. (c)	124. (d)	125. (c)
126. (b)	127 (d)	128. (a)	129. (d)	130. (b)
131. (b)	132. (c)	133. (c)	134. (a)	135. (a)
136. (a)	137. (b)	138. (c)	139. (d)	140. (d)
141. (d)	142. (b)	143. (a)	144. (b)	145. (b)
146. (a)	147. (a)	148. (c)	149. (c)	150. (c)
151. (a)	152. (b)	153. (a)	154. (d)	155. (d)
156. (d)	157. (b)	158. (a)	159. (c)	160. (a)
161. (a)	162. (c)	163. (c)	164. (b)	165. (a)
166. (a)	167. (a)	168. (d)	169. (a)	170. (c)
171. (d)	172. (a)	173. (d)	174. (b)	175. (c)
176. (b)	177. (a)	178. (c)	179. (b)	180. (d)
181. (a)	182. (c)	183. (a)	184. (d)	185. (c)
186. (d)	187. (c)	188. (a)	189. (d)	190. (d)
191. (b)	192. (d)	193. (a)	194. (a)	195. (d)
196. (a)	197. (b)	198. (a)	199. (b)	200. (a)
201. (b)	202. (a)	203. (d)	204. (d)	205. (a)
206. (d)	207. (a)	208. (b)	209. (d)	210. (b)
211. (b)	212. (a)	213. (b)	214. (b)	215. (a)
216. (b)	217. (b)	218. (d)	219. (a)	220. (d)
221. (c)	222. (d)	223. (d)	224. (a)	225. (a)
226. (a)	227. (d)	228. (a)	229. (a)	230. (a)
231. (c)	232. (d)	233. (b)	234. (a)	235. (b)

236. (a)	237. (b)	238. (a)	239. (b)	240. (d)
241. (b)	242. (c)	243. (b)	244. (b)	245. (a)
246. (a)	247. (d)	248. (b)	249. (c)	250. (b)
251. (a)	252. (c)	253. (c)	254. (a)	255. (c)
256. (d)	257. (b)	258. (a)	259. (b)	260. (a)
261. (a)	262. (d)	263. (a)	264. (c)	265. (c)
266. (b)	267. (b)	268. (c)	269. (d)	270. (d)
271. (a)	272. (d)	273. (d)	274. (d)	275. (a)
276. (a)	277. (b)	278. (b)	279. (a)	280. (a)
281. (a)	282. (a)	283. (b)	284. (b)	285. (b)
286. (a)	287. (b)	288. (c)	289. (d)	290. (a)
291. (b)	292. (a)	293. (d)	294. (c)	295. (b)
296. (a)	297. (a)	298. (a)	299. (c)	300. (d)
301. (c)	302. (a)	303. (b)	304. (a)	305. (b)
306. (b)	307. (d)	308. (a)	309. (c)	310. (c)
311. (a)	312. (b)	313. (a)	314. (a)	315. (b)
316. (a)	317. (b)	318. (a)	319. (a)	320. (d)
321. (d)	322. (a)	323. (a)	324. (d)	325. (b)
326. (c)	327. (a)	328. (d)	329. (b)	330. (b)
331. (b)	332. (b)	333. (a)	334. (a)	335. (b)
336. (a)	337. (a)	338. (b)	339. (b)	340. (b)
341. (d)	342. (a)	343. (b)	344 (b)	345. (c)
346. (c)	347. (b)	348. (a)	349. (d)	350. (b)
351. (c)	352. (c)	353. (b)	354. (d)	355. (b)

356. (a)	357. (b)	358. (a)	359. (b)	360. (c)
361. (b)	362. (a)	363. (b)	364. (a)	365. (c)
366. (b)	367. (c)	368. (a)	369. (b)	370. (d)
371. (a)	372. (a)	373. (d)	374. (c)	375. (c)
376. (b)	377. (c)	378. (a)	379. (a)	380. (a)
381. (b)	382. (d)	383. (d)	384. (b)	385. (b)
386. (d)	387. (c)	388. (b)	389. (c)	390. (d)
391. (d)	392. (c)	393. (b)	394. (a)	395. (a)
396. (b)	397. (b)	398. (a)	399. (d)	400. (a)
401. (d)	402. (a)	403. (c)	404. (d)	405. (c)
406. (a)	407. (a)	408. (d)	409. (a)	410. (a)
411. (b)	412. (c)	413. (d)	414. (b)	415. (a)
416. (d)	417. (a)	418. (a)	419. (a)	420. (b)
421. (c)	422. (c)	423. (a)	424. (a)	425. (a)
426. (a)	427. (c)	428. (a)	429. (b)	430. (c)
431. (d)	432. (b)	433. (d)	434. (a)	435. (c)
436. (d)	437. (c)	438. (a)	439. (a)	440. (a)
441. (d)	442. (c)	443. (c)	444. (c)	445. (a)
446. (a)	447. (a)	448. (b)	449. (a)	450. (c)
451. (a)	452. (c)	453. (a)	454. (c)	455. (a)
456. (c)	457. (a)	458. (a)	459. (b)	460. (b)
461. (c)	462. (d)	463. (b)	464. (b)	465. (b)
466. (a)	467. (d)	468. (c)	469. (c)	470. (b)
471. (a)	472. (c)	473. (b)	474. (c)	475. (b)

476. (b)	477. (b)	478. (a)	479. (b)	480. (d)
481. (a)	482. (a)	483. (b)	484. (c)	485. (d)
486. (b)	487. (c)	488. (d)	489. (a)	490. (b)
491. (c)	492. (a)	493. (a)	494. (c)	495. (a)
496. (b)	497. (c)	498. (a)	499. (a)	500. (b)
501. (a)	502. (b)	503. (c)	504. (a)	505. (d)
506. (c)	507. (c)	508. (a)	509. (b)	510. (d)
511. (c)	512. (b)	513. (d)	514. (a)	515. (c)
516. (c)	517. (b)	518. (b)	519. (a)	520. (c)
521. (b)	522. (a)	523. (a)	524. (a)	525. (a)
526. (d)	527. (d)	528. (a)	529. (c)	530. (b)
531. (b)	532. (a)	533. (c)	534. (d)	535. (a)
536. (b)	537. (c)	538. (b)	539. (a)	540. (c)
541. (a)	542. (b)	543. (c)	544. (a)	545. (a)
546. (b)	547. (a)	548. (c)	549. (a)	550. (a)
551. (b)	552. (c)	553. (a)	554. (a)	555. (b)
556. (a)	557. (b)	558. (a)	559. (b)	560. (a)
561. (d)	562. (a)	563. (b)	564. (a)	565. (b)
566. (d)	567. (a)	568. (a)	569. (a)	570. (a)
571. (d)	572. (c)	573. (b)	574. (a)	575. (b)
576. (b)	577. (a)	578. (c)	579. (b)	580. (a)
581. (d)	582. (c)	583. (a)	584. (a)	585. (b)
586. (d)	587. (a)	588. (a)	589. (b)	590. (a)
591. (d)	592. (b)	593. (a)	594. (a)	595. (a)

596. (a)	597. (a)	598. (b)	599. (a)	600. (c)
601. (a)	602. (b)	603. (d)	604. (d)	605. (d)
606. (a)	607. (a)	608. (a)	609. (b)	610. (a)
611. (a)	612. (a)	613. (b)	614. (a)	615. (a)
616. (a)	617. (b)	618. (b)	619. (a)	620. (a)
621. (b)	622. (a)	623. (b)	624. (b)	625. (d)
626. (a)	627. (a)	628. (c)	629. (d)	630. (d)
631. (c)	632. (d)	633. (d)	634. (a)	635. (a)
636. (c)	637. (b)	638. (a)	639. (a)	640. (c)
641. (c)	642. (d)	643. (a)	644. (c)	645. (a)
646. (d)	647. (c)	648. (b)	649. (b)	650. (c)
651. (c)	652. (c)	653. (a)	654. (b)	655. (b)
656. (d)	657. (a)	658. (b)	659. (a)	660. (b)
661. (b)	662. (a)	663. (b)	664. (b)	665. (b)
666. (b)	667. (a)	668. (a)	669. (c)	670. (a)
671. (d)	672. (d)	673. (a)	674. (a)	675. (a)
676. (d)	677. (d)	678. (d)	679. (c)	680. (b)
681. (b)	682. (a)	683. (d)	684. (b)	685. (a)
686. (a)	687. (c)	688. (d)	689. (a)	690. (b)
691. (d)	692. (a)	693. (c)	694. (a)	695. (a)
696. (a)	697. (d)	698. (c)	699. (d)	700. (a)
701. (c)	702. (d)	703. (a)	704. (b)	705. (c)
706. (b)	707. (d)	708. (a)	709. (a)	710. (c)
711. (a)	712. (d)	713. (b)	714. (a)	715. (b)

716. (b)	717. (c)	718. (c)	719. (d)	720. (a)
721. (a)	722. (a)	723. (d)	724. (c)	725. (b)
726. (c)	727. (b)	728. (a)	729. (a)	730. (c)
731. (b)	732. (a)	733. (c)	734. (d)	735. (b)
736. (b)	737. (a)	738. (a)	739. (d)	740. (b)
741. (c)	742. (b)	743. (b)	744. (d)	745. (a)
746. (b)	747. (a)	748. (d)	749. (b)	750. (a)
751. (d)	752. (c)	753. (d)	754. (c)	755. (a)
756. (d)	757. (d)	758. (c)	759. (c)	760. (d)
761. (a)	762. (b)	763. (b)	764. (d)	765. (d)
766. (a)	767. (a)	768. (c)	769. (d)	

V   OTHERS

1. What is the other name for UV-Visible Spectroscopy?
   (a) Electromagnetic radiation
   (b) Electromagnetic spectroscopy
   (c) Electronic spectroscopy
   (d) Electrochemical spectroscopy

2. For UV- Visible spectrum electronic excitation occur in the range of
   (a) 200-800 mμ (b) 400-800 mμ
   (c) 400-700 mμ (d) 300-600 mμ

3. The wavelength of a radiation can be expressed in terms of
   (a) Frequency or energy in kcal/mol
   (b) Wave number or energy in kcal/ mol
   (c) Frequency or energy in k joule/ mol
   (d) Wave number or energy in k joule/mol

4. If a substance is exposed to certain different value of frequency then, what happens to energy and intensity of radiation?
   (a) Energy is not absorbed, loss in intensity respectively
   (b) Energy is not absorbed, no loss in intensity respectively
   (c) Energy is absorbed, loss in intensity respectively
   (d) Energy is absorbed, no loss in intensity respectively

5. Calculate the energy associated with radiation having wavelength 280mμ?
   (a) 110 kcal / mol
   (b) 100 kjoule / mol
   (c) 100 kcal / mol
   (d) 180 kcal / mol

6. A record of amount of light absorbed by the sample as a function of the wavelength of light is called as
   (a) Excitation band
   (b) Adsorption band
   (c) Electronic band
   (d) Absorption band

7. Which of the following is a far UV region?
   (a) Above 200 mμ
   (b) Below 200 mμ
   (c) 200 mμ
   (d) 400 mμ

8. Which of the following expression is related to Lambert's law?
   (a) $dI/dx = kI$ (b) $dI/dx = -kI$
   (c) $-dx/dI = kI$ (d) $-dI/dx = kI$

9. The value k = absorption coefficient depends upon
   (a) Nature of the absorbing medium
   (b) Thickness of the absorbing medium
   (c) Intensity of the absorbing medium
   (d) Radiation

10. The value a = extinction coefficient of the absorbing medium is written as
    (a) $a = I_0 e^{-kx}$
    (b) $a = I/2.303$
    (c) $a = k/2.303$
    (d) $a = I_0 10^{-ax}$

11. Beer's law depends upon
    (a) Intensity of incident light
    (b) Concentration of the solution
    (c) Intensity of incident light & radiation
    (d) Intensity of incident light & concentration of the solution

12. Which of the following compounds for which beer's & lambert's law is obeyed?
    (a) Tautomers
    (b) Conjugated double bonds, Aromatic compounds
    (c) Fluorescent compounds
    (d) Complexes

13. Calculate the E_{max} for this transition for $2.5 \times 10^{-4} M$ solution of a substance in a 1cm length cell at λ_{max} 245nm has absorbance 1.17
    (a) $0.468 \times 10^7 cm^2/mole$
    (b) $0.568 \times 10^7 cm^2/mole$
    (c) $0.668 \times 10^7 cm^2/mole$
    (d) $0.768 \times 10^7 cm^2/mole$

14. Spectrophotometer is used to detect the
    (a) Refraction
    (b) % Absorbance
    (c) % Transmittance
    (d) Diffraction

15. Which of the following is most suitable light source for UV – Visible spectroscopy?
    (a) Hydrogen deuterium discharge lamp
    (b) Carbon arc lamp source
    (c) Nernst glower
    (d) Radio frequency source

16. The region below 200 mµ is also called as
    (a) Flushing UV region
    (b) Forbidden UV region
    (c) Vacuum UV region
    (d) Dispersion UV region

17. In higher energy state, if spin of electrons are paired then it is called as
    (a) Excited doublet state
    (b) Excited singlet state
    (c) Excited quadruplet state
    (d) Excited triplet state

18. Triplet state is more stable than excited singlet state due to
    (a) Electron-Electron attraction is low
    (b) Electron-Orbital repulsion is low
    (c) Electron-Electron repulsion is high
    (d) Electron-Electron repulsion is low

19. $\sigma \rightarrow \sigma^*$ transition requires
    (a) Very short wavelength, high energy
    (b) Very short wavelength, low energy
    (c) Very high wavelength, high energy
    (d) Very high wavelength, low energy

20. $n{\rightarrow}\sigma^*$ transition takes places in which type of compounds?
    (a) Saturated compounds
    (b) Unsaturated compounds with one hetero atom
    (c) Saturated compounds with one hetero atom
    (d) Unsaturated compounds

21. Which of the following functional groups does not undergo $n{\rightarrow}\sigma^*$ transition?
    (a) Alcohols   (b) Esters
    (c) Ethers   (d) Ketones

22. Which of the following halo compounds require high energy to excite?
    (a) Methyl Fluoride
    (b) Methyl Iodide
    (c) Methyl Chloride
    (d) Methyl Bromide

23. Arrange the increasing order of energy required for the following various transitions
    (a) $\sigma{\rightarrow}\sigma^* > n{\rightarrow}\sigma^* > \pi{\rightarrow}\pi^* > n{\rightarrow}\pi^*$
    (b) $n{\rightarrow}\sigma^* < n{\rightarrow}\pi^* < \sigma{\rightarrow}\sigma^* < \pi{\rightarrow}\pi^*$
    (c) $n{\rightarrow}\pi^* < n{\rightarrow}\sigma^* < \pi{\rightarrow}\pi^* < \sigma{\rightarrow}\sigma)^*$
    (d) $n{\rightarrow}\pi^* < \pi{\rightarrow}\pi^* < n{\rightarrow}\sigma^* < \sigma{\rightarrow}\sigma^*$

24. The color yellow is produced for which type of compounds?
    (a) Halogens
    (b) Nitro compounds
    (c) Alcohols
    (d) Aldehydes

25. If ethylene acts as chromophore then which of the following type of transition will occur?
    (a) $\pi{\rightarrow}\pi^*$ (b) $n{\rightarrow}\pi^*$

(c) $\pi{\rightarrow}\pi$ (d) $\pi^*{\rightarrow}n$

26. Which of the following function groups will not acts as auxochrome?
    (a) $-OH$ (b) $- C{=}0$
    (c) $-OR$ (d) $-NH_2$

27. (a) Auxochrome does not acts as chromophore, it brings the shift of the absorption bond towards the red end of the spectrum
    (b) Ability to extend the conjugation of a chromophore by the sharing of non-bonding electrons
    (a) A& B are incorrect
    (b) A is correct & B is wrong
    (c) A & B are correct
    (d) A is wrong & B is correct

28. Shift in absorption maximum towards longer wavelength is called as
    (a) Bathochromic shift
    (b) Hypsochromic shift
    (c) Hyperchromic shift
    (d) Hypochromic shift

29. Removal of conjugation and change in polarity of solvent causes
    (a) Hyperchromic shift
    (b) Hypsochromic shift
    (c) Bathochromic shift
    (d) Hypochromic shift

30. Increase in intensity of absorption maximum and decrease in intensity of absorption maximum are called as
    (a) Hyper & Hyper chromic shift respectively
    (b) Hypo & Hypo chromic shift respectively

    (c) Hypo & Hyper chromic shift respectively

    (d) Hyper & Hypo chromic shift respectively

31. In enones which type of bands will occur?
    (a) E band   (b) R band
    (c) K band   (d) B band

32. In $\pi \rightarrow \pi^*$ transition in conjugated system which of the following bands will occur?
    (a) K band   (b) R band
    (c) B band   (d) E band

33. If a compound having a single chromophore and having at least one lone pair of electrons on hetero atom experience then which of the following bands will occur?
    (a) B band   (b) E band
    (c) R band   (d) K band

34. What is the other name for R band?
    (a) Forbidden bands
    (b) Transition bands
    (c) Step up bands
    (d) Cyclic bands

35. In $\pi \rightarrow \pi^*$ transition in aromatic or hetero- aromatic molecules experience which type of band?
    (a) K band   (b) B band
    (c) E band   (d) R band

36. Out of K, B, R bands which of the following bands appears at longer wavelength in the spectrum of an aromatic compound?
    (a) K band   (b) R band
    (c) E band   (d) B band

37. E_2 band of E- Band appears at
    (a) Longer wavelength
    (b) Shorter wavelength
    (c) Longer wave number
    (d) Shorter wave number

38. Commercial ethanol contains?
    (a) Phenanthracene
    (b) Anthracene
    (c) Benzene
    (d) Terpenes

39. Judge the following statements
    (a) Commercial ethanol is not used as a solvent in UV-Visible spectroscopy.
    (b) It contains benzene which absorbs strongly in UV region.
    (a) A is correct, B is wrong
    (b) A is incorrect, B is correct
    (c) A & B are incorrect
    (d) A & B are correct

40. In $n \rightarrow \pi^*$ transition for α, β-unsaturated carbonyl compounds, the ground which states will be______ compared to excited state.
    (a) Non polar
    (b) More polar
    (c) Polar
    (d) Less polar

41. In $\pi \rightarrow \pi^*$ transition for α, β unsaturated carbonyl compounds the absorption band will be move to
    (a) Longer wavelength
    (b) Same wavelength
    (c) Shorter wavelength
    (d) None

42. By increasing the polarity of solvents the $n \rightarrow \pi^*$, $n \rightarrow \sigma^*$, $\pi \rightarrow \pi^*$ experience which type of wavelengths.
    (a) Shorter, longer, shorter wavelengths respectively
    (b) Shorter, longer, longer wavelengths respectively
    (c) Shorter, shorter, longer wavelengths respectively
    (d) Longer, longer, shorter wavelengths respectively

43. The conjugated polyene system appears colored to the naked eye, the number of double bonds present in those system will be
    (a) More than two
    (b) More than one
    (c) More than three
    (d) More than five

44. Calculate the absorption maximum in the UV spectrum of 2, 4 octadiene.
    (a) 227mμ
    (b) 237mμ
    (c) 217mμ
    (d) 247mμ

45. Calculate the absorption maximum in the UV spectrum of
    (a) 232mμ
    (b) 220mμ
    (c) 221mμ
    (d) 262mμ

46. Calculate the λ_{max} for
    (a) 255mμ
    (b) 225mμ
    (c) 245mμ
    (d) 235mμ

47. Calculate the absorption maximum for the compound given
    (a) 263mμ
    (b) 273mμ
    (c) 283mμ
    (d) 293mμ

48. Calculate the λ_{max} for the given structure.
    (a) 239mμ
    (b) 249mμ
    (c) 259mμ
    (d) 269mμ

49. If the spectrum is transparent above 200mμ, it indicates absence of
    (a) Enol
    (b) Conjugation
    (c) Dienes
    (d) Alkyl group

50. If the number of double bonds increases in a compound then, the compound experiences which type of wavelength?
    (a) Shorter
    (b) More shorter
    (c) Less shorter
    (d) Longer

51. The region between $2000A^0$ to $4000A^0$ is called as
    (a) Far UV region
    (b) Near UV region
    (c) UV region
    (d) End UV region

52. The region below $2000A^0$ is called as
    (a) Near UV region
    (b) UV region
    (c) Far Vacuum UV region
    (d) Step up UV region

53. (a) The UV spectroscopy is called as Electronic Spectroscopy.
    (b) Longer wavelength region of Visible and the near UV region of electromagnetic radiation cause electronic transition in the molecule and produces electronic spectrum.

(a) A & B are correct
(b) A is correct, B is wrong
(c) A is wrong, B is correct
(d) A & B are incorrect

54. According to Born-Oppenheimer approximation, the total energy of the molecule is given by
(a) $E_{Total}=E_{Transitional}+E_{Vibrational}+E_{Electronic}$
(b) $E_{Total}=E_{Vibrational}+E_{Transitional}+E_{Electronic}$
(c) $E_{Total}=E_{Transitional}+E_{Vibrational}+E_{Rotational}+E_{Electronic}$
(d) $E_{Total}=E_{Transitional}+E_{Rotational}+E_{Electronic}$

55. The UV region extending from 100-200 nm is called as
(a) Vacuum region
(b) Visible region
(c) Near UV region
(d) Far UV region

56. The UV region at 200-400nm and below 200 nm are called as
(a) Near UV & vacuum UV region respectively
(b) Vacuum UV & near UV region respectively
(c) Far UV & vacuum region respectively
(d) Far UV & near UV region respectively

57. When carbonyl compounds are placed in a suitable solvent and by gradually increasing the polarity of the solvent, the $n\rightarrow\pi^*$, $\pi\rightarrow\pi^*$ transition undergoes
(a) Red & blue shift respectively
(b) Blue & red shift respectively
(c) Black & blue shift respectively
(d) Pink &red shift respectively

58. (a) Sharp peaks are rarely observed than broad peaks
(b) Due to vibrational & rotational effects are superimposed on the electronic transitions
(a) A &B are wrong
(b) A is correct, B is wrong
(c) A & B are correct
(d) A is wrong & B is correct

59. Isomer of benzene which is yellow in color?
(a) Flavaonoids   (b) Fulvene
(c) Terpenes   (d) Dienes

60. Which information will you get for a compound to be identified by IR spectroscopy?
(a) Molecular weight
(b) Structure
(c) Number of signals
(d) Number of peaks

61. The ordinary IR region extends from
(a) 2.5μ-15μ (b) 0.8μ-2.5μ
(c) 15μ-200μ (d) 2.5μ-200μ

62. The near IR region extends from
(a) $1200 \text{ cm}^{-1} - 4000 \text{ cm}^{-1}$
(b) $12100 \text{cm}^{-1} - 4000 \text{ cm}^{-1}$
(c) $12500 \text{cm}^{-1} - 4000 \text{ cm}^{-1}$
(d) $667 \text{cm}^{-1} - 50 \text{ cm}^{-1}$

63. The region 15μ- 200μ is called as
(a) Far IR region
(b) Near IR region
(c) IR region
(d) Shorter IR region

64. Convert the given wavelength (15μ) for a compound to wave number?
    (a) 4000 cm^{-1} (b) 667 cm^{-1}
    (c) 50 cm^{-1} (d) 12500 cm^{-1}

65. For a compound to be observed in IR region it should possess
    (a) Change in wave length
    (b) Change in wave number
    (c) Change in dipole moment
    (d) Change in frequency

66. Absorption in the IR region is due to changes in which energies in the molecule
    (a) Vibrational, rotational
    (b) Vibrational, electronic
    (c) Rotational, translational
    (d) Electronic, vibrational

67. In IR region, the absorbed energy does not depend upon the
    (a) Masses of atom in molecule
    (b) Strength of atom in molecule
    (c) Structure of atom
    (d) Arrangements of atoms within the molecule

68. Which of the following are the types of fundamental vibrations?
    (a) Stretching & bending
    (b) Scissoring & bending
    (c) Wagging & bending
    (d) Symmetric & asymmetric stretching

69. The distance between the two atoms increases or decreases but the atom remain the same bond axis is
    (a) Bending   (b) Stretching
    (c) Rocking   (d) Twisting

70. If the position of the atoms change with respect to the original bond axis is called as
    (a) Stretching   (b) Rocking
    (c) Scissoring   (d) Bending

71. Stretching absorption of a bond appear at _______ frequencies as compounds to bending absorption of the same bond
    (a) High   (b) Low
    (c) Medium   (d) Lesser

72. How many types of stretching vibrations will occur?
    (a) Scissoring & rocking
    (b) Scissoring & symmetric stretching
    (c) Rocking & asymmetric stretching
    (d) Symmetric & asymmetric stretching

73. If one atom approaches the central atom while the other departs from it then, which type of vibrations will occur?
    (a) Asymmetric stretching
    (b) Symmetric stretching
    (c) Scissoring
    (d) Twisting

74. In which type of bending vibrations two atoms approach each other?
    (a) Symmetric   (b) Rocking
    (c) Scissoring   (d) Twisting

75. If moment of atoms takes place in same direction then which type of bending vibrations will occur?
    (a) Scissoring   (b) Rocking
    (c) Wagging   (d) Twisting

76. If two atoms move up and down the plane with respect to central atom then which type of bending vibrations will occur?
    (a) Scissoring   (b) Rocking
    (c) Wagging   (d) Twisting

77. If the movement of atoms with respect to a particular atoms in a molecule in the same direction then which type of stretching vibrations will occur?
    (a) Asymmetric stretching
    (b) Rocking stretching
    (c) Symmetric stretching
    (d) Twisting stretching

78. In which type of bending vibrations, one of the atoms moves up the plane while the other moves down the plane with respect to the central atoms?
    (a) Twisting   (b) Scissoring
    (c) Rocking   (d) Wagging

79. Bending vibrations differ from stretching vibrations in what aspects?
    (a) Requires more energy
    (b) Requires less energy
    (c) Requires medium energy
    (d) None of the above

80. Which of the following expression is correct for Hooke's law?
    (a) $\upsilon = 1/2\pi c[k/m_1 m_2 / m_1 + m_2]^{1/2}$
    (b) $\upsilon = 1/2\pi c[k/m_1 m_2 / m_1 + m_2]^{2/3}$
    (c) $\upsilon = 1/2\pi c[k/m_1 m_2 / m_1 + m_2]^{1/2}$
    (d) $\upsilon = 1/2\pi c[k/m_1 + m_2 / m_1 m_2]^{1/2}$

81. From the Hooke's law the value of 'k' represents
    (a) Planks constant
    (b) Wavelength constant
    (c) Bond strength
    (d) Force constant

82. For single bond the value of 'k' will be
    (a) 5×10^5 gm/sec^2
    (b) 10×10^5 gm/sec^2
    (c) 5×10^5 gm/sec^2
    (d) 20×10^5 gm/sec^2

83. The value of force constant is _____ if double bond is present
    (a) 5×10^5 gm/sec^2
    (b) 10×10^5 gm/sec^2
    (c) 5×10^5 gm/sec^2
    (d) 20×10^5 gm/sec^2

84. The value of vibrational frequency depends upon
    (a) Bond strength
    (b) Reduced mass
    (c) Bond strength & reduced mass
    (d) Force constant

85. Bond strength & vibrational frequency both are
    (a) Directly proportional to each other
    (b) Same
    (c) Different
    (d) Inversely proportional to each other

86. Calculate the wave number of stretching vibrational of a carbon-carbon double bond. Force constant $(k=10 \times 10^5$ dynes/cm)
    (a) 1680 cm^{-1} (b) 1690 cm^{-1}
    (c) 1780 cm^{-1} (d) 1880 cm^{-1}

87. Calculate the wave number of stretching vibrational of a carbon-hydrogen single bond. Force constant $(k=5 \times 10^5$ dynes/cm)
    (a) 2500 cm^{-1} (b) 2100 cm^{-1}
    (c) 4100 cm^{-1} (d) 3100 cm^{-1}

88. C=C stretching absorbs at frequency than C-C stretching
    (a) Higher   (b) Lower
    (c) Medium   (d) Faster

89. For linear molecules, the vibrational degrees of freedom will be
    (a) 3n-4   (b) 3n-5
    (c) 3n-6   (d) 3n-7

90. For non- linear molecules, the vibrational degrees of freedom will be
    (a) 3n-5   (b) 3n-4
    (c) 3n-6   (d) 3n-7

91. For CO_2, the numbers of vibrational degrees of freedom will be
    (a) Six   (b) Seven
    (c) Five   (d) Four

92. For C_6H_6, the numbers of vibrational degrees of freedom will be
    (a) 30   (b) 20
    (c) 25   (d) 40

93. The region below $1500cm^{-1}$ is called as
    (a) Infrared active region
    (b) Functional group region
    (c) Finger print region
    (d) Dipole moment region

94. For detecting functional group like esters, ethers, which type of region is required?
    (a) Finger print region
    (b) Dipole moment region
    (c) Functional group region
    (d) Forbidden region

95. If molecule is infrared inactive in nature, then it having which type of symmetry?
    (a) Plane of symmetry
    (b) Centre of symmetry
    (c) Sign of symmetry
    (d) Centro symmetry

96. Which of the following is an important source in IR spectroscopy?
    (a) H_2 discharge lamp
    (b) Deuterium lamp
    (c) Nernst source
    (d) Carbon arc lamp

97. Sintered mixture of oxides of zirconium, yttrium & erbium together called as which type of source?
    (a) Globar source
    (b) Carbon arc lamp
    (c) Nernst glower
    (d) Deuterium lamp

98. If Nernst glower is heated, at which of the following temperature to produce IR radiations?
    (a) $200°c$
    (b) $1000°c$
    (c) $2500°c$
    (d) $1500°c$

99. Globar source is
    (a) Silicon carbide
    (b) Titanium carbide
    (c) Zirconium carbide
    (d) Nernst carbide

100. Which of the following prism material is used in IR region?
    (a) Alkaline metal halides & Nacl
    (b) Potassium chloride

(c) Barium chloride

(d) Nacl or certain alkali metal halides

101. Finger print region is
(a) 1600 cm^{-1} to 300 cm^{-1}
(b) 1500 cm^{-1} to 400 cm^{-1}
(c) 1500 cm^{-1} to 300 cm^{-1}
(d) 1000 cm^{-1} to 400 cm^{-1}

102. Calibration of IR can be done by using
(a) Polyethylene
(b) Polypropylene
(c) Polyphenyl
(d) Polystyrene

103. For solids which substance is mixed with sample substance to form discs
(a) NaBr
(b) KBr
(c) FBr
(d) KCl

104. The solid sample can be made in to a paste like substance by adding is
(a) Mulling agents
(b) Nulling agents
(c) Absorbing agents
(d) Refracting agents

105. Which of the following is not an example for Mulling agents?
(a) Nujol
(b) Hexachlorobutadiene
(c) Chlorobromide carbon oil
(d) Chloroflouro carbon oil

106. Nujol is a mixture of a
(a) Liquid paraffinic hydrocarbons with high molecular weights
(b) Liquid paraffinic hydrocarbons with low molecular weights
(c) Hydrocarbons with high molecular weights
(d) Liquid paraffinic with low molecular weights

107. For liquids, the liquid sample is squeezed in between which of the following plates?
(a) KCl plates
(b) RbCl plates
(c) NaCl plates
(d) CeCl plates

108. Which of the following solvents are used in IR spectroscopy?
(a) CCl$_4$
(b) Hexane
(c) Toluene
(d) Acetone

109. In H-bonding, broad bands arise due to which type of bonding?
(a) Intra molecular hydrogen bonding
(b) Inter molecular hydrogen bonding
(c) Molecular hydrogen bonding
(d) Covalent bonding

110. Which type of ion is produced, when a molecule is bombarded with high energetic electrons?
(a) Parent molecule
(b) Molecular ion
(c) Negative ion
(d) Positive ion

111. If charge (e) is 1, then m/e ratio is same for which type of ion?
(a) Negative ion
(b) Parent ion
(c) Molecular mass of ion
(d) Daughter ion

112. In mass spectroscopy intensity of each signal represents
     (a) Relative abundance
     (b) Base peak
     (c) Parent abundance
     (d) Molecular mass abundance

113. The largest peak in mass spectrum is
     (a) Parent peak
     (b) Molecular ion peak
     (c) Base peak
     (d) Meta stable peak

114. The intensity for base peak is taken as
     (a) 110   (b) 100
     (c) 90   (d) 120

115. The bombarding electrons are produced from which type of source?
     (a) Tungsten filament
     (b) Heated tungsten filament
     (c) Radium filament
     (d) Heated Silicon filament

116. The operating pressure in ion source is
     (a) 10^{-5} mm   (b) 10^{-8} mm
     (c) 10^{-7} mm   (d) 10^{-6} mm

117. The minimum amount of energy required for the electrons to bombard with molecule is
     (a) 50 ev   (b) 40 ev
     (c) 70 ev   (d) 80 ev

118. If 10ev of energy is made to bombarded with molecule then
     (a) Fragmentation occurs
     (b) No fragmentation occurs
     (c) Produces heat
     (d) No effect on the molecule

119. Which type of ions are detected in mass spectrometer
     (a) Positive ions with even or odd electrons
     (b) Negative ions with even or odd electrons
     (c) Neutral ions with even electron species
     (d) Neutral ions with odd electron species

120. After ionization step, the ions will enter in to which of the following chamber
     (a) Detector
     (b) Amplifier
     (c) Mass analyzer
     (d) Collector slit

121. The fragmented ions are differentiated based on which of the following ratio?
     (a) m/e ratio   (b) e/m ratio
     (c) M^{+}/m ratio   (d) m/M^{+} ratio

122. The positive ions travel in a circular path at
     (a) $110°$ (b) $120°$
     (c) $160°$ (d) $180°$

123. Double focusing mass spectrometers is used to detect
     (a) Ions having kinetic energy
     (b) Ions having close kinetic energy
     (c) Ions having close potential energy
     (d) Ions having far kinetic energy

124. In order to get 3-5 records of same peak, which additional device is used in mass spectroscopy
     (a) Ohmmeter   (b) Ammeter
     (c) Galvanometer   (d) Thermopile

125. In mass spectroscopy, if the rate of decomposition is too high then
    (a) Parent ion peak is formed
    (b) Parent ion peak is not formed
    (c) Base ion peak is formed
    (d) Base ion peak is not formed

126. How the rate of decomposition and molecular size are related to each other
    (a) Directly proportional to each other
    (b) Inversely proportional to each other
    (c) Both are same
    (d) Not related to each other

127. In mass spectrum, the peak on extreme right corresponds to
    (a) Base peak on original molecule
    (b) Parent peak on original molecule
    (c) Parent mass on original molecule
    (d) Molecular mass of original molecule

128. In Mc Lafferty rearrangement elimination of neutral molecules takes place from
    (a) Aldehydes   (b) Benzene
    (c) Hexane   (d) Amide

129. Which of the following compounds to do not follow Mc Lafferty rearrangement?
    (a) Amides   (b) Aldehydes
    (c) Ketones   (d) Amines

130. In mass spectrum, the metastable peaks can be detected by
    (a) Absence of peak
    (b) Absence of narrow peak
    (b) Parent ion peak is not formed

    (c) Base ion peak is formed
    (d) Base ion peak is not formed

131. Which of the following is not an important characteristic to metastable peak?
    (a) No integral m/e value
    (b) Integral m/e value
    (c) Broad peak
    (d) Low abundance

132. If molecule has even number molecular mass then it contains
    (a) Nitrogen atom
    (b) No nitrogen atom
    (c) Less nitrogen atom
    (d) More nitrogen atom

133. In retro-diel's alder reaction is a characteristic for which type of compounds?
    (a) Cyclic olefins
    (b) Cyclic polyfines
    (c) Olefins
    (d) Polyfines

134. In retro-diels's alder reaction, which compounds are formed?
    (a) Three stable unsaturated fragments
    (b) Two stable saturated fragments
    (c) Two stable unsaturated fragments
    (d) Three stable saturated fragments

135. In Mc Lafferty rearrangement which of the following cleavage patterns will occur?
    (a) Cleavage of α-bond occurs
    (b) Cleavage of β-bond occurs
    (c) Cleavage of β-bond followed by γ- hydrogen transfer
    (d) Cleavage of α-bond followed by γ-hydrogen transfer

136. Which of the following solvents in which the molecular ion peak is not visible?
    (a) Amines
    (b) Aldehyde
    (c) Acetone
    (d) Alcohol

137. Which of the following peak has highest m/e value?
    (a) Metastable peak
    (b) Isotopic peak
    (c) Base peak
    (d) Molecular ion peak

138. In mass spectrum, which of the following peaks occur at very low abundance?
    (a) Isotopic peak
    (b) Base peak
    (c) Metastable peak
    (d) Molecular ion peak

139. In Mc Lafferty rearrangement, which of the following molecule is lost?
    (a) Alkenes
    (b) Alkynes
    (c) Styrene
    (d) Alkanes

140. Mass spectroscopy is also called as
    (a) Narrow spectra
    (b) Broad spectra
    (c) Positive ion spectra
    (d) Negative ion spectra

141. For excitation of neutral atom we use
    (a) Electromagnetic radiation
    (b) Electron bombardment
    (c) Vibrational energy
    (d) Visible radiation

142. When magnetic field is applied between two positive fragments then they travel in which path?
    (a) Straight line path
    (b) Parabolic path
    (c) Curved path
    (d) Circular path

143. Which of the following mass spectrometer has high resolution?
    (a) Double focusing mass spectrometer
    (b) Single focusing mass spectrometer
    (c) Chemical ionization mass spectrometer
    (d) Field ionization mass spectrometer

144. M+1 peak occurs for which type of isotopes?
    (a) ^{18}O
    (b) ^{34}S
    (c) ^{13}C
    (d) ^{81}Br

145. M+2 peak occurs for which type of isotopes?
    (a) ^{13}C
    (b) ^{2}H
    (c) ^{33}S
    (d) ^{18}O

146. Which of the following detectors are used in mass spectroscopy?
    (a) Photomultiplier tube
    (b) Photo tube
    (c) Photo voltaic cell
    (d) Thermopile

147. Why metastable peaks are broader in mass spectrum?
    (a) Conversion of some relaxation energy to additional potential energy
    (b) Conversion of some excitation energy to additional kinetic energy

(c) Conversion of some relaxation energy to additional kinetic energy

(d) Conversion of some excitation energy to additional potential energy

148. If the parent ion mass is 20 amu and the daughter ion mass is 40 amu then calculate the metastable ion?
    (a) 50 amu   (b) 60 amu
    (c) 70 amu   (d) 80 amu

149. In chemical ionization most commonly used reactant gas is
    (a) Chloroform
    (b) Carbon tetrachloride
    (c) Methane
    (d) CH_3

150. In fast atom bombardment the sample is dispersed in
    (a) Hexane   (b) Glycerol
    (c) Toluene   (d) Acetone

151. In quadruple mass spectrometer between 4 rods which energy is supplied?
    (a) Radio frequency potential
    (b) Cosmic rays potential
    (c) X-rays potential
    (d) γ- rays potential

152. In NMR spectroscopy which energy is absorbed?
    (a) Cosmic energy
    (b) Vibrational energy
    (c) Radio frequency energy
    (d) Rotational energy

153. The Radio frequency energy is absorbed in the presence of which of the following field?
    (a) Magnetic field
    (b) Electric field
    (c) Rotational field
    (d) Electrostatic field

154. Which type of nuclei will give NMR spectra?
    (a) Odd mass number
    (b) Even mass number
    (c) Odd & Even mass number
    (d) None of the above

155. Which type of quantum number is preferred in NMR spectra?
    (a) Plank quantum number
    (b) Absorption quantum number
    (c) Azimuthal quantum number
    (d) Spin quantum number

156. Nuclei with odd mass number give which type of charge distribution?
    (a) Symmetrical charge distribution
    (b) Asymmetrical charge distribution
    (c) Binomial charge distribution
    (d) Polynomial charge distribution

157. Nuclei with even mass number give which type of charge distribution?
    (a) Asymmetrical charge distribution
    (b) Symmetrical charge distribution
    (c) Integral value distribution
    (d) Binomial distribution

158. When external magnetic field (H_o) is applied to odd mass number species, it spins on its own axis & magnetic moment is created, it produces
    (a) Precessional frequency

(b) Applied frequency
(c) Radio frequency
(d) Vibrational frequency

159. Precessional frequency is obtained at which state?
(a) Exited state
(b) Spin state
(c) Ground state
(d) Magnetic state

160. NMR signal is obtained when
(a) Applied frequency = radio frequency
(b) Applied frequency = precessional frequency
(c) Precessional frequency = radio frequency
(d) Precessional frequency = microwave frequency

161. The nucleus from ground state to exited state will be moved which causes?
(a) Spin reversal
(b) Parallel orientation
(c) Spin-Spin reversal
(d) Spin-Electron reversal

162. If magnetic field is not applied then there are
(a) No two spin states
(b) Only one average spin
(c) Three spin states
(d) Four spin states

163. In ground state, the nuclei is
(a) Aligned with the external applied magnetic field
(b) Aligned against the external applied magnetic field
(c) Aligned with the internal applied magnetic field
(d) Aligned against the internal applied magnetic field

164. Absorbed energy can be lost by
(a) Spin-Lattice relaxation process
(b) Spin- Spin relaxation process
(c) Both a and b
(d) None

165. Solvent used in NMR Spectroscopy should not contains
(a) Hydrogen atom
(b) Helium atom
(c) Sodium atom
(d) Lithium atom

166. Which of the following solvent is not used in NMR spectroscopy?
(a) Carbon tetrachloride
(b) Deuterium oxide
(c) $CDCl_3$
(d) Methane

167. Which of the following is not the property of the solvent used in NMR spectroscopy?
(a) Chemical inertness
(b) Dipole moment
(c) Magnetic isotropy
(d) Volatility

168. Precession due to earth's gravity is called as
(a) Gyroscopic motion
(b) Gravitational motion
(c) Orbital motion
(d) Displacement motion

169. Which of the following is the expression for gyroscopic ratio?
(a) $\gamma = 2\pi / hI$
(b) $\gamma = 2\pi M/hI$
(c) $\gamma = 2\pi \upsilon/hI$
(d) $\gamma = 2\pi/h\upsilon$

170. In Gyroscopic ratio 'h' represents
(a) Plank's constant
(b) Gravitational constant
(c) Orbital constant
(d) Displacement constant

171. In $\omega = 2\pi\upsilon$, 'υ' represents
(a) Gyroscopic frequency
(b) Frequency
(c) Wave number
(d) Precessional frequency

172. The transition from one energy state to other is called as
(a) Jumping of protons
(b) Flipping of protons
(c) Curve path of protons
(d) Straight line path of protons

173. The energy required to bring the transition of protons depends upon
(a) Radio frequency waves
(b) Strength of external filed
(c) Precessional frequency
(d) Angular frequency

174. Which of the following expression is suitable for frequency of radiation?
(a) $\upsilon = \gamma H_O / 2\pi$
(b) $\upsilon = \gamma H / 2\pi$
(c) $\upsilon = H_O \acute{\upsilon} / 2\pi$
(d) $\upsilon = H_O / 2\pi$

175. Electromagnetic radiation is supplied at which frequency?
(a) 1000 MHZ
(b) 60 MHZ
(c) 80 MHZ
(d) 100 MHZ

176. If precesised proton will absorb energy from radio frequency source only if
(a) Precessing frequency is same as frequency of radio frequency beam
(b) Precessing frequency is same as frequency of magnetic frequency beam
(c) Precessing frequency is different from frequency of radio frequency beam
(d) Precessing frequency is same as frequency of external applied magnetic frequency beam

177. Nuclear magnetic resonance spectrum occurs when?
(a) Radio frequency is kept constant and strength of the magnetic field is varied
(b) Radio frequency is varied and strength of the magnetic field is kept constant
(c) Precessional frequency is kept constant and strength of magnetic field is varied
(d) Precessional frequency is varied and strength of magnetic field is kept constant

178. Which of the following is not a kind of relaxation processes?
(a) Spin-Spin relaxation
(b) Spin-Electron relaxation
(c) Spin-Lattice relaxation
(d) Quadruple relaxation

179. Transfer of energy from one nucleus to the other causes
(a) Spin-Lattice relaxation
(b) Quadruple relaxation

(c) Spin-Spin relaxation
(d) Spin-Electron relaxation

180. In spin-lattice relaxation
(a) Transfer of energy from the nucleus in its higher energy state to the molecular lattice
(b) Transfer of energy from the nucleus in its ground state to the molecular lattice
(c) Release of energy from molecular lattice to higher energy state
(d) Release of energy from atomic lattice to higher energy state

181. The other name for spin-lattice relaxation process
(a) Spin-Electron relaxation
(b) Vertical relaxation
(c) Transverse relaxation
(d) Longitudinal relaxation

182. In NMR spectrum, the number of signals represents
(a) Number of different sets of equivalent electrons in a molecule
(b) Number of different sets of equivalent protons in a molecule
(c) Number of different sets of equivalent positrons in a molecule
(d) None of the above

183. Number of signals in acetone molecule
(a) Zero signals   (b) Two signals
(c) Three signals   (d) One signal

184. Number of signals in cyclobutane molecule
(a) Three signals   (b) Two signals
(c) One signal   (d) Zero signal

185. In tetra methyl methane how many number of signals present?
(a) One signal   (b) Zero signal
(c) Three signals   (d) Two signals

186. In methyl alcohol how many number of signals present?
(a) Two signals
(b) Three signals
(c) Zero signal
(d) One signal

187. In p-Xylene how many number of signals present?
(a) Zero signal
(b) One signal
(c) Two signals
(d) Three signals

188. In methyl acetate, how many number of signals present?
(a) Two signals
(b) Three signals
(c) Zero signal
(d) One signal

189. Calculate the number of signals in methyl cyclopropane?
(a) Two signals
(b) Three signals
(c) Zero signal
(d) Four signals

190. Calculate the number of signals in tetra-butyl amine?
(a) Two signals
(b) Zero signals
(c) One signal
(d) Three signals

191. Calculate the number of signals in 1,2- dibromoethane
    (a) Two signals   (b) One signal
    (c) Three signals   (d) One signal

192. Calculate the number of signals in propanal?
    (a) Two signals
    (b) Zero signals
    (c) One signal
    (d) Three signals

193. Calculate the number of signals in ethyl benzene?
    (a) Three signals   (b) Two signals
    (c) One signal   (d) Zero signal

194. If the field by the proton, is diminished and the proton is said to be
    (a) Deshielded
    (b) Shielded
    (c) Resonance
    (d) Chemical shift

195. If the field by the proton, is induced and the proton is said to be
    (a) Chemical shift
    (b) Shielded
    (c) Deshielded
    (d) Resonance

196. Shielding shifts the absorption towards
    (a) Down field   (b) High field
    (c) Up field   (d) Low field

197. Down field is felt due to
    (a) Shielding
    (b) Deshielding
    (c) Resonance
    (d) Chemical shift

198. In NMR spectroscopy, the reference compound is taken as
    (a) Tetra methylsilane
    (b) Tri methylsilane
    (c) Tetra methylstrontium
    (d) Tri methylstrontium

199. Which of the following is the correct expression?
    (a) $\delta = 10 - \upsilon$ (b) $\upsilon = 10 - \delta$
    (c) $\delta = 10 - \Gamma$ (d) $\Gamma = 10 - \delta$

200. For deshielding protons, the value of δ will be
    (a) Smaller
    (b) Larger
    (c) Thicker
    (d) None of the above

201. Calculate the value of chemical shift if observed shift from TMS is 250 MHZ and operating frequency from the instrument is 100 MHZ?
    (a) 2.5×10^{-6} (b) 3.5×10^{-6}
    (c) 4.5×10^{-6} (d) 1.5×10^{-6}

202. Calculate the value of chemical shift if observed shift from TMS is 150MHZ and operating frequency from the instrument is 100MHZ?
    (a) 1.5×10^{-6} (b) 2.5×10^{-6}
    (c) 3.5×10^{-6} (d) 4.5×10^{-6}

203. Chemical shift is depends upon
    (a) Operating frequency
    (b) Deshielding effects
    (c) Shielding effects
    (d) Solvents

204. Deshielding effect depends upon
    (a) Electro chemical activity
    (b) Vander wall forces
    (c) Electro positivity of atom
    (d) Electro negativity of atom

205. The distance between the centers of two adjacent peaks in a multiplet is called as
    (a) Spin-Spin coupling
    (b) Coupling constant
    (c) Spin-lattice coupling
    (d) Relaxation constant

206. Nuclear over Hauser effect is used to study
    (a) Molecular geometry of the compounds
    (b) Structure of molecule
    (c) Electronic transition of molecule
    (d) Molecular mass of the molecule

207. Which of the following factors will cause deshielding of protons?
    (a) Dipole moment
    (b) Electro positivity
    (c) Hydrogen bonding
    (d) Ionization potential

208. Spin-Spin splitting occurs only
    (a) Between nuclei with same chemical shift
    (b) Between nuclei with different chemical shift
    (c) Between atoms with same chemical shift
    (d) Between atoms with different chemical shift

209. The strength of earth's magnetic field is about
    (a) 0.67gauss   (b) 0.47gauss
    (c) 0.57gauss   (d) 0.37gauss

210. How many spin states present in ^1H nucleus
    (a) One   (b) Four
    (c) Three   (d) Two

211. The strength of applied magnetic field is in the range of
    (a) 1.4-14 tesla   (b) 1.0-10 tesla
    (c) 1.3-13 tesla   (d) 1.2-12 tesla

212. The study of measurement of emitted radiation of electrons undergo transition from singlet excited to singlet ground state is
    (a) Phosphorescence
    (b) Flame photometry
    (c) Fluorometry
    (d) Excitation

213. The wavelength of absorbed radiation is called as
    (a) Phosphorescence
    (b) Fluorescence
    (c) Emission wavelength
    (d) Excitation wavelength

214. The emitted radiation in fluorescence will be
    (a) Longer
    (b) Shorter
    (c) Longer and shorter
    (d) None of the above

215. The phenomenon of emission of light radiation by substance, when excitation occurs is called as
    (a) Fluorescence
    (b) Luminescence
    (c) Phosphorescence
    (d) Absorption

216. If the wavelength of emitted radiation is shorter than the absorbed radiation is called as
    (a) Raleigh fluorescence
    (b) Stokes fluorescence
    (c) Anti-stokes fluorescence
    (d) Resonance fluorescence

217. If the wavelength of emitted radiation is equal to the absorbed radiation is called as
 (a) Anti-stokes fluorescence
 (b) Resonance fluorescence
 (c) Stokes fluorescence
 (d) Raleigh fluorescence

218. Which of the following groups enhance fluorescence intensity?
 (a) Electron donating groups
 (b) Electron negativity groups
 (c) Electron with drawing groups
 (d) Hydrogen bonding groups

219. Which of the following are the examples for electron donating groups?
 (a) $-COOH$
 (b) $-NO_2$
 (c) $-OH$
 (d) $-CH_3$

220. Which of the following are the examples for electron with drawing groups?
 (a) $-NH_2$
 (b) $-NO_2$
 (c) $-OH$
 (d) $-CH_3$

221. Which groups reduce fluorescence intensity?
 (a) Hydrogen bonding groups
 (b) Electron donating groups
 (c) Electro negativity groups
 (d) Electron with drawing groups

222. If flexible structures are present then
 (a) Less phosphorescence intensity
 (b) More fluorescence intensity
 (c) Less fluorescence intensity
 (d) More phosphorescence intensity

223. If temperature is increased, what happens to fluorescence intensity?
 (a) Decrease in fluorescence intensity
 (b) Increase in fluorescence intensity
 (c) Both a & b are correct answers
 (d) None of the above

224. If viscosity of the molecule is increased then fluorescence intensity will be
 (a) No change in fluorescence intensity
 (b) Decrease in fluorescence intensity
 (c) Increase in fluorescence intensity
 (d) None of the above

225. Fluorescence intensity is directly proportional to
 (a) Concentration of substance
 (b) Radiation from the sources
 (c) Temperature
 (d) Viscosity

226. Self quenching occurs when
 (a) Low concentration is present
 (b) High concentration is present
 (c) Medium concentration is present
 (d) None of the above

227. Which of the following is used as source in flouriometry?
 (a) Carbon arc lamp
 (b) H_2 discharge lamp
 (c) Deuterium lamp
 (d) Tungsten lamp

228. Primary filter absorbs
 (a) Visible & transmits IR radiation
 (b) UV & transmits IR radiation

(c) Visible & transmits UV radiation

(d) IR & transmits visible radiation

229. The filter which absorbs UV & transmits visible radiation is
(a) Excitation filter
(b) Emission filter
(c) Primary filter
(d) Secondary filter

230. The sample cells in Fluorometry should be
(a) Only two surfaces to be polished
(b) All surfaces should be polished
(c) No polished surfaces should be present
(d) None of the above

231. Which of the following is used as detectors in Fluorometry?
(a) Golay cells
(b) Photovoltaic cells
(c) Photo tubes
(d) Photomultiplier tubes

232. In Single beam flourometer, the primary filter is kept at which angle to the secondary filter
(a) 360° (b) 180°
(c) 60° (d) 90°

233. In Spectroflourometer the filter in double beam flourometer is replaced by
(a) Monochromators
(b) Gratings
(c) Prisms
(d) Detectors

234. The materials which exhibits fluorescence intensity can emit excess radiation
(a) $10^{-4} - 10^{-6}$ sec
(b) $10^{-3} - 10^{-2}$ sec
(c) $10^{-5} - 10^{-3}$ sec
(d) $10^{-6} - 10^{-4}$ sec

235. Which of the following gas should not be present when fluorescence phenomenon is conducted?
(a) H_2 (b) He
(c) O_2 (d) N_2

236. Which of the following compound is well susceptible to oxygen?
(a) Naphthalene
(b) Anthracene
(c) Phenanthcene
(d) Benzene

237. Which of the following salts can be detected in Fluorometry in the field of nuclear research?
(a) Francium   (b) Radium
(c) Uranium   (d) Thallium

238. Oxidation product of vitamin – B_1 is
(a) Thiamine diketone
(b) Thiamine diphenyl
(c) Thiamine
(d) Thiochrome

239. Most commonly used substance to perform Fluorometry is
(a) Quinine   (b) Squill
(c) Cinchona   (d) Nux vomica

240. Which of the following vitamin's can be detected by Fluorometry?
(a) Vit –B_3 (b) Vit –B_2

   (c) Vit $-B_{12}$ (d) Vit $-B_6$

241. Which of the following is not used as fluorescent indicator in Fluorometry?
   (a) Eosin
   (b) Acridines
   (c) 3-Napthoquinone
   (d) 2-Napthoquinone

242. What is the other name for flame photometry?
   (a) Flame absorption spectroscopy
   (b) Flame emission spectroscopy
   (c) Flame diffraction spectroscopy
   (d) Flame reflection spectroscopy

243. Which of the following sequence is correct in flame photometry?
   (a) Exited state atoms→ neutral atoms→residue→fine droplets solutions of metal salt
   (b) Residue→ solutions of metal salt→ neutral atoms→ exited state atoms
   (c) Exited state atoms→ residue fine droplets→ neutral atoms→ solutions of metal salt
   (d) Solutions of metal salt fine droplets residue→ neutral atoms→ exited state atoms

244. Wavelength of radiation in flame photometry is used to determine?
   (a) Thermal energy of the element
   (b) Identification of elements
   (c) Concentration of element
   (d) Dielectric constant of element

245. For quantitative analysis which parameter is used to determine?
   (a) Concentration of element
   (b) Dielectric constant of element
   (c) Identification of element
   (d) Hydrogen bonding of atoms

246. Flame photometry is used to analyze which type of elements?
   (a) Group IV elements
   (b) Group IA & IIA elements
   (c) Group IA elements
   (d) Group IIA elements

247. Intensity of radiation depends upon the
   (a) Temperature of the flame & concentration of element
   (b) Temperature of the substance & concentration of element
   (c) Concentration of solution & temperature of the flame
   (d) Concentration of solution & temperature of the substance

248. Which of the following is correct expression?
   (a) $N^*/No = Ae^{-\Delta E}/KT$
   (b) $No/N^* = Ae^{-\Delta E}/KT$
   (c) $N^*/No = Ae^{-\Delta e}/KT$
   (d) $N^*/No = Ae^{-\Delta K}/ET$

249. The wavelength of light emitted depends upon the
   (a) Difference in energy level of atoms from exited state to ground state
   (b) Sum of energy level of atoms from exited state to ground state
   (c) Difference in energy level of atoms from ground state to exited state
   (d) Sum of energy level of atoms from ground state to exited state

250. Yellow color radiation is emitted by

    (a) Calcium   (b) Sodium
    (c) Lithium   (d) Potassium

251. Calcium emits which color radiation?
    (a) Brick red color
    (b) Yellow color
    (c) Orange color
    (d) Red color

252. Which of the following burner is most widely used in flame photometry?
    (a) Consumption burner
    (b) Total consumption burner
    (c) Laminar burner
    (d) Laminar flow burner

253. Laminar flow (Premix) burner is most commonly used burner in flame photometry because
    (a) Uniform flame intensity
    (b) Un-Uniform flame intensity
    (c) High pressure
    (d) Fuel and oxidant are mixed before reaching the burner tip

254. Which type of monochromators is used in flame photometry?
    (a) Filters (with Ca, Li, Na, K filters)
    (b) Gratings
    (c) Prisms
    (d) Filter wheel (with Ca, Li, Na, K filters)

255. Which of the following detectors are used in flame spectrophotometer?
    (a) Phototube
    (b) Photovoltaic cells
    (c) Photomultiplier tube
    (d) Golay cells

256. From the read out device which readings are displayed?
    (a) % Flame length

    (b) Concentration of element
    (c) Wavelength of light
    (d) % Flame Intensity

257. For therapeutic drug monitoring which element is analyzed?
    (a) Lithium
    (b) Lithium fluoride
    (c) Lithium chloride
    (d) Lithium bromide

258. Flame photometry is used to determine
    (a) Alkali earth metals
    (b) Alkaline earth metals
    (c) Halides
    (d) Lanthanides

259. Which of the following material is used as internal standard?
    (a) Potassium   (b) Calcium
    (c) Sodium   (d) Lithium

260. Which of the following is the oldest burner?
    (a) Mecker burner
    (b) Total consumption burner
    (c) Laminar flow burner
    (d) Lundergraph burner

261. To increase the emission intensity which device is used?
    (a) Collimating mirror
    (b) Mirror
    (c) Detector
    (d) Solvent

262. Atomic absorption spectroscopy is also called as
    (a) Flame emission spectroscopy
    (b) Flame spectroscopy

(c) Flame absorption spectroscopy
(d) Flame diffraction spectroscopy

263. Specific wavelength of radiation is generated by using
(a) Hollow anode lamp
(b) Hollow cathode lamp
(c) Hollow lamp
(d) Filter wheel

264. Intensity of light absorbed by neutral atoms is directly proportional to the
(a) Wavelength of light emitted
(b) Concentration of the element
(c) Absorption of radiation
(d) Emission of radiation

265. Excitation of neutral atoms is brought by
(a) Radiation of hollow cathode lamp
(b) Radiation of hollow anode lamp
(c) Emission of hollow cathode lamp
(d) Emission of hollow anode lamp

266. Source of light used in atomic absorption spectroscopy is
(a) Hollow anode lamp
(b) Hollow cathode lamp
(c) Hollow lamp
(d) Filter wheel

267. The filter gas used in hollow cathode lamp is
(a) Argon   (b) Helium
(c) Nitrogen   (d) Hydrogen

268. In Atomic absorption spectroscopy, chopper is used for
(a) To measure the concentration of elements
(b) To measure the wavelength of light emitted by the substance

(c) To measure intensity of light absorbed by elements
(d) To measure radiation from the source

269. Which of the following spectrometers having more advantages?
(a) Double beam atomic absorption spectroscopy
(b) Single beam atomic absorption spectroscopy
(c) Spectrometers
(d) Spectro flourometers

270. The atomic absorption spectroscopy is used for
(a) Qualitative purpose
(b) Quantitative purpose
(c) Both a & b
(d) None of the above

271. Mercury in thiomersal solution is detected by using which technique?
(a) Fluorometry
(b) IR spectroscopy
(c) UV- Visible spectroscopy
(d) Atomic absorption spectroscopy

272. Zinc in zinc Insulin Injection is detected by using which technique?
(a) Flame photometry
(b) Atomic absorption spectroscopy
(c) IR spectroscopy
(d) Fluorometry

273. Which of the following spectroscopy is temperature dependent?
(a) Fluorometry
(b) Flame photometry
(c) Atomic absorption spectroscopy
(d) IR spectroscopy

274. Which law is obeyed over a wide range of substances?
    (a) Atomic absorption spectroscopy
    (b) Flame photometry
    (c) Fluorometry
    (d) SpectroFluorometry

275. Which of the following techniques is more sensitive & can detect concentration below 1ppm?
    (a) Flame photometry
    (b) Atomic absorption spectroscopy
    (c) Fluorometry
    (d) SpectroFluorometry

276. The process of conversion of liquid sample to sample droplets is called as
    (a) Nebulisation
    (b) Flame photometry
    (c) Spectrometry
    (d) Atomic absorption spectroscopy

277. Photomultiplier tube is most commonly used detector because of which of the following reason?
    (a) We get stable power supply
    (b) We get stable ion-source
    (c) We get stable voltage supply
    (d) High sensitivity

278. Series of electrodes in photomultiplier tube is
    (a) Anode
    (b) Cathode
    (c) Dynodes
    (d) Photocathode

279. If radiation is overlapped, then which type of interferences will occur?
    (a) Ionization interference
    (b) Matrix interference
    (c) Solvent interference
    (d) Spectral interference

280. Ionization interference occurs when
    (a) Flame temperature is too high
    (b) Flame temperature is too low
    (c) Photo voltaic cell is used
    (d) Filter wheel is used

281. If the solvent is changed then which type of interference will occur?
    (a) Matrix interference
    (b) Ionization interference
    (c) Solvent interference
    (d) Spectral interference

282. Solvent plays a major role in recording which type of readings?
    (a) Absorbance   (b) Emission
    (c) Diffraction   (d) Reflection

283. In calibration curve the absorbance value depends upon
    (a) Concentration of the element
    (b) Wavelength of light emitted
    (c) Freezing point of the element
    (d) Radiation source of the element

284. Determination of lead in petrol is analyzed by which of the following technique?
    (a) Flame photometry
    (b) Atomic absorption spectroscopy
    (c) Fluorometry
    (d) IR Spectroscopy

285. In x-ray diffraction methods which phenomenon will occur?
    (a) Scattering of x-rays by crystals will occur
    (b) Refraction of x-rays by crystals will occur

    (c) Reflection of x-rays by crystals will occur

    (d) Diffraction of x-rays by crystals will occur

286. Crystal structures can be studied by using which technique?
    (a) X-ray absorption method
    (b) X-ray diffraction method
    (c) X-ray fluorescence method
    (d) X-ray emission method

287. The range of x-rays in the electro-magnetic spectrum
    (a) $0.1\text{-}10\ A^0$ (b) $0.1\text{-}100\ A^0$
    (c) $0.01\text{-}100\ A^0$ (d) $0.01\text{-}10\ A^0$

288. For analytical purpose, the range of x-rays should be
    (a) $0.7\text{-}0.9\ A^0$ (b) $0.17\text{-}2.0\ A^0$
    (c) $0.7\text{-}2.0\ A^0$ (d) $0.7\text{-}1.0\ A^0$

289. In X-ray spectrum of a copper target consists of sharp & intense lines superimposed on polychromatic back ground are called as
    (a) Both white & black radiation
    (b) VIBGYOR radiation
    (c) Black body radiation
    (d) White radiation

290. Which of the following is correct expression?
    (a) $\lambda_{min} = he/Vc$
    (b) $\lambda_{min} = hc/Ve$
    (c) $\lambda_{min} = h/Vc$
    (d) $\lambda_{min} = hV/ec$

291. The λ_{min} is inversely proportional to
    (a) Voltage applied
    (b) Speed of light
    (c) Planks constant
    (d) Accelerating voltage applied

292. Which type of interferences will occur when scattered waves are coming from electrons?
    (a) Destructive interference
    (b) Constructive interference
    (c) Both a & b
    (d) None of the above

293. The conditions of diffractions are governed by which law?
    (a) Beer's law
    (b) Lambert's law
    (c) Bragg's law
    (d) Ohm's law

294. Which of the following is the correct expression for Bragg's law?
    (a) $n\upsilon = 2d\sin\theta$ (b) $n\lambda = 2d\sin\theta$
    (c) $n\acute{\upsilon} = 2d\sin\theta$ (d) $n = 2d\sin\theta$

295. For Miller's indices, which of the following is the correct expression?
    (a) $n\lambda = 2d_{hkl}\sin\theta$
    (b) $n\upsilon = 2d_{hkl}\sin\theta$
    (c) $n\acute{\upsilon} = 2d_{hkl}\sin\theta$
    (d) $n = 2d_{hkl}\sin\theta$

296. Which of the following filament is used for producing of x-rays?
    (a) Sodium filament
    (b) Tungsten filament
    (c) Calcium filament
    (d) Lithium filament

297. To get a narrow beam of x-rays which system is used?
    (a) Collimator   (b) Filter
    (c) Gratings   (d) Prisms

298. Which of the following monochromators is most used?
 (a) Filter
 (b) Prism
 (c) Crystal monochromators
 (d) Emission monochromators

299. The other name for crystalline monochromator is
 (a) Analysing crystal
 (b) Emission crystal monochromator
 (c) Absorption crystal monochromator
 (d) Diffraction crystal monochromator

300. The Rotating crystal method was developed by which scientist?
 (a) Schiebold
 (b) Fermi
 (c) Debye and Scherrer
 (d) Hull

301. Which of the following arrranagement is in correct order in rotating crystal method?
 (a) Photographic plate→crystal→ collimating system→ X-ray source
 (b) X-ray source→collimating system →crystal→ photographic plate
 (c) Crystal→ photographic plate→ collimating system→ X-ray source
 (d) None of the above

302. In Powder crystal method, the amount of sample required is?
 (a) 1mg   (b) 10 mg
 (c) 100 mg   (d) 1000 mg

303. X-Ray diffraction is used to study
 (a) Structure of wavelength
 (b) Structure of crystal
 (c) Concentration of element
 (d) Radiation source

304. Which of the following can be detected by using x-ray diffraction method?
 (a) Polymer characterisation
 (b) State of anneal in metals
 (c) Detection of Na, K in urine
 (d) Tooth enamel & dentine

305. Which of the following detector is used in x-rays is?
 (a) Phototubes
 (b) Photomultiplier tubes
 (c) Photovoltaic cell
 (d) Photographic film

306. RIA is used for measuring which type of complexes?
 (a) Unlabelled antigen
 (b) Antigen complexes
 (c) Radioactivity of labelled antigen-antibody complex
 (d) Antibody

307. The principle of RIA is based on
 (a) Antigen-Antibody reaction
 (b) Antigen- Antibody complex
 (c) Unlabelled antigen
 (d) Antibody

308. The labeled antigen – antibody complex is measured by using
 (a) Scintillation counter
 (b) Counter-coulter
 (c) Phototubes
 (d) Photomultiplier tubes

309. The measured radioactivity is inversely proportional to
     (a) Concentration of antigen-antibody complex
     (b) Concentration of ligand
     (c) Concentration of antibody
     (d) None of the above

310. For Calibration which agent is used for RIA
     (a) Antigen
     (b) Antibody
     (c) Antigen- Antibody complex
     (d) Radio labeled antigen

311. The radio labelling is done by using which isotopes for antigen?
     (a) ^{125}I (b) ^{13}C
     (c) ^{2}H (d) ^{1}H

312. Specific antibodies are produced by injecting
     (a) Radio labeled antigen
     (b) Antigen
     (c) Antigen–Antibody complex
     (d) Radio labeled antibody

313. In case of drugs, like morphine they are injected by using
     (a) Albumin
     (b) Bilirubin
     (c) Bile pigments
     (d) Adipose tissue

314. Which of the following sequence is correct regarding RIA?
     (a) Validation→ development of assay methodology→preparation of specific antibody→radio labelling antigen
     (b) Preparation and characterisation of antigen→preparation of specific antibody→radio labeling antigen→ development of assay methodology→validation of method
     (c) Preparation and characterisation of antigen→radio labeling antigen→preparation of specific antibody→ development of assay methodology→validation of method
     (d) None of the above

315. The inner wall of plates is coated with
     (a) Antigen – Antibody complex
     (b) Radio labeled antigen
     (c) Antigen
     (d) Antibody

316. The Radio labelled antigen is bound to antibody is separated by
     (a) Chromatography
     (b) Filtration
     (c) Vaccum pump
     (d) None of the above

317. Which of the following cannot be detected by using RA technique?
     (a) Insulin in human plasma
     (b) β-HCG levels in females
     (c) Digoxin levels in patients
     (d) Concentration of Na^+, K^+ in urine

318. Polarography is developed by which of the following scientist?
     (a) Hull
     (b) Jaroslav heyrovsky
     (c) Schiebold
     (d) Einstein

319. The graph in polarography is drawn between
    (a) Current Vs Voltage
    (b) Current Vs Absorbance
    (c) Current Vs Concentration
    (d) Current Vs Electrolyte

320. How many electrodes are used in polarography?
    (a) One　　　　(b) Two
    (c) Three　　　(d) Five

321. The electrodes are made up of which metal?
    (a) Silicon　　(b) Aurum
    (c) Tungsten　(d) Mercury

322. The small electrode in polarography is called as
    (a) Electro chemical electrode
    (b) Dropping silicon electrode
    (c) Dropping mercury electrode
    (d) Dropping electrode

323. The function of base electrolyte is used to
    (a) Carry the bulk of the current and raise the conductivity of the solution
    (b) Carry the bulk of the voltage
    (c) Decrease the conductivity of the solution
    (d) Detect functional group in the sample

324. From the current-voltage curve we get information regarding
    (a) Electrolyte of the solution
    (b) Nature of the material
    (c) Concentration of the material
    (d) Both b & c

325. Polarography is used to determine
    (a) Functional group in solution
    (b) Organic functional groups in solution
    (c) In organic functional groups in solution
    (d) None of the above

326. Dropping mercury electrode acts as
    (a) Dynode
    (b) Anode
    (c) Cathode
    (d) None of the above

327. The other name for dropping mercury electrode is
    (a) Macro electrode
    (b) Reference electrode
    (c) Micro electrode
    (d) None of the above

328. The reference electrode acts as
    (a) Cathode
    (b) Anode
    (c) Dynode
    (d) None of the above

329. The applied voltage can be changed by using
    (a) Potentiometer wire
    (b) Galvanometer wire
    (c) Ammeter wire
    (d) Current wire

330. Galvanometer is used to measure
    (a) Current
    (b) Voltage
    (c) Current strength
    (d) Conductivity of the solution

331. Shunt is used for
    (a) Adjusting sensitivity of potentio-meter
    (b) Adjusting sensitivity of galvano-meter
    (c) To record current Vs Voltage graphs
    (d) None of the above

332. In Polarographic cell, which of the following solution is analyzed?
    (a) Strontium chloride
    (b) Barium chloride
    (c) Lithium chloride
    (d) Cadmium chloride

333. The positive ions in solution will be attracted towards which electrode?
    (a) Micro electrode
    (b) Macro electrode
    (c) Both a & b
    (d) None of the above

334. The total current flowing through the cell is
    (a) Diffusive force
    (b) Electrical force
    (c) Diffusive & electrical force
    (d) None of the above

335. The concentration gradient occurs due to which force?
    (a) Electrical force
    (b) Diffusive force
    (c) Force constant
    (d) All of the above

336. In current-voltage graph which of the following is not present?
    (a) Residual current
    (b) Migration current
    (c) Diffusion current
    (d) Potential current

337. The supporting electrolyte will carry which type of current?
    (a) Migration current
    (b) Residual current
    (c) Diffusion current
    (d) Kinetic current

338. The decomposition potential occurs due to
    (a) Concentration of electrolyte
    (b) Potential of electrode is not equal to decomposition potential
    (c) Diffusive force
    (d) Potential of electrode is equal to decomposition potential

339. Limiting current occurs due to
    (a) When no increase in current occurs
    (b) When increase in current occurs
    (c) When no voltage increase will occur
    (d) None of the above

340. The diffusion current is the difference between which two currents?
    (a) Residual & migrating current
    (b) Migrating & diffusion current
    (c) Residual & limiting current
    (d) Diffusion & kinetic current

341. The drop formation can be minimized by using which device?
    (a) High capacity condenser
    (b) Galvanometer
    (c) Shunt
    (d) Potentiometer

342. The mercury drop has which charge?
    (a) Positive charge
    (b) Negative charge
    (c) Neutral charge
    (d) None of the above

343. Residual current occurs due to
    (a) Migration of electrolyte solution
    (b) Migration of mercury drop
    (c) Migration of negative ions from electrolyte solution toward mercury drop
    (d) Migration of positive ions from electrolyte solution toward mercury drop

344. If electrolyte contains small impurities then which type of current will occurs?
    (a) Residual current
    (b) Kinetic current
    (c) Faradic current
    (d) Condenser current

345. Which of the following expression is correct regarding residual current?
    (a) Residual current = faradic current + condenser current
    (b) Residual current = migration current + diffusion current
    (c) Residual current = diffusion current + faradic current
    (d) Residual current = faradic current + kinetic current

346. The potassium atoms can be reduced to potassium in potassium chloride solution by raising which potential?
    (a) Neutral potential
    (b) Positive potential
    (c) Negative potential
    (d) All of the above

347. The migration current occurs by
    (a) Migration followed by diffusion of particles
    (b) Diffusion of charged particles
    (c) Migration of charged particles
    (d) None of the above

348. The maximum current occurs due to which type of current?
    (a) Kinetic current
    (b) Residual current
    (c) Migration current
    (d) Diffusion current

349. Which of the following is correct expression for ilkovic expression?
    (a) $id = 607nD^{½} m^{2/3} t^{1/6}$
    (b) $id = 607nCD^{½} m^{2/3} t^{1/6}$
    (c) $id = 607nCD^{2/3} m^{1/2} t^{1/6}$
    (d) $id = 609nCD^{½} m^{2/3} t^{1/6}$

350. The id current is directly proportional to
    (a) Voltage
    (b) Concentration of electrolyte
    (c) Potential difference across the electrode
    (d) Nature of the electrode

351. Kinetic current occurs due to
    (a) None electrode reaction
    (b) Concentration of electrode
    (c) Nature of the electrode
    (d) Potential difference across the electrode

352. The kinetic current occurs due to which type of current?
    (a) Faradic current
    (b) Condenser current
    (c) Residual current
    (d) Limiting current

353. Ilkovic equation is used for which purpose?
    (a) Qualitative purpose
    (b) Quantitative purpose
    (c) Both a & b
    (d) None of the above

354. Half wave potential is the characteristic property of
    (a) Current
    (b) Voltage
    (c) Electrolyte solution
    (d) None of the above

355. Half wave potential occurs due to
    (a) Steeply rising portion of current-voltage curve & is one half the distance between residual & migration current
    (b) Steeply rising portion of current-voltage curve & is one half the distance between Residual & Limiting current
    (c) Steeply rising portion of current-voltage curve & is one half the distance between residual & diffusion current
    (d) Steeply rising portion of current-voltage curve & is one half the distance between kinetic & residual current

356. The importance of half wave potential is due to
    (a) Increase in current-voltage curve
    (b) Reduction of electrolyte
    (c) Reduction at macro electrode
    (d) Reduction at micro electrode

357. Which of the following expression is correct for half wave potential?
    (a) $E_{1/2} = E^0 + 0.0590/n \log [D_{ox}/D_{red}]^{1/2}$
    (b) $E_{1/2} = E^0 + 0.0591/n \log [D_{red}/D_{ox}]^{1/2}$
    (c) $E_{1/2} = E^0 + 0.0591/n \log [D_{red}/D_{ox}]^{2/3}$
    (d) $E_{1/2} = E^0 + 0.0691/n \log [D_{red}/D_{ox}]^{1/2}$

358. Organic polarography is used for which purpose?
    (a) Quantitative purpose
    (b) Qualitative purpose
    (c) Both a & b
    (d) Determination of functional groups

359. In Organic polarography, which considerations are given more priority?
    (a) Solvent
    (b) Solute
    (c) Solution
    (d) None of the above

360. Which of the following solvents is not given much priority?
    (a) Alcohol   (b) Dioxane
    (c) Glycols   (d) Water

361. Which of the following supporting electrolytes are used in organic polarography?
    (a) Lithium salts
    (b) Silica salts
    (c) Sodium salts
    (d) Potassium salts

362. In estimation of sugars, which of the following is used as supporting electrolyte?
    (a) Hydrazine
    (b) Hydrazine sulphate

(c) Hydrazine chloride

(d) Hydro benzoin

363. The oxidized product of epinephrine is iodoadrenochrome it is oxidized by
(a) Perchloric acid
(b) Acetic acid
(c) Perbromate
(d) Periodate

364. Which of the following drugs is not analyzed by polarography?
(a) Chloramphenicol
(b) Nifedipine
(c) Amlodeipine
(d) Nitrobenzene

365. The size of the capillary in the DME is
(a) 20-30 μ   (b) 20-50 μ
(c) 20-40 μ   (d) 10-40 μ

366. Why supporting electrolyte is added in polarographic method?
(a) To eliminate kinetic current
(b) To eliminate diffusion current
(c) To eliminate migration current
(d) To eliminate residual current

367. If oxygen is present in electrolyte solution, it is removed by using which gas
(a) He   (b) H_2
(c) Ar   (d) N_2

368. The electrochemical method which is used to measure electro motive force is called as
(a) Amperometry
(b) Conductometry
(c) Polarography
(d) Potentiometry

369. The electrode whose potential does not change is called as?
(a) Reference electrode
(b) Indicator electrode
(c) Dropping mercuric electrode
(d) None of the above

370. Example for indicator electrode is
(a) Hydrogen electrode
(b) Saturated calomel electrode
(c) Glass electrode
(d) Silver- Silver chloride electrode

371. Silver- Silver chloride electrode is an example for
(a) Reference electrode
(b) Indicator electrode
(c) Dropping mercuric electrode
(d) None of the above

372. Antimony electrode is an example for
(a) Reference electrode
(b) Indicator electrode
(c) Residual electrode
(d) Kinetic electrode

373. The most commonly used Reference electrode is
(a) Hydrogen electrode
(b) Antimony electrode
(c) Saturated calomel electrode
(d) Silver-Silver chloride electrode

374. The potential of metal electrode is measured at a temperature of
(a) 25°C   (b) 35°C
(c) 45°C   (d) 65°C

375. Which of the following is the correct expression for nernst equation?
(a) $E = E^0 + 0.0692 / n \log C$
(b) $E = E^0 + 0.0592 / C \log n$

(c) $E = E^0 + 0.0592 / n \log C$
(d) $E = E^0 + 0.0592 / k \log C$

376. Which of the following electrodes can be used over wide pH range?
(a)   Hydrogen electrode
(b)   Glass electrode
(c)   Saturated calomel electrode
(d)   Silver- Silver chloride electrode

377. Which of the following electrode can be used as both reference and indicator electrode?
(a)   Glass electrode
(b)   Hydrogen electrode
(c)   Saturated calomel electrode
(d)   Antimony electrode

378. When hydrogen electrode dipped in a standard acid solution it acts as
(a)   Micro electrode
(b)   Dropping mercuric electrode
(c)   Reference electrode
(d)   Indicator electrode

379. When hydrogen electrode dipped in sample solution it acts as
(a)   Indicator electrode
(b)   Reference electrode
(c)   Dropping mercuric electrode
(d)   Glass electrode

380. In saturated calomel electrode, the inner jacket is plugged with mixture of
(a)   Hg & chloride
(b)   Chlorine & potassium chloride
(c) Hg_2cl_2 & potassium chloride
(d)   Kcl & Nacl

381. The potential of the silver-silver chloride electrode depends upon
(a)   Temperature
(b)   Concentration   &   potassium chloride
(c)   Both a & b
(d)   None of the above

382. In glass electrode the inner wire is made up of
(a)   Silver-chloride wire
(b)   Silver-Silver chloride wire
(c)   Antimony - chloride wire
(d)   Antimony- fluoride wire

383. Calculate the potential of unknown solution whose standard potential is 100mv and length of the wire in standard cell and sample is 50 & 20 respectively
(a)   200 mv   (b)   350 mv
(c)   250 mv   (d)   450 mv

384. In commercial potentiometer the calibration is done by using which type of buffers
(a)   pH 7 & pH 4   (b)   pH 7 & pH 3
(c)   pH 4 & pH 6   (d)   pH 3 & pH 9

385. In potentiometric titrations, the end point of titration is determined by
(a)   Changes in potential of the solution by addition of titrant
(b)   No changes in potential of the solution by addition of titrant
(c)   No changes in potential of the solution by addition of titrate
(d)   Changes in concentration of the solution by addition of titrant

386. In potentiometric titration, at the end point
    (a) The rate of change of concentration of solution is maximum
    (b) The rate of change of current of solution is maximum
    (c) The rate of change of voltage of solution is maximum
    (d) The rate of change of potential of solution is maximum

387. In acid-base titrations, the indicator and reference electrodes are
    (a) Saturated calomel & glass electrode
    (b) Glass & saturated calomel electrode
    (c) Saturated calomel & hydrogen electrode
    (d) Antimony chloride & silver-silver chloride electrode

388. In redox titrations the reference electrode is
    (a) Glass electrode
    (b) Hydrogen electrode
    (c) Saturated calomel electrode
    (d) Antimony electrode

389. In diazotization titrations, examples for titrate & titrant are
    (a) Sodium nitrite & aromatic primary amino group
    (b) Aromatic primary amino group & sodium nitrite in acidic medium
    (c) Aliphatic primary amino group & sodium nitrite in acidic medium
    (d) Aromatic primary amino group & sodium nitrite in basic medium

390. Which of the following reference electrode is used in diazotization titrations?
    (a) Saturated calomel electrode
    (b) Glass electrode
    (c) Hydrogen electrode
    (d) Antimony electrode

391. Which of the following drugs cannot be used in diazotization titrations?
    (a) Sulfa drugs   (b) Alkaloids
    (c) Amines   (d) Glycosides

392. Which of the following ions cannot be used as precipitants in precipitation titrations?
    (a) Mercury   (b) Lead
    (c) Silver   (d) Aurum

393. In complexometric titrations, the metallic ions are titrated against
    (a) Disodium EDTA
    (b) Dipotassium EDTA
    (c) Trisodium EDTA
    (d) Tripotassium EDTA

394. Biamperometry titrations are used to determine
    (a) Alcohol   (b) Water
    (c) Ether   (d) Glycol

395. The moisture content is determined by using which reagents?
    (a) Draggen droff's reagent
    (b) Liebermann burchard reagent
    (c) Karl Fischer reagent
    (d) None of the above

396. From the following equation which is an oxidizing agent
    $$Ce^{4+} + Fe^{2+} \rightarrow Ce^{3+} + Fe^{3+}$$
    (a) Fe^{2+} (b) Fe^{3+}
    (c) Ce^{3+} (d) Ce^{4+}

397. Which of the following expression is correct for redox titrations?
    (a) $E = E^0 + 0.0592/n \log [ox /red]$
    (b) $E = E^0 + 0.0692/n \log [red /ox]$
    (c) $E = E^0 + 0.0792/n \log [red /ox]$
    (d) $E^0 = E + 0.0592/n \log [ox /red]$

398. In acid-base titrations changes in concentration of which ion will takes place?
    (a) H^+ ions
    (b) OH^- ions
    (c) H^+ & OH^- ions
    (d) None of the above

399. Conductometry is the measurement of
    (a) Conductivity of the solution
    (b) EMF of the solution
    (c) Current across the solution
    (d) Voltage across the solution

400. Conductivity is inversely proportional to which parameter
    (a) Potential   (b) Current
    (c) Voltage   (d) Resistance

401. The unit of conductivity is
    (a) Ohm   (b) Mho
    (c) Ohm meter   (d) Mho cm^{-1}

402. Conductivity of solution depends upon
    (a) Concentration of ions
    (b) Charge of ions
    (c) Size & temperature of ions
    (d) All of the above

403. Units for specific conductivity is
    (a) Mho cm^{-1} (b) Ohm cm^{-1}
    (c) Mho m^{-1} (d) Ohm m^{-1}

404. Equivalent conductivity is the conductivity of the solution containing
    (a) Concentration of solute
    (b) Molecular weight of solute
    (c) Specific conductivity of the solution
    (d) Equivalent weight of the solute

405. Which of the following is correct for equivalent conductivity?
    (a) Equivalent conductivity = molar conductivity × Volume of solution containing 1gm equivalent weight of solute
    (b) Equivalent conductivity = Specific conductivity × Volume of solution containing 1gm equivalent weight of solute
    (c) a & bare correct
    (d) None of the above

406. For conducting conductivity of the solution which cells are required?
    (a) Conductivity cell
    (b) Conductivity and wheat stone bridge circuit
    (c) Wheat stone bridge circuit
    (d) Cell constant

407. The conductivity cell is made up of
    (a) Aluminum   (b) Aurum
    (c) Platinum   (d) Mercury

408. If electrodes are very old enough platinisation can be done by using
    (a) 3% Solution of chloroplatinic acid
    (b) 0.02%-0.03% lead acetate
    (c) Both a & b are correct
    (d) 4% Solution of chloroplatinic acid

409. Calculate the conductivity of unknown solution whose resistance of known and unknown solution is 200 ohm and known solution is 400 ohm and the standard resistance is of 400 ohms?
(a) 80 ohms   (b) 80 mhos
(c) 8.0 mhos   (d) 0.08 ohms

410. Calculate the cell constant whose surface area of electrode is 25 sq.cm?
(a) 4   (b) 0.4
(c) 0.04   (d) 0.004

411. Which of the following expression is correct for specific conductivity?
(a) Specific conductivity = cell constant × observed conductivity
(b) Specific conductivity = cell constant × molar conductivity
(c) Specific conductivity = cell constant × equivalent conductivity
(d) All are correct

412. Cell constant is used to determine
(a) Specific conductivity
(b) Conductivity
(c) Molar conductivity
(d) Equivalent conductivity

413. The cell constant is determined at which solution?
(a) Nacl   (b) Kcl
(c) Bacl$_2$ (d) Becl$_2$

414. The concentration of Kcl is required to determine cell constant is
(a) 0.2   (b) 0.002
(c) 0.02   (d) 2

415. The cell constant is determined at which temperature?
(a) 15°c   (b) 24°c
(c) 35°c   (d) 25°c

416. Which of the following expression is correct for cell constant at 25°c?
(a) Cell constant = 2765/observed conductivity of 0.02 Kcl at 25°c in μmhos
(b) Cell constant = 2765/observed conductivity of 0.02 Kcl at 25°c in μmhos
(c) Cell constant = 2665/observed conductivity of 0.2 Kcl at 25°c in μmhos
(d) All are correct

417. Calculate the specific conductivity of the solution whose cell constant is 400 ohm and observed conductivity is 80 μmhos?
(a) 69.1   (b) 66.1
(c) 67.1   (d) 64.1

418. Calculate the cell constant of the solution who's observed conductivity of 0.02 Kcl at 25°C is 40 μmhos?
(a) 69.1   (b) 66.1
(c) 67.1   (d) 64.1

419. The conductivity of the solution changes due to
(a) Change in number of ions
(b) Mobility of ions
(c) Both a & b are correct
(d) Concentration of ions

420. Which of the following is not an example for acid base titrations?
(a) Strong acid Vs Strong base
(b) Strong acid Vs Weak base

(c) Weak acid Vs Strong base

(d) Strong acid Vs Weak acid

421. Examples for Strong acid Vs Strong base titrations
(a) Hcl Vs NaoH
(b) Hcl Vs NH_4OH
(c) CH_3COOH Vs NaoH
(d) CH_3COOH Vs NH_4OH

422. In every titration, the solution in burette is called as
(a) Electrolyte solution
(b) Titrant
(c) Electrochemical solution
(d) Titrate

423. The solution in beaker / conical flask is called as
(a) Titrate
(b) Titrant
(c) Indicator
(d) None of the above

424. Which of the following is an example for weak acid Vs strong base titrations?
(a) Hcl Vs NaoH
(b) CH_3COOH Vs NaoH
(c) Hcl Vs NH_4OH
(d) CH_3COOH Vs NH_4OH

425. In Hcl Vs NaoH, the H+ ions completely dissociates then the conductivity
(a) Gradually increases
(b) Gradually decreases
(c) Remains same
(d) None of the above

426. Example for precipitation titrations is
(a) Kcl Vs Agcl
(b) Kcl Vs $AgNo_3$
(c) Nacl Vs $AgNo_3$
(d) $Bacl_2$ Vs $AgNo_3$

427. Which of the following is an example for displacement titrations?
(a) $NH_4Cl+NaOH \rightarrow NH_4OH+NaCl$
(b) $NH_4OH+NaCl \rightarrow NH_4Cl+NaOH$
(c) $NaCl+NaoH \rightarrow NaOH+H_2O$
(d) All are incorrect

428. Redox titrations are conducted in which medium?
(a) Alkaline medium
(b) Acidic medium
(c) Neutral medium
(d) None of the above

429. Which of the following is not an example for non-aqueous solvents?
(a) Methanol
(b) Pyridine
(c) Dimethyl formamide
(d) Water

430. The other name for amperometric titrations is
(a) Conductometry
(b) Potentiometry
(c) Polarography
(d) Spectropolarography

431. Which current is measured in amperometric titrations?
(a) Diffusion current
(b) Kinetic current
(c) Limiting current
(d) Residual current

432. The diffusion current depends upon
    (a) Nature of electro reducible ion
    (b) Concentration of electro reducible ion
    (c) Size of electro reducible ion
    (d) All of the above

433. In order to perform amperometric titrations
    (a) The titrate should be electro-reducible
    (b) The titrant should be electro-reducible
    (c) Both titrate & titrant should be electroreducible
    (d) None of the above

434. The reference electrode in amperometric titrations is
    (a) Saturated calomel electrode
    (b) Silver–Silver chloride electrode
    (c) Hydrogen electrode
    (d) Antimony chloride electrode

435. The example for reference electrode is
    (a) Polarisable electrode
    (b) Non polarisable electrode
    (c) Electro chemical electrode
    (d) None of the above

436. The Example for polarisable electrode is
    (a) Dropping mercury electrode
    (b) Rotating platinum micro electrode
    (c) Both a & b are correct
    (d) Electro chemical electrode

437. The rotating platinum electrode consists of wire, it is made up which of the following material
    (a) Platinum wire (b) Aurum wire
    (c) Steel wire   (d) Sliver wire

438. To remove excess of oxygen which gas is pumped?
    (a) Helium   (b) Hydrogen
    (c) Nitrogen   (d) Neon

439. Which of the following is an example for supporting electrolyte?
    (a) Nacl   (b) Kcl
    (c) $Cacl_2$ (d) $Bacl_2$

440. If titrate is electro reducible, then examples for titrate are
    (a) Lead ions
    (b) Sulphate ions
    (c) Chloride ions
    (d) Silver ions

441. If titrate is electro reducible then lead ions is the titrate, then titrant used is
    (a) Chloride ions
    (b) Silver ions
    (c) Sulphate ions
    (d) Dichromate ions

442. If titrant is electro reducible then the examples for titrant is
    (a) Dichromate ions
    (b) Silver ions
    (c) Titanous ions
    (d) Ferric ions

443. If both titrate & titrant are electroreducible then which of the following ions are used?
    (a) Lead ions & dichromate ions respectively
    (b) Dichromate ions & lead ions respectively
    (c) Lead ions & trichromate ions respectively
    (d) Trichromate ions & lead ions respectively

444. In dead stop end point technique what happens?
    (a) Diffusion current is maximum
    (b) Diffusion current is minimum
    (c) Diffusion current is zero
    (d) None of the above

445. The amperometric detector is used in which type of chromatography?
    (a) HPLC
    (b) GC
    (c) Paper chromatography
    (d) TLC

446. Composition of Karl Fischer reagent is
    (a) Solution of iodine & sulphur trioxide in pyrimidine and ethanol
    (b) Solution of potassium & sulphur trioxide in pyridine and methanol
    (c) Solution of iodine & sulphur dioxide in pyridine and methanol
    (d) Solution of iodine & sulphur dioxide in pyrimidine and methanol

447. Coulometric method of analysis is used to measure
    (a) Concentration of electrolyte
    (b) Nature of material
    (c) Size of material
    (d) Quantity of electrolyte

448. In primary coulometric method of analysis the substance is
    (a) Oxidized at one electrode
    (b) Reduced at another electrode
    (c) Oxidized or Reduced at one electrode
    (d) All are in correct

449. In the coulometric titrations the primary standard is
    (a) Electron
    (b) Positron
    (c) Neutron
    (d) Molecular ion

450. The coulometric titrations is used to determine
    (a) Gaseous chemicals
    (b) Volatile material
    (c) Unstable chemicals
    (d) All are correct

451. In primary coulometric titration, which of the following is the correct expression?
    (a) $Q = mt$
    (b) $Q = ct$
    (c) $Q = it$
    (d) $Q = dt$

452. In secondary coulometric titrations
    (a) The active intermediate is first produced
    (b) It has quantitative applications
    (c) The active intermediate reacts with sample solution quantitatively
    (d) All the above

453. In neutralization titrations, in platinum cathode which ions are generated?
    (a) H^+ IONS
    (b) OH^- ions
    (c) H_3O^+ ions
    (d) None of the above

454. Which compounds are analyzed by organic titrations?
    (a) Trichloroacetic acid
    (b) Tetrachloroacetic acid

(c) Dichloroacetic acid

(d) Formic acid

455. The GLP principles were published in which year?
(a) 1982
(b) 1971
(c) 1981
(d) 1991

456. The OECD principles of good laboratory practice is incorporated under the membership of
(a) European Directive 87/18/EEC
(b) American Directive 87/18/EEC
(c) European Directive 88/18/EEC
(d) European Directive 87/18/ECE

457. In USA, the GLP regulations was incorporated into the national legislation under
(a) Code of pharmaceutical regulations
(b) Code of federal regulations
(c) Code of economic regulations
(d) Code of industry regulations

458. GLP is a type of which system
(a) Quantity system
(b) Quality system
(c) Both a & b
(d) None of the above

459. Which studies are given in GLP?
(a) Clinical health studies
(b) Environmental safety studies
(c) Nonclinical & Environmental safety studies
(d) None of the above

460. The non clinical safety data is submitted to which regulatory body
(a) FDA

(b) ICH
(c) CFR
(d) All of the above

461. The ISO stands for
(a) International standard organization
(b) Inter regulation standard organization
(c) Inter spacious standard organization
(d) Inter regulation standard, sample organization

462. ISO 9000 was issued in which year
(a) 1987
(b) 1997
(c) 1967
(d) 1989

463. The ISO is made up of
(a) Three standards
(b) Four standards
(c) Two standards
(d) Five standards

464. The design part is included in which part of ISO 9000
(a) ISO 9003
(b) ISO 9004
(c) ISO 9002
(d) ISO 9001

465. Which of the following ISO 9000 standards has less value?
(a) ISO 9003
(b) ISO 9002
(c) ISO 9001
(d) ISO 9004

466. For calibration of laboratories what is the other standard mentioned?
(a) ISO/IEC 17035: 2005
(b) ISO/IEC 16025: 2005
(c) ISO/IEC 18025: 2005
(d) ISO/IEC 17025: 2005

467. For medical laboratories the standards are incorporated in
    (a) ISO 16189: 2003
    (b) ISO 15189: 2003
    (c) ISO 14189: 2003
    (d) ISO 15289: 2003

468. The requirements of both ISO 9001 and ISO/IEC 17025 are incorporated in
    (a) ISO 16189: 2003
    (b) ISO 15187: 2003
    (c) ISO 15186: 2003
    (d) ISO 15189: 2003

469. OECD stands for
    (a) Organization for economic co-operation and development
    (b) Organization for economic commerce and development
    (c) Organization for education co-operation and development
    (d) None of the above

470. Analytical laboratories has selected certification to
    (a) ISO 9014   (b) ISO 9001
    (c) ISO 17025   (d) ISO 15189

471. TQM stands for
    (a) Total quantity management
    (b) Total quality management
    (c) Total quantity maintenance
    (d) Total quality middle management

472. TQM approach originated in which year?
    (a) 1950's   (b) 1960's
    (c) 1970's   (d) 1980's

473. The word "TQM" means
    (a) All in one

    (b) By Everyone
    (c) Every body
    (d) All of the above

474. TQM is used to satisfy which people
    (a) Customers
    (b) Government
    (c) National regulatory body
    (d) ISO standards

475. In documentation which product specifications should be readily available?
    (a) Raw materials
    (b) Intermediate products
    (c) Finished products
    (d) All of the above

476. Sampling procedures is one for which products
    (a) Raw materials
    (b) Intermediate products
    (c) Finished products
    (d) All of the above

477. Control samples of raw material must be maintained for how many years?
    (a) 1yr   (b) 3yrs
    (c) 4yrs   (d) 5yrs

478. When there is no expiry date, the documents are retained for about
    (a) 1yr   (b) 2yrs
    (c) 3yrs   (d) 6yrs

479. Validation activity team members are taken from which of the following department?
    (a) R & D department
    (b) Quality department
    (c) Production & engineering department
    (d) All of the above

480. URS stands for
   (a) User requirement specification
   (b) User random specification
   (c) User requirement standards
   (d) User random standards

481. URS is done for
   (a) Buildings in manufacture of pharmaceutical formulation
   (b) Facilities in manufacture of pharmaceutical formulation
   (c) Both a & b
   (d) Production department

482. Design qualification specifications are to be finalized by team members from
   (a) Production
   (b) Engineering
   (c) Quality management
   (d) All of the above

483. Installation qualification is done for
   (a) Instrument
   (b) Equipment of pharmaceutical manufacturing
   (c) Engineering department
   (d) Production department

484. In order to perform Equipment validation which of the following process should be covered?
   (a) User requirement specification
   (b) Preparation of design qualification
   (c) Installation qualification
   (d) All of the above

485. F.A.T stands for
   (a) Factory acceptance test
   (b) Foreign acceptance test
   (c) Formulation acceptance test
   (d) Factory assurance test

486. D.Q is agreeable for
   (a) Purchaser
   (b) Manufacturers
   (c) Both a & b
   (d) Customer

487. F.A.T is performed at which stage of validation?
   (a) Design qualification
   (b) Installation qualification
   (c) Operational qualification
   (d) Performance qualification

488. After D.Q what is the next stage of qualification?
   (a) Operational qualification
   (b) Design qualification
   (c) Manufacturer qualification
   (d) Design qualification

489. Which of the following is correct in validation process?
   (a) User requirement specification → design qualification → installation qualification → operational qualification→ performance qualifycation
   (b) User requirement specification→ installation qualification → design qualification → operational qualification → performance qualification
   (c) User requirement specification→ design qualification→ operational qualification→ installation qualifycation → performance qualifycation
   (d) User requirement specification → design qualification→ performance qualification→ installation qualification→ operational qualification

490. An established documented evidence which provides a high degree of assurance that the specific process will consistently produce product meetings its predetermined specification and quality characteristics is called as
    (a) Validation
    (b) Equipment validation
    (c) Cleaning validation
    (d) Analytical validation

491. The closeness of true value to observed value is called as
    (a) Precision   (b) Robustness
    (c) Ruggedness   (d) Accuracy

492. Accuracy is calculated by
    (a) Accuracy = mean value–true value
    (b) % Recovery
    (c) Both a & b
    (d) Signal to noise ratio

493. In order to determine % recovery of analyte
    (a) Spiking of analyte to standard is done
    (b) Removal of sample from standard is done
    (c) Both a & b
    (d) Signal to error ratio

494. The closeness of agreement between a series of measurement obtained from multiple sampling of the homogenous sample is
    (a) Accuracy   (b) Precision
    (c) Ruggedness   (d) Robustness

495. Precision is usually expressed in terms of
    (a) Variance
    (b) Standard deviation
    (c) Sigma method
    (d) % RSD

496. Repeatability also called as
    (a) Intra assay precision
    (b) Inter assay precision
    (c) Assay precision
    (d) Intermediate precision

497. The precision under the same operating conditions over a short-interval of time is called as
    (a) Reproducibility
    (b) Intermediate precision
    (c) Repeatability
    (d) Robustness

498. Intermediate precision is done by
    (a) Different analysts
    (b) Different days
    (c) Different equipment
    (d) All of the above

499. Collaborative studies are expressed by which precision?
    (a) Repeatability
    (b) Reproducibility
    (c) Intermediate precision
    (d) Precision

500. Ability to determine analyte in the presence of other components is called as
    (a) Precision   (b) Accuracy
    (c) Specificity   (d) Security

501. Identification test, purity tests and assay tests can comes under
    (a) Precision   (b) Accuracy
    (c) Specificity   (d) LOD

502. LOD means
  (a) Limit of detection
  (b) Lower limit of detection
  (c) Upper limit of detection
  (d) Limit of degradation

503. LOD can be determined based on
  (a) Visual evaluation
  (b) Signal to noise approach
  (c) Standard deviation & slope
  (d) All of the above

504. Which of the following expression is correct for detection limit?
  (a) $DL = 3.3S/\sigma$
  (b) $DL = 3.3\sigma/S$
  (c) $DL = 4.3\sigma/S$
  (d) $DL = 3.3\sigma^2/S$

505. LOQ means
  (a) Limit of quality
  (b) Limit of quantity
  (c) Limit of quantification
  (d) Lower of the quantification

506. Which of the following expression is correct for quantification limit?
  (a) $QL = 10\sigma/S$
  (b) $QL = 10S/\sigma$
  (c) $QL = 9\sigma/S$
  (d) $QL = 10S^2/\sigma$

507. Linearity graph is obtained by
  (a) Concentration Vs absorbance
  (b) Directly proportional to concentration Vs absorbance
  (c) Inversely proportional to freezing point Vs absorbance
  (d) None of the above

508. Calculate the detection limit, when standard deviation is 1.01 & slope is 4.1
  (a) 0.812
  (b) 0.712
  (c) 0.612
  (d) 0.912

509. Calculate the quantification limit, when standard deviation is 1.09 & slope is 3.12
  (a) 3.156
  (b) 3.493
  (c) 3.312
  (d) 3.021

510. The correlation coefficient is expressed for which parameters
  (a) Accuracy
  (b) Linearity
  (c) Precision
  (d) Robustness

511. System suitability parameters are applicable for which chromatographic conditions?
  (a) Gas chromatography
  (b) Liquid chromatography
  (c) Solid chromatography
  (d) Both a & b are correct

512. Range is defined as
  (a) Interval between upper & lower limit
  (b) Interval between lower & upper limit
  (c) Interval between upper & most upper limit
  (d) Interval between lower & most upper limit

513. Range is expressed in terms of
  (a) % (Percentage)
  (b) Parts per million
  (c) Both a & b are correct
  (d) Microgram per mL

514. "The analysis of sample under different conditions like laboratories, analysts, instruments, reagents, times, temperature, days" is called as
  (a) Ruggedness
  (b) Repeatability
  (c) Robustness
  (d) Reproducibility

515. "A measure of capacity to remain unaffected by small but deliberate variations in method parameters & provides & indication of its reliability during normal usage"
(a) Ruggedness
(b) Repeatability
(c) Robustness
(d) Reproducibility

516. The process of separation of mixture into individual components using stationary phase and mobile phase is called as
(a) Chromatography
(b) Resolution
(c) Retention factor
(d) Adsorption

517. If stationary phase is solid then which phenomenon will occur?
(a) Partition
(b) Adsorption
(c) Counter current
(d) Reverse phase chromatography

518. In adsorption chromatography, the compounds and stationary phase are called as
(a) Adsorbent & adsorption
(b) Adsorbent & adsorbate
(c) Adsorption & adsorbate
(d) All are correct

519. In the adsorption chromatography the compound which has more affinity towards stationary phase will travels
(a) Faster
(b) Slower
(c) Medium
(d) Remains there itself

520. Which of the following chromatography techniques where adsorption phenomenon occur?
(a) Gas solid chromatography
(b) Thin layer chromatography
(c) Gas liquid chromatography
(d) Only a & b are correct

521. When two immiscible liquids are present then which phenomenon will takes place?
(a) Adsorption   (b) Partition
(c) Permeation   (d) Ion exchange

522. Which of the following chromatographic techniques where partition phenomenon will occur?
(a) Gas liquid chromatography
(b) Paper chromatography
(c) Column chromatography
(d) All are correct

523. If the stationary phase is polar then which type of chromatography it is?
(a) Reverse phase chromatography
(b) Normal phase chromatography
(c) Adsorption chromatography
(d) Partition chromatography

524. If mobile phase is polar then which type of chromatography it is?
(a) Adsorption chromatography
(b) Partition chromatography
(c) Reverse phase chromatography
(d) Normal phase chromatography

525. Which of the following is most widely used chromatography in pharmaceutical analysis?
(a) Reverse phase chromatography
(b) Normal phase chromatography

(c) Adsorption chromatography

(d) Partition chromatography

526. When stationary phase is solid it is called as which type of column chromatography?
(a) Column partition chromatography
(b) Column adsorption chromatography
(c) Column column chromatography
(d) Column chromatography

527. If stationary phase is liquid coated on solid support it is called as
(a) Column adsorption chromatography
(b) Column column chromatography
(c) Column chromatography
(d) Column partition chromatography

528. The compound which has more affinity towards stationary phase travels?
(a) Slower
(b) Faster
(c) Medium
(d) Remains there itself

529. The stationary phase particle size there itself should be around
(a) $60 - 250\ \mu$ (b) $60 - 200\ \mu$
(c) $100 - 150\ \mu$ (d) $200 - 400\ \mu$

530. Which of the following is a weak adsorbent?
(a) Fuller's earth
(b) Activated magnesia
(c) Mgo
(d) Starch

531. Which of the following is a medium adsorbent?
(a) Sucrose   (b) Talc
(c) Mgo   (d) $Mg\ (OH)_2$

532. Which of the following is not a strong adsorbent?
(a) Fuller's earth
(b) Activated charcoal
(c) Activated alumina
(d) Mgo

533. Which of the following is not a medium adsorbent?
(a) $CaCo_3$ (b) $Ca_3\ (PO_4)_2$
(c) $Ca\ (OH)_2$ (d) Talc

534. Which of the following is not a weak adsorbent?
(a) Sucrose   (b) Fuller's earth
(c) Talc   (d) Starch

535. Which of the following is not a strong adsorbent?
(a) Fuller's earth
(b) Activated charcoal
(c) Activated magnesium silicate
(d) $MgCo_3$

536. Which of the following is most commonly used stationary phase?
(a) Silica gel   (b) Fuller's earth
(c) Silica   (d) $Caco_3$

537. The adsorbate : adsorbent ratio should be
(a) $1:20$ (b) $20:1$
(c) $2:10$ (d) $1:30$

538. Mobile phase acts as
     (a) Solvent
     (b) Eluent
     (c) Developer
     (d) All the above

539. To remove pure component out of the column the mobile phase acts as
     (a) Solvent
     (b) Eluent
     (c) Developing agent
     (d) Polarity

540. To introduce mixture into column mobile phase acts as
     (a) Solvent
     (b) Eluent
     (c) Developing agent
     (d) Polarity

541. Column is made up of
     (a) Quartz
     (b) Kcl
     (c) Lithiumflouride
     (d) Glass

542. In order to get more efficiency, the length: diameter of the column should be in the ratio of
     (a) 10 : 1   (b) 20 :1
     (c) 100 :1   (d) 50 :1

543. The air bubbles are entrapped in which packing technique?
     (a) Wet Packing technique
     (b) Dry Packing technique
     (c) Both a & b are correct
     (d) Solvent packing technique

544. Which of the following is most efficient packing technique?
     (a) Wet Packing technique

(b) Solvent packing technique
(c) Dry Packing technique
(d) Both a & c are correct

545. The bottom portion of column is packed with which material?
     (a) Cotton wool
     (b) Glass wool
     (c) Asbestos pad
     (d) All the above

546. In isocratic elution technique, the solvent is having same
     (a) Concentration
     (b) Polarity
     (c) Viscosity
     (d) Dipolar moment

547. In gradient elution technique, the solvents of increasing
     (a) Polarity
     (b) Concentration
     (c) Viscosity
     (d) Dipolar moment

548. Which of the following is correct order for gradient elution technique?
     (a) Methanol→ethylacetatechloro-from→ benzene
     (b) Benzene→chlorofrom→ethyl-acetate → methanol
     (c) Chlorofrom→ethylacetate→methanol→benzene
     (d) All are correct

549. Which of the following detectors are used in column chromatography?
     (a) UV/Visible detector
     (b) FID detector
     (c) Fluorescence detector
     (d) All of the above

550. The recovery of components can be done by using
     (a) Adsorption (b) Partition
     (c) Elution (d) Eluate

551. Which of the following factors increases column efficiency?
     (a) Increase in particle size
     (b) Decrease in particle size
     (c) Using more viscous solvents
     (d) Applying low temperature

552. Separation of geometrical isomers can be done by using which type chromatography?
     (a) Column chromatography
     (b) Thin layer chromatography
     (c) High pressure liquid chromatography
     (d) Gas chromatography

553. Separation of tautomers can be done by using which chromatography technique?
     (a) GC
     (b) HPLC
     (c) TLC
     (d) Column chromatography

554. If original solution is used for the displacement it is called as
     (a) Elution analysis
     (b) Displacement analysis
     (c) Frontal analysis
     (d) Tailing analysis

555. For separation of racemetes which adsorbent is used?
     (a) Starch (b) Sucrose
     (c) Cellulose (d) Fructose

556. If the stationary phase is silica impregnated on filter paper then it is called as
     (a) Paper chromatography
     (b) Paper adsorption chromatography
     (c) Paper partition chromatography
     (d) Paper – Paper chromatography

557. Paper partition chromatography is due to
     (a) Pores of cellulose fibers
     (b) Pores of silica fibers
     (c) Moisture present in pores of cellulose fibers
     (d) None of the above

558. Which of the phenomenon occurs mainly in paper chromatography?
     (a) Partition
     (b) Adsorption
     (c) Normal phase
     (d) Reverse phase

559. Which of the following stationary phase is not used in paper chromatography?
     (a) α- cellulose (b) β-cellulose
     (c) Silica (d) Pentosans

560. Hydrophilic papers are modified with which agent?
     (a) α- cellulose (b) Pentosans
     (c) β-cellulose (d) Glycol

561. Hydrophobic papers are used for
     (a) Normal phase chromatography
     (b) Reverse phase chromatography
     (c) Partition chromatography
     (d) Adsorption chromatography

562. Sample is applied with the help of
    (a) Pipette
    (b) Burette
    (c) Micro pipette
    (d) Measuring cylinder

563. Which of the following is an example for hydrophilic mobile phases?
    (a) Isopropanol : ammonia : water
    (b) Isopropanol : water
    (c) Isopropanol : ammonia
    (d) Dimethyl ether : cyclohexane

564. In ascending development technique the solvent flows
    (a) Towards gravity
    (b) Against gravity
    (c) Both a & b
    (d) All the above

565. In descending development technique the solvent flows
    (a) Against gravity
    (b) Towards gravity
    (c) Both a & b
    (d) All the above

566. Which of the following development technique is faster?
    (a) Two dimensional development
    (b) Circular development
    (c) Ascending development
    (d) Descending development

567. If the spot is kept at the centre then which type of development will occur?
    (a) Two dimensional development
    (b) Descending development
    (c) Circular development
    (d) Descending development

568. Which of the following is a non-specific method?
    (a) Ferric chloride method
    (b) Dragendroff's method
    (c) Ninhydrin method
    (d) Iodine chamber method

569. In specific method for detection of cardiac glycosides which of the following reagent is used?
    (a) 2, 4 DNP
    (b) Ninhydrin
    (c) 3, 5-Dinitro Phenyl hydrazine
    (d) 3, 5-Dinitro benzoic acid

570. Ferric chloride reagent is used to detect
    (a) Cardiac glycosides
    (b) Amino acids
    (c) Tannins
    (d) Alkaloids

571. In densitometric method, sample is
    (a) Destroyed
    (b) Not destroyed
    (c) Remains as same
    (d) None of the above

572. Which of the following is a destructive technique?
    (a) UV chamber method
    (b) Iodine chamber method
    (c) Ninhydrin method
    (d) Densitometric method

573. Densitometry is a ______ method
    (a) Qualitative technique
    (b) Quantitative technique
    (c) Both a & b are correct
    (d) All are in correct

574. Spectrophotometry is a

(a) Direct method
(b) In direct method
(c) Qualitative technique
(d) Quantitative technique

575. Rf stands for
(a) Retention factor
(b) Resolution factor
(c) Retardation factor
(d) All are incorrect

576. Which of the following is correct?
(a) Rf = Distance travelled by solvent/ distance travelled by solute
(b) Rf = Distance travelled by solute / distance travelled by solvent
(c) Rf = Distance travelled by solution/ distance travelled by solute
(d) Rf = Distance travelled by solution/ distance travelled by solvent

577. R_x is
(a) Ratio of distance travelled by sample by standard
(b) Ratio of distance travelled by standard by sample
(c) Ratio of distance travelled by solute by solvent
(d) Ratio of distance travelled by solvent by solute

578. Which of the following antibiotics can be detected by paper chromatography?
(a) Penicillin
(b) Gentamicin
(c) Amikacin
(d) Streptomycin

579. The choice of development techniques depends upon
(a) Nature of substance
(b) Concentration of substance
(c) Size of substance
(d) Molecular weight of substance

580. The TLC was developed by which scientist?
(a) Stahl
(b) Consden
(c) Gorden
(d) Martin

581. In TLC the principle of separation is
(a) Partition
(b) Adsorption
(c) Normal phase
(d) Reverse phase

582. The mobile phase flows through adsorbent by
(a) Capillary action
(b) Macro capillary action
(c) Micro capillary action
(d) Gravitational action

583. The component with more affinity towards stationary phase travels
(a) Faster
(b) Medium
(c) Slower
(d) Remains there itself

584. Which of the following is the composition for kieselghur G
(a) Silica gel + $CaSO_4$
(b) Al_2O + $CaSO_4$
(c) Cellulose + $CaSO_4$
(d) Diatomaceous earth + Binder

585. Which of the following plates are used in TLC?
(a) Alumina plates
(b) Steel plates
(c) Glass plates
(d) Platinum plates

586. The slurry, is a mixture of
 (a) Stationary phase & Water
 (b) Adsorbent & Water
 (c) Both a & b are correct
 (d) All are in correct

587. TLC plates are prepared by which of the following techniques?
 (a) Pouring
 (b) Dipping
 (c) Spraying & spreading
 (d) All the above

588. Which of the following is the best technique for preparation of TLC plates?
 (a) Pouring   (b) Dipping
 (c) Spraying   (d) Spreading

589. The thickness of stationary phase for analytical purpose is
 (a) 0.35 mm   (b) 1 mm
 (c) 0.25 mm   (d) 0.9 mm

590. TLC plates are activated due to
 (a) Removal of active constituents from adsorbent
 (b) Removal of analyte from adsorbent
 (c) Removal of moisture from adsorbent
 (d) Removal of mobile phase from adsorbent

591. Activation is done due to
 (a) Retain adsorption activity
 (b) Retain adsorbent activity
 (c) Retain adsorbate activity
 (d) All the above

592. Which of the following quantity of sample to be spotted on TLC plates?
 (a) 10 µL   (b) 1-9 µL
 (c) 20 µL   (d) 2-5 µL

593. In order to saturate the atmosphere in the development chamber
 (a) Adsorbent is kept
 (b) Filter paper is kept
 (c) Mobile phase is kept
 (d) None of the above

594. If saturation of atmosphere is not done
 (a) Edge effect
 (b) Non edge effect
 (c) Activation effect
 (d) Partition effect

595. Which of the following factors depends upon the selection of mobile phase?
 (a) Nature of substances to be separated
 (b) Nature of stationary phase used
 (c) Mode of chromatography
 (d) All of the above

596. In which development technique the plates are kept vertical?
 (a) 1-D development technique
 (b) 2-D development technique
 (c) Horizontal development technique
 (d) Multiple development technique

597. Which of the following detection technique used for colorless spots?
 (a) Specific method
 (b) Non specific method
 (c) 1-D technique
 (d) 2 –D technique

598. Which of the following is not a non-specific method for detection?
 (a) Iodine chamber method
 (b) Sulphuric acid spray method

(c) Ferric chloride method

(d) UV method

599. Ninhydrin reagent is used as a
 (a) Specific method of detection
 (b) Non-specific method of detection
 (c) In specific method of detection
 (d) UV method

600. Ninhydrin reagent is used to detect
 (a) Alkaloids
 (b) Amino acids
 (c) Tannins
 (d) Cardiac glycosides

601. Which of the following expression is correct for R_m Value?
 (a) $R_m = \log (1/R_x - 1)$
 (b) $R_m = \log (1/R_f - 1)$
 (c) $R_m = \log (1/R_x)$
 (d) $R_m = \log (R_f - 1/100)$

602. What is the detecting agent for drug methyl dopa?
 (a) UV 254nm
 (b) Iodine vapour
 (c) Trichloroacetic acid
 (d) Potassium ferricyanide

603. What is the detecting agent for the drug carbimazole?
 (a) $FeCl_3$
 (b) Phosphomolybdic acid
 (c) Potassium iodobismuthate
 (d) Ninhydrin

604. For cimetidine what is the detecting agent?
 (a) UV 254nm
 (b) Potassium ferricyanide
 (c) Iodine vapour

(d) Trichloroacetic acid + chloramine T

605. Ferric chloride reagent is used to detect
 (a) Alcohol
 (b) Phenols
 (c) Tannins
 (d) Both b & c

606. In HPTLC the particle size of the stationary phase is
 (a) Less than 100 μ
 (b) Less than 1000 μ
 (c) Less than 10 μ
 (d) More than 10 μ

607. For Normal phase HPTLC, the stationary phase used is
 (a) C8
 (b) C18
 (c) C4
 (d) Silica gel

608. For Reverse Phase HPTLC, the stationary phase used is
 (a) Alumina
 (b) $CaSO_4$
 (c) Diatomaceous earth
 (d) Silica gel

609. In HPTLC, the thickness of the adsorbent layer is
 (a) 2 mm (b) 4 mm
 (c) 1 mm (d) 10 mm

610. Which type of detecting system is used in HPTLC?
 (a) UV
 (b) Visible
 (c) Fluorescence
 (d) All the above

611. In HPTLC, which type of detecting system is used?
    (a) Destructive detecting system
    (b) Non destructive detecting system
    (c) Both a & b
    (d) Specific method

612. Which of the following nondestructive detection techniques is used in HPTLC?
    (a) UV
    (b) Iodine chamber method
    (c) Both a & b are correct
    (d) Sulphuric acid method

613. HPTLC is more efficient because
    (a) Smaller particle size of adsorbents
    (b) Uniform size of adsorbents
    (c) Both b & c
    (d) All the above

614. Which of the following compounds is detected by HPTLC?
    (a) Ranitidine
    (b) Digoxin
    (c) Carbidopa
    (d) Cimetidine

615. Other name for high performance liquid chromatography
    (a) High pressure liquid chromatography
    (b) High pressure laser chromatography
    (c) High partition liquid chromatography
    (d) High partition laser chromatography

616. The particle size of stationary phase in HPLC is
    (a) 100 μ
    (b) 60-200 μ
    (c) 3-20 μ
    (d) 20-40 μ

617. The length and diameter of the column should be around
    (a) 5-50 ×1-100 mm i.d
    (b) 5-50 ×1-10 mm i.d
    (c) 5-100 × 1-10 mm i.d
    (d) 100-150 × 1-20 mm i.d

618. Column is made up of which material
    (a) Glass
    (b) Carbon
    (c) Aluminum
    (d) Any metal

619. Operating pressure of HPLC is
    (a) 500 – 3000 psi
    (b) 500 – 1000 psi
    (c) 500 – 2000 psi
    (d) 500 – 5000 psi

620. The flow rates of mobile phase should be
    (a) Greater than 3mL/min
    (b) Less than 1mL/min
    (c) 3 mL/min
    (d) None of the above

621. Which of the following is correct for sample load in HPLC?
    (a) ng
    (b) gm
    (c) mg
    (d) μg

622. In Normal phase HPLC, the mobile phase and stationary phase should be
    (a) Non polar & polar
    (b) Polar & non polar
    (c) Polar & polar
    (d) Non polar & non polar

623. In Normal phase HPLC, non polar &
polar compounds travels
    (a) Slower and faster respectively
    (b) Faster and slower respectively
    (c) Slower and slower respectively
    (d) Faster and faster respectively

624. In normal phase HPLC, the non polar
compounds
    (a) Elute first
    (b) Travel faster
    (c) Both a & b
    (d) Retained longer

625. Normal   phase   HPLC,   is   not
advantageous because
    (a) Most of drug molecules are
         nonpolar
    (b) Most of drug molecules are Polar
    (c) Both a & b
    (d) None of the above

626. In reverse phase HPLC, the mobile
phase & stationary phase should be
    (a) Polar & polar
    (b) Nonpolar & nonpolar
    (c) Polar & nonpolar
    (d) Nonpolar & polar

627. In Reverse phase HPLC, the polar &
nonpolar compounds travel
    (a) Faster, slower respectively
    (b) Faster, faster respectively
    (c) Slower, slower respectively
    (d) Slower, faster respectively

628. Which of the following is not an
example for non-polar column?
    (a) Octa decyl silane
    (b) C_4

    (c) C_8
    (d) Slicagel

629. ODS stands for
    (a) Octa decyl silane
    (b) Ortho decyl silane
    (c) Octa decyl support
    (d) Octa damage silane

630. Ion exchange chromatography is due
to
    (a) Irreversible exchange of
         functional groups
    (b) Reversible exchange of
         functional groups
    (c) Both a & b
    (d) All the above

631. In Ion pair chromatography, which of
the following is used as ion pairing
agents?
    (a) Toluene   (b) Pentane
    (c) Acetone   (d) Ether

632. In Ion pair chromatography, which
column is temporarily converted to
ion exchange column?
    (a) Reverse phase column
    (b) Normal phase column
    (c) Partition column
    (d) Adsorption column

633. Which of the following soft gels is
used   in   gel   permeation
chromatography?
    (a) Polystyrene
    (b) Dextran
    (c) Alkyl dextran
    (d) Styrene

634. Which of the following semi rigid gels is used in gel permeation chromatography?
    (a) Styrene
    (b) Dextran
    (c) Agarose
    (d) Polystyrene

635. In the field of biotechnology which chromatographic technique is used?
    (a) Affinity chromatography
    (b) Ion exchange chromatography
    (c) Ion pair chromatography
    (d) Size exclusion chromatography

636. For separation of optical isomers which chromatographic technique is used?
    (a) Size exclusion chromatography
    (b) Chiral chromatography
    (c) Ion pair chromatography
    (d) Ion exchange chromatography

637. In analytical HPLC the sample concentration is about
    (a) μg
    (b) ng
    (c) mg
    (d) kg

638. Qualitative analysis is used to determine
    (a) Concentration of analyte
    (b) Identification of analyte
    (c) Identify impurities
    (d) Peak area of standard

639. The principle of separation in normal phase and reverse phase mode is
    (a) Adsorption
    (b) Partition
    (c) Adsorption & partition
    (d) None of the above

640. Which pumps operate at constant flow rates?
    (a) Pneumatic pump
    (b) Check pump
    (c) Mechanical pump
    (d) Pulser pump

641. The solvents used must pass through which filter
    (a) 0.45 μ
    (b) 0.10 μ
    (c) 0.19 μ
    (d) 0.55 μ

642. Which device in solvent delivery system is used to control flow rate of solvent?
    (a) Check valve
    (b) Pneumatic valve
    (c) Pulse dampness
    (d) Mechanical valve

643. In low pressure mixing chamber which gas is used for degassing solvents?
    (a) H_2
    (b) N_2
    (c) Ar
    (d) He

644. Which type of mixer operates under high pressure?
    (a) Static mixer
    (b) Pulse mixer
    (c) Mechanical mixer
    (d) Dynamic mixer

645. Solvent degassing is done by which of the following techniques?
    (a) Mechanical mixer
    (b) Dynamic mixer
    (c) Helium purging
    (d) Filtration

646. In which type of injector systems the flow of mobile phase is stopped and sample is injected through a valve device?
    (a) Septum injectors
    (b) Stop flow
    (c) Rheodyne injector
    (d) Ultrasonication

647. Which of the following is the most popular injector?
    (a) Septum injector
    (b) Stop flow
    (c) Rheodyne injector
    (d) Ultrasonication

648. Which of the following column is used to remove impurities?
    (a) Guard column
    (b) Analytical column
    (c) Packed column
    (d) Capillary column

649. Which of the following material is used to make Analytical column?
    (a) Platinum   (b) Aluminum
    (c) Carbon   (d) Polyethylene

650. Which of the following column material is used to withstand high pressure?
    (a) Polyethylene
    (b) PEEK
    (c) Glass
    (d) Stainless steel

651. Which of the following functional group responsible for normal phase chromatography?
    (a) C_8 (b) C_{18}
    (c) Silanol group   (d) CN

652. Which of the following is the universal detector?
    (a) UV detector
    (b) Flourometric detector
    (c) Conductivity detector
    (d) Refractive Index detector

653. In which detector both excitation and emission wavelengths can be detected?
    (a) UV detector
    (b) Conductivity detector
    (c) Flourometric detector
    (d) Amperometric detector

654. Which detector is used to detect cations & anions?
    (a) Flourometric detector
    (b) Conductivity detector
    (c) Amperometric detector
    (d) Refractive index detector

655. If the compounds have both oxdizable & reducible functional groups then which type of detector is used?
    (a) Photo diode array detector
    (b) Conductivity detector
    (c) Amperometric detector
    (d) UV detector

656. Which of the following is a 3D detector?
    (a) UV detector
    (b) Amperometric detector
    (c) Conductivity detector
    (d) Photo diode array detector

657. Which of the following detector detects compounds of wide wave length range?
    (a) Refractive index detector

(b) Photo diode array detector

(c) Amperometric detector

(d) Conductivity detector

658. In Photo diode array detector, a 3D plot of which parameters takes place?

(a) Response Vs Time Vs Wavelength

(b) Response Vs Concentration Vs Time

(c) Response Vs Wavelength Vs Concentration

(d) Time Vs Concentration Vs Wavelength

659. In Qualitative analysis sample and standard is compared with which factor

(a) Retention time

(b) Response factor

(c) Retardation factor

(d) Resolution factor

660. Which of the following method is an example for quantitative analysis?

(a) Comparison method

(b) Curve method

(c) Internal standard method

(d) Standard method

661. Which of the following drugs is not analyzed by HPLC?

(a) Cefadroxil

(b) Norfloxacin

(c) Omeprazole

(d) Penicillin

662. Cyanocobalamine is determined by which of the following technique?

(a) HPLC   (b) GC

(c) HPTLC   (d) TLC

663. In gas solid chromatography the principle of separation is

(a) Partition

(b) Adsorption

(c) Normal phase

(d) Reverse phase

664. In gas liquid chromatography the principle of separation is

(a) Partition

(b) Normal phase

(c) Reverse phase

(d) Adsorption

665. The sample components in GC separated according to their

(a) Nature of substance

(b) Concentration of substance

(c) Partition coefficient

(d) Dipolar moment

666. Which of the following criteria is essential for the compounds to be analyzed by GC?

(a) Volatility

(b) Thermostability

(c) Both a & b

(d) All the above

667. Which of the following is not an example for carrier gas?

(a) H_2 (b) Helium

(c) Nitrogen   (d) Neon

668. The choice of the carrier gas depends upon

(a) Detector

(b) Column

(c) Injection devices

(d) Oven

669. Hydrogen is used for which type of detectors?
    (a) Argon ionization detector
    (b) Electron capture detector
    (c) UV detector
    (d) Thermal conductivity & flame ionization detector

670. Helium is used for which detector?
    (a) UV detector
    (b) Electron capture detector
    (c) Thermal conductivity detector
    (d) Flame ionization detector

671. Flow meter is used to measure flow rate of
    (a) Mobile phase
    (b) Carrier gas
    (c) Stationary phase
    (d) Column

672. Which of the following is an example for flow meters?
    (a) Rotameter
    (b) Soap bubble meter
    (c) Both a & b
    (d) All the above

673. Injection devices are used to inject sample into the
    (a) Column
    (b) Detector
    (c) Flow regulators
    (d) Oven

674. Gases can be introduced into the column by which of the following techniques?
    (a) Loop devices
    (b) Septum devices
    (c) Valve devices
    (d) None of the above

675. Liquids can be introduced into the column by which of the following devices?
    (a) Septum devices
    (b) Valve devices
    (c) Both a & b are correct
    (d) Rotameter

676. Separation of components takes place in
    (a) Injection devices
    (b) Column
    (c) Detector
    (d) Recorder

677. If only small quantity of ample is used then which type of column is used?
    (a) Preparative column
    (b) Packed column
    (c) Analytical column
    (d) Capillary column

678. If only large amounts of sample to be loaded then which type of column is used?
    (a) Capillary column
    (b) Analytical column
    (c) Packed column
    (d) Preparative column

679. Open tubular capillary column comes under the type of
    (a) Analytical column
    (b) Packed column
    (c) Capillary column
    (d) Preparative column

680. Which of the following column is having more advantages?
    (a) Support coated open tubular column

(b) Wall coated open tubular column
(c) Packed column
(d) Capillary column

681. Pre heaters are attached to
(a) Column
(b) Injecting devices
(c) Detector
(d) Septum devices

682. Temperature of the oven depends upon
(a) Concentration of solute
(b) Partition coefficient
(c) Solubility of solute
(d) Both b & c

683. Which of the following parts in GC are maintained at constant temperature?
(a) Column
(b) Injecting devices
(c) Detector
(d) Both a & b

684. The capillary columns are in coiled due to which material?
(a) Polyethylene
(b) Polypropylene
(c) Polyether
(d) Polyamide

685. In oven if same temperature is maintained throughout the process of separation is called as
(a) Linear programming
(b) Isothermal programming
(c) Thermal programming
(d) Nonlinear programming

686. If sample have a mixture of low boiling and high boiling point mixtures then which type of programming system is operated?
(a) Isothermal programming
(b) Linear programming
(c) Thermal programming
(d) Nonlinear programming

687. Which of the following detectors used in GC?
(a) Phototubes
(b) Photomultiplier tubes
(c) Thermal conductivity detector
(d) Photovoltaic cell

688. Thermal conductivity detector works under the principle of
(a) Thermal conductivity
(b) Electrical conductivity
(c) Both a & b
(d) All the above

689. Katharometer is an example for which detector?
(a) Flame ionization detector
(b) Argon ionization detector
(c) Thermal conductivity detector
(d) Electron capture detector

690. In Thermal conductivity detector the wires are made up of
(a) Platinum wire
(b) Aluminum wire
(c) Carbon wire
(d) Sodium wire

691. Which of the following is best carrier gas?
(a) Hydrogen   (b) Helium
(c) Nitrogen   (d) Hexane

692. Flame ionization detector works under the principle of
     (a) Thermal conductivity
     (b) Electrical conductivity
     (c) Chemical conductivity
     (d) Potential conductivity

693. In FID detector the most commonly used carrier gas is
     (a) Hydrogen   (b) Helium
     (c) Nitrogen   (d) Argon

694. The anode in FID detector is made up of
     (a) Platinum gauze
     (b) Silver gauze
     (c) Steel gauze
     (d) Aurum gauze

695. In FID, the potential difference across due to
     (a) Ionization of pure carrier gas and analyte
     (b) Non ionization of pure carrier gas and analyte
     (c) Ionization of pure carrier gas
     (d) Ionization of analyte

696. In Flame ionization detector, which parameter is measured?
     (a) Potential difference
     (b) Current
     (c) Voltage
     (d) Chemical reaction between anode & cathode

697. Which of the following detector is most commonly used?
     (a) Thermal conductivity detector
     (b) Flame ionization detector
     (c) Argon ionization detector
     (d) Electron capture detector

698. Argon capture detector which type of energy source is irradiated with carrier gas?
     (a) α-particles
     (b) β-particles
     (c) Both a & b are correct
     (d) γ particles

699. α Particles are obtained from which compound?
     (a) Strontium   (b) Tritium
     (c) Radium – D   (d) Radium

700. In Electron capture detector, the electrode is treated with
     (a) Radio isotope
     (b) Active isotope
     (c) Radioactive isotope
     (d) All the above

701. The electrons emitted from radioactive isotope produces
     (a) Primary electrons
     (b) Secondary electrons
     (c) Tertiary electrons
     (d) All the above

702. The secondary electrons are collected at
     (a) Cathode
     (b) Dyanode
     (c) Anode
     (d) All the above

703. Which of the following compounds cannot be detected by electron capture detector?
     (a) Chlorine
     (b) Fluorine
     (c) Bromine
     (d) Sodium

704. Which of the following parameter is recorded in recorder?
    (a) Peak area
    (b) % area
    (c) Width of the peaks
    (d) Retention time

705. In which of the derivatization techniques in which the compounds are converted to more volatile?
    (a) Post column derivatization
    (b) Pre column derivatization
    (c) Column derivatization
    (d) Integrator derivatization

706. In which of the following conditions does the precolumn derivatization is done?
    (a) Components is less volatile
    (b) Components are thermostabile
    (c) To reduce tailing factor
    (d) All of the above

707. Examples of compounds which undergoes precolumn derivatization technique?
    (a) Tannins
    (b) Aldehydes
    (c) Ketones
    (d) Alcohols

708. In precolumn derivatization technique carboxylic acids, phenolic compounds are converted into
    (a) Ester derivative
    (b) Amine derivative
    (c) Amide derivative
    (d) Acetyl derivative

709. Post column derivatisation is done for
    (a) Column
    (b) Integrator
    (c) Oven
    (d) Detector

710. If pretreatment of solid support is not done for stationary phase then
    (a) Tailing of peaks will occur
    (b) Fronting of peaks will occur
    (c) Degassing will occur
    (d) Less resolution

711. Which of the following agents are used in pretreatment of solid support?
    (a) Hexa ethyl disilazone
    (b) Hexa methyl disilazone
    (c) Penta methyl disilazone
    (d) Penta ethyl disilazone

712. Chromatography was first discovered which scientist?
    (a) Siebold
    (b) Hull
    (c) Tswett
    (d) Warsaw

713. Who introduced gas chromatography?
    (a) Siebold
    (b) Einstein & martin
    (c) Faraday & synge
    (d) Martin & synge

714. Plate theory of chromatogarphy was developed by
    (a) Martin
    (b) Synge
    (c) Martin & synge
    (d) Siebold & hull

715. According to plate theory the horizontal layers in column are nothing but
    (a) Theoretical cups
    (b) Plates
    (c) Theoretical plates
    (d) None of the above

716. The efficiency of separation in column increased due to
    (a) Increase in number of theoretical plate
    (b) Decrease in number of theoretical plate
    (c) Both a & b
    (d) None

717. The number of theoretical plates is given as
    (a) L
    (b) H
    (c) K
    (d) N

718. Which of the following is correct expression for calculation of number of theoretical plates?
    (a) $N = L/H$
    (b) $L = N/H$
    (c) $H = L/N$
    (d) $H = N/L$

719. HETP stands for
    (a) High equivalent theoretical plate
    (b) Height equivalent theoretical plate
    (c) High equilibrium theoretical plate
    (d) High equilibrium theory plate

720. HETP refers to
    (a) Height of layer of column
    (b) Height of layer of column

(c) Height of layer of stationary
(d) Height of layer of mobile phase

721. If HETP is less, column is
    (a) More efficient
    (b) Less efficient
    (c) No effect
    (d) All the above

722. If HETP is more, the column is
    (a) Less efficient
    (b) More efficient
    (c) No effect
    (d) All the above

723. Efficiency of column depends upon
    (a) No. of theoretical plates
    (b) Length of column
    (c) Surface area of stationary phase
    (d) Height Equivalent theoretical plate

724. Which of the following is correct expression for calculation of number of theoretical plates?
    (a) $n = 14\, Rt^2/w^2$
    (b) $n = 6\, Rt^2/w^2$
    (c) $n = 16\, Rt^2/w^2$
    (d) $n = 16\, Rw^2/t^2$

725. For the column to be more efficient,
    (a) The number of theoretical plates should be high
    (b) Increase in length of column
    (c) HETP s more
    (d) None

726. Fronting is done due to
    (a) Saturation of mobile phase
    (b) Saturation of stationary phase
    (c) Both a & b
    (d) None

727. Tailing is done due to
   (a) Less active adsorption sites
   (b) More active adsorption sites
   (c) Decrease in length of column
   (d) Increase in length of column

728. The difference in time between point of injection and appearance of peak maxima is called as
   (a) Retention factor
   (b) Retardation factor
   (c) Resolution factor
   (d) Retention time

729. The volume of carrier gas required to elute 50% of component from the column is
   (a) Retention volume
   (b) Void volume
   (c) Resolution volume
   (d) Retardation volume

730. Product of Retention time and flow rate gives
   (a) Retention volume
   (b) Resolution
   (c) Separation factor
   (d) Retardation factor

731. The ratio of partition coefficients of two components to be separated is
   (a) Retention time
   (b) Retardation factor
   (c) Resolution
   (d) Separation factor

732. If Partition coefficient of two compounds are same the
   (a) Separation factor is less
   (b) Separation factor is more
   (c) Separation factor is medium
   (d) None

733. The extent of separation of two components with base line separation is called as
   (a) Retardation factor
   (b) Resolution factor
   (c) Resolution
   (d) Retention time

734. Which of the following is the correct expression for resolution?
   (a) $R_S = 2\,(Rt_2 - Rt_1) / w_1 + w_2$
   (b) $R_S = (Rt_2 - Rt_1) / w_1 + w_2$
   (c) $R_S = w_1 + w_2 / 2\,(Rt_2 - Rt_1)$
   (d) $R_S = w_1 + w_2 / (Rt_2 - Rt_1)$

735. Column resolution depends upon
   (a) Selectivity factor
   (b) Separation factor
   (c) Retardation factor
   (d) Retention factor

736. The Selectivity factor is the relative magnitude of
   (a) Concentration of two species
   (b) Partition coefficient of two species
   (c) Nature of any of two substances
   (d) Size of the substance

737. Which of the following expression is correct for van deemter equation for GLC?
   (a) $HETP = B + A/u + C_u$
   (b) $HETP = A + B/u + C_u$
   (c) $HETP = A + B/C_u + u$
   (d) $HETP = A + B/R + C_u$

738. In van deemter equation "A" represents
   (a) Longitudinal Diffusion
   (b) Flow rate of mobile phase

(c) Eddy diffusion

(d) Effect of mass transfer

739. In van deemter equation B, C, u represents
  (a) Longitudinal diffusion, effect of mass transfer, flow rate of mobile phase respectively
  (b) Flow rate of mobile phase, effect of mass transfer, longitudinal diffusion respectively
  (c) Flow rate of mobile phase, longitudinal diffusion, effect of mass transfer respectively
  (d) All the above

740. Eddy diffusion can be minimized by
  (a) Uniform flow rate of mobile phase
  (b) Non uniform flow rate of mobile phase
  (c) Uniform packing of column
  (d) Non uniform packing of column

741. Longitudinal diffusion depends upon
  (a) Mass transfer
  (b) Uniform packing of column
  (c) Flow rate
  (d) Charge transfer

742. If Eddy diffusion occurs then we get
  (a) Narrow bands
  (b) Broad bands
  (c) Less resolution chromatography
  (d) b & c are correct

743. Longitudinal diffusion occurs most commonly in
  (a) Gases   (b) Liquids
  (c) Solids   (d) Semisolids

744. In the van deemter equation for HPLC then H represents
  (a) Resolution of column
  (b) Retardation of column
  (c) Efficiency of column
  (d) Separation factor for column

745. C_s term depends upon
  (a) Eddy diffusion
  (b) Number of theoretical plates
  (c) Thickness of stationary phase
  (d) Velocity of mobile phase

746. If thinner and more uniform stationary phase is present the value of C_s will be
  (a) More
  (b) Less
  (c) Medium
  (d) No effect

747. In X, Y substances, X substance is having thin layer and Y substance having thick layer, then which substance will have less C_s value?
  (a) X   (b) Y
  (c) Both X & Y   (d) No effect

748. In X, Y substances, X substance is having more regular shape, Y substance is having irregular shape, then which substance will elute first?
  (a) X   (b) Y
  (c) Both X & Y   (d) No effect

KEY

1.	(c)	2.	(a)	3.	(a)	4.	(b)	5.	(c)
6.	(d)	7.	(b)	8.	(d)	9.	(a)	10.	(c)
11.	(d)	12.	(b)	13.	(a)	14.	(c)	15.	(a)
16.	(c)	17.	(b)	18.	(d)	19.	(a)	20.	(c)
21.	(b)	22.	(c)	23.	(d)	24.	(b)	25.	(b)
26.	(b)	27.	(c)	28.	(a)	29.	(b)	30.	(d)
31.	(b)	32.	(a)	33.	(c)	34.	(a)	35.	(b)
36.	(b)	37.	(a)	38.	(c)	39.	(d)	40.	(b)
41.	(c)	42.	(c)	43.	(d)	44.	(b)	45.	(a)
46.	(d)	47.	(b)	48.	(a)	49.	(b)	50.	(d)
51.	(b)	52.	(c)	53.	(b)	54.	(c)	55.	(d)
56.	(a)	57.	(b)	58.	(c)	59.	(b)	60.	(b)
61.	(a)	62.	(c)	63.	(a)	64.	(b)	65.	(c)
66.	(a)	67.	(c)	68.	(a)	69.	(b)	70.	(d)
71.	(a)	72.	(d)	73.	(a)	74.	(c)	75.	(d)
76.	(c)	77.	(c)	78.	(a)	79.	(b)	80.	(c)
81.	(d)	82.	(a)	83.	(b)	84.	(c)	85.	(d)
86.	(a)	87.	(d)	88.	(a)	89.	(b)	90.	(c)
91.	(d)	92.	(a)	93.	(c)	94.	(a)	95.	(b)
96.	(c)	97.	(c)	98.	(d)	99.	(a)	100.	(d)
101.	(b)	102.	(d)	103.	(b)	104.	(a)	105.	(c)
106.	(a)	107.	(c)	108.	(a)	109.	(b)	110.	(d)
111.	(c)	112.	(a)	113.	(c)	114.	(b)	115.	(a)
116.	(d)	117.	(c)	118.	(b)	119.	(a)	120.	(c)
121.	(a)	122.	(d)	123.	(b)	124.	(c)	125.	(b)
126.	(a)	127.	(d)	128.	(b)	129	(a)	130.	(d)
131.	(b)	132.	(b)	133.	(a)	134.	(c)	135.	(c)
136.	(d)	137.	(d)	138.	(a)	139.	(d)	140.	(c)
141.	(b)	142.	(c)	143.	(a)	144.	(c)	145.	(d)
146.	(a)	147.	(b)	148.	(d)	149.	(c)	150.	(b)

151.	(a)	152.	(c)	153.	(a)	154.	(a)	155.	(d)
156.	(b)	157.	(b)	158.	(a)	159.	(b)	160.	(b)
161.	(a)	162.	(b)	163.	(a)	164.	(c)	165.	(a)
166.	(d)	167.	(b)	168.	(a)	169.	(b)	170.	(a)
171.	(d)	172.	(b)	173.	(b)	174.	(a)	175.	(c)
176.	(a)	177.	(a)	178.	(b)	179.	(c)	180.	(a)
181.	(d)	182.	(b)	183.	(d)	184.	(c)	185.	(a)
186.	(a)	187.	(c)	188.	(a)	189.	(d)	190.	(a)
191.	(b)	192.	(d)	193.	(a)	194.	(b)	195.	(c)
196.	(c)	197.	(b)	198.	(a)	199.	(d)	200.	(b)
201.	(a)	202.	(a)	203.	(d)	204.	(d)	205.	(b)
206.	(a)	207.	(c)	208.	(b)	209.	(c)	210.	(d)
211.	(a)	212.	(c)	213.	(d)	214.	(a)	215.	(b)
216.	(c)	217.	(b)	218.	(a)	219.	(c)	220.	(b)
221.	(d)	222.	(c)	223.	(a)	224.	(c)	225.	(a)
226.	(b)	227.	(d)	228.	(c)	229.	(d)	230.	(b)
231.	(d)	232.	(d)	233.	(a)	234.	(d)	235.	(c)
236.	(b)	237.	(c)	238.	(d)	239.	(a)	240.	(b)
241.	(c)	242.	(b)	243.	(d)	244.	(b)	245.	(a)
246.	(b)	247.	(a)	248.	(a)	249.	(c)	250.	(b)
251.	(a)	252.	(d)	253.	(a)	254.	(d)	255.	(c)
256.	(d)	257.	(a)	258.	(c)	259.	(d)	260.	(a)
261.	(a)	262.	(c)	263.	(b)	264.	(b)	265.	(a)
266.	(b)	267.	(a)	268.	(c)	269.	(a)	270.	(b)
271.	(d)	272.	(b)	273.	(c)	274.	(a)	275.	(b)
276.	(a)	277.	(a)	278.	(c)	279.	(d)	280.	(a)
281.	(a)	282.	(a)	283.	(a)	284.	(b)	285.	(a)
286.	(b)	287.	(b)	288.	(c)	289.	(d)	290.	(b)
291.	(a)	292.	(b)	293.	(c)	294.	(b)	295.	(a)
296.	(b)	297.	(a)	298.	(c)	299.	(a)	300.	(a)
301.	(b)	302.	(a)	303.	(b)	304.	(c)	305.	(d)
306.	(c)	307.	(a)	308.	(a)	309.	(b)	310.	(a)

311.	(a)	312.	(b)	313.	(a)	314.	(c)	315.	(d)
316.	(a)	317.	(d)	318.	(b)	319.	(a)	320.	(b)
321.	(d)	322.	(c)	323.	(a)	324.	(d)	325.	(b)
326.	(c)	327.	(c)	328.	(b)	329.	(a)	330.	(c)
331.	(b)	332.	(d)	333.	(a)	334.	(c)	335.	(b)
336.	(d)	337.	(b)	338.	(d)	339.	(a)	340.	(c)
341.	(a)	342.	(b)	343.	(d)	344.	(c)	345.	(a)
346.	(c)	347.	(a)	348.	(d)	349.	(b)	350.	(b)
351.	(a)	352.	(d)	353.	(b)	354.	(c)	355.	(b)
356.	(d)	357.	(b)	358.	(c)	359.	(a)	360.	(d)
361.	(a)	362.	(b)	363.	(d)	364.	(d)	365.	(b)
366.	(c)	367.	(d)	368.	(d)	369.	(a)	370.	(c)
371.	(a)	372.	(b)	373.	(c)	374.	(a)	375.	(c)
376.	(a)	377.	(b)	378.	(c)	379.	(a)	380.	(c)
381.	(c)	382.	(b)	383.	(c)	384.	(a)	385.	(a)
386.	(d)	387.	(b)	388.	(c)	389.	(b)	390.	(a)
391.	(d)	392.	(d)	393.	(a)	394.	(b)	395.	(c)
396.	(d)	397.	(a)	398.	(c)	399.	(a)	400.	(d)
401.	(b)	402.	(d)	403.	(a)	404.	(d)	405.	(b)
406.	(a)	407.	(c)	408.	(a)	409.	(b)	410.	(c)
411.	(a)	412.	(b)	413.	(b)	414.	(c)	415.	(d)
416.	(a)	417.	(d)	418.	(a)	419.	(c)	420.	(d)
421.	(a)	422.	(c)	423.	(a)	424.	(b)	425.	(a)
426.	(b)	427.	(a)	428.	(a)	429.	(d)	430.	(c)
431.	(a)	432.	(b)	433.	(c)	434.	(a)	435.	(b)
436.	(c)	437.	(a)	438.	(c)	439.	(b)	440.	(a)
441.	(c)	442.	(b)	443.	(a)	444.	(c)	445.	(a)
446.	(c)	447.	(d)	448.	(c)	449.	(a)	450.	(d)
451.	(c)	452.	(c)	453.	(b)	454.	(a)	455.	(c)
456.	(a)	457.	(b)	458.	(b)	459.	(c)	460.	(a)
461.	(a)	462.	(a)	463.	(a)	464.	(d)	465.	(a)
466.	(d)	467.	(b)	468.	(d)	469.	(a)	470.	(b)

471.	(b)	472.	(a)	473.	(b)	474.	(a)	475.	(d)
476.	(d)	477.	(a)	478.	(d)	479.	(d)	480.	(a)
481.	(c)	482.	(d)	483.	(b)	484.	(d)	485.	(a)
486.	(c)	487.	(a)	488.	(d)	489.	(a)	490.	(a)
491.	(d)	492.	(c)	493.	(a)	494.	(b)	495.	(d)
496.	(a)	497.	(c)	498.	(d)	499.	(b)	500.	(c)
501.	(c)	502.	(a)	503.	(d)	504.	(c)	505.	(c)
506.	(a)	507.	(b)	508.	(a)	509.	(b)	510.	(b)
511.	(d)	512.	(a)	513.	(c)	514.	(a)	515.	(a)
516.	(a)	517.	(b)	518.	(b)	519.	(b)	520.	(d)
521.	(b)	522.	(d)	523.	(b)	524.	(c)	525.	(a)
526.	(b)	527.	(d)	528.	(a)	529.	(b)	530.	(d)
531.	(c)	532.	(d)	533.	(b)	534.	(a)	535.	(d)
536.	(a)	537.	(a)	538.	(d)	539.	(b)	540.	(a)
541.	(d)	542.	(c)	543.	(b)	544.	(a)	545.	(d)
546.	(b)	547.	(a)	548.	(b)	549.	(d)	550.	(c)
551.	(a)	552.	(a)	553.	(d)	554.	(c)	555.	(a)
556.	(b)	557.	(c)	558.	(a)	559.	(c)	560.	(d)
561.	(b)	562.	(c)	563.	(a)	564.	(b)	565.	(b)
566.	(d)	567.	(c)	568.	(d)	569.	(d)	570.	(c)
571.	(b)	572.	(c)	573.	(b)	574.	(b)	575.	(c)
576.	(b)	577.	(a)	578.	(b)	579.	(a)	580.	(a)
581.	(b)	582.	(a)	583.	(c)	584.	(d)	585.	(c)
586.	(c)	587.	(d)	588.	(d)	589.	(c)	590.	(c)
591.	(b)	592.	(d)	593.	(b)	594.	(a)	595.	(d)
596.	(a)	597.	(b)	598.	(c)	599.	(a)	600.	(b)
601.	(b)	602.	(d)	603.	(c)	604.	(c)	605.	(c)
606.	(c)	607.	(d)	608.	(d)	609.	(a)	610.	(d)
611.	(b)	612.	(c)	613.	(c)	614.	(d)	615.	(a)
616.	(c)	617.	(b)	618.	(d)	619.	(a)	620.	(a)
621.	(d)	622.	(a)	623.	(b)	624.	(c)	625.	(b)
626.	(c)	627.	(a)	628.	(d)	629.	(a)	630.	(b)

631.	(c)	632.	(a)	633.	(c)	634.	(d)	635.	(a)
636.	(b)	637.	(a)	638.	(b)	639.	(a)	640.	(c)
641.	(a)	642.	(a)	643.	(d)	644.	(d)	645.	(c)
646.	(b)	647.	(c)	648.	(a)	649.	(d)	650.	(d)
651.	(c)	652.	(d)	653.	(c)	654.	(b)	655.	(c)
656.	(d)	657.	(b)	658.	(a)	659.	(a)	660.	(c)
661.	(d)	662.	(a)	663.	(b)	664.	(a)	665.	(c)
666.	(c)	667.	(d)	668.	(a)	669.	(d)	670.	(c)
671.	(b)	672.	(c)	673.	(a)	674.	(c)	675.	(a)
676.	(b)	677.	(c)	678.	(d)	679.	(c)	680.	(a)
681.	(b)	682.	(d)	683.	(d)	684.	(d)	685.	(b)
686.	(b)	687.	(c)	688.	(a)	689.	(c)	690.	(a)
691.	(b)	692.	(b)	693.	(a)	694.	(b)	695.	(a)
696.	(b)	697.	(b)	698.	(c)	699.	(c)	700.	(c)
701.	(b)	702.	(c)	703.	(d)	704.	(d)	705.	(b)
706.	(d)	707.	(d)	708.	(d)	709.	(d)	710.	(a)
711.	(b)	712.	(c)	713.	(d)	714.	(c)	715.	(c)
716.	(a)	717.	(d)	718.	(a)	719.	(b)	720.	(a)
721.	(a)	722.	(b)	723.	(a)	724.	(c)	725.	(a)
726.	(b)	727.	(b)	728.	(d)	729.	(a)	730.	(a)
731.	(d)	732.	(a)	733.	(c)	734.	(a)	735.	(a)
736.	(b)	737.	(b)	738.	(c)	739.	(a)	740.	(c)
741.	(c)	742.	(d)	743.	(a)	744.	(c)	745.	(c)
746.	(b)	747.	(a)	748.	(a)				